Keratitis: An Issue of Ophthalmology Clinics

Keratitis: An Issue of Ophthalmology Clinics

Editor: Abigail Gipe

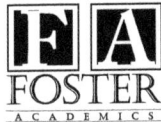

FA
FOSTER
ACADEMICS

www.fosteracademics.com

www.fosteracademics.com

FA
FOSTER
ACADEMICS

Cataloging-in-Publication Data

Keratitis : an issue of ophthalmology clinics / edited by Abigail Gipe.
     p. cm.
Includes bibliographical references and index.
ISBN 978-1-63242-509-6
1. Keratitis. 2. Glaucoma. 3. Cornea--Diseases. 4. Ophthalmology. 5. Eye--Diseases. I. Gipe, Abigail.
RE338 .K47 2017
617.719--dc23

Foster Academics,
118-35 Queens Blvd., Suite 400,
Forest Hills, NY 11375, USA

ISBN 978-1-63242-509-6 (Hardback)

Printed and bound in the United States of America.

Contents

Preface

In my initial years as a student, I used to run to the library at every possible instance to grab a book and learn something new. Books were my primary source of knowledge and I would not have come such a long way without all that I learnt from them. Thus, when I was approached to edit this book; I became understandably nostalgic. It was an absolute honor to be considered worthy of guiding the current generation as well as those to come. I put all my knowledge and hard work into making this book most beneficial for its readers.

Keratitis is defined as a condition where the cornea of the eye becomes inflamed. This book on keratitis discusses diagnosis and treatment methods for keratitis. Acute keratitis may result in the scarring of the cornea, perforation of the cornea or even eye loss. Infectious keratitis must be treated rapidly and requires antibacterial, antifungal or antiviral therapy. This book is a compilation of chapters that discuss the most vital concepts and emerging trends in this field. It aims to shed light on some of the unexplored aspects of keratitis and the recent researches in this area. This book will serve as a reference to a broad spectrum of readers such as researchers, students, ophthalmogists, etc. In this book, using case studies and examples, constant effort has been made to make the understanding of difficult concepts of keratitis as easy and informative as possible for the readers.

I wish to thank my publisher for supporting me at every step. I would also like to thank all the authors who have contributed their researches in this book. I hope this book will be a valuable contribution to the progress of the field.

Editor

Changes in the choroidal thickness in reproductive-aged women with iron-deficiency anemia

Erhan Yumusak[1,5*], Aydin Ciftci[2], Selim Yalcin[3], Cemile Dayangan Sayan[4], Nevin Hande Dikel[1] and Kemal Ornek[1]

Abstract

Background: The aim of this study was to investigate the potential significance of the central macular thickness (foveal thickness-FT) and choroidal thickness (CT) in the eyes of patients with iron-deficiency anemia, the most common form of the anemia, via enhanced-depth imaging optical coherence tomography (EDI-OCT). We also investigated whether such changes might serve as an early indicator of underlying hematological disease.

Methods: This prospective clinical study compared 96 female patients with iron-deficiency anemia and 60 healthy female control subjects. The macular and choroidal thicknesses in the temporal and nasal subfoveal areas were measured using enhanced-depth imaging optical coherence tomography (EDI-OCT) at 500 and 1500 microns and in five different regions (FCT, T_{1500}, T_{500}, N_{500}, and N_{1500}).

Results: The mean ages of the patients and healthy controls were 34.08 ± 10.39 years and 32.29 ± 8.28 years, respectively ($P = 0.232$). There were no significant changes in macular thickness between the groups (225.58 ± 19.76 vs. 222.45 ± 13.51, $P = 0.2$). The choroidal thickness was significantly reduced in the patient group relative to the controls at all measured points (foveal choroidal thickness, $P = 0.042$; nasal–500 microns, $P = 0.033$; temporal–500 microns, $P = 0.033$; and temporal–1500 microns, $P = 0.019$). At some points, the choroidal thickness findings correlated with the hemoglobin values (temporal–500 microns, $r = -0.287$, $P = 0.001$; nasal–500 microns, $r = -0.287$, $P = 0.005$; nasal–1500 microns, $r = -0.245$, $P = 0.016$; and temporal–1500 microns, $r = -0.280$, $P = 0.06$).

Conclusions: Patients with iron-deficiency anemia had a significantly reduced choroidal thickness.

Keywords: Choroidal thickness, Iron-deficiency anemia, Enhanced-depth imaging optical coherence tomography

Background

The development of optical coherence tomography (OCT) technology has revolutionized the diagnostic, monitoring, and therapeutic approaches to many retinal and systemic diseases. Spectral domain OCT offers improved axial resolution (3 μm), reduces examination times, and accordingly reduces both patient exposure and artifacts by allowing 19,000 A-scans per second. The latest development in OCT technology, swept-source longer wavelength OCT, better penetrates the retinal pigment epithelium (RPE) and thus allows better visualization of the choroid; however, its use is currently limited to research purposes.

Similar to swept-source OCT, enhanced-depth imaging (EDI), which was recently introduced by Spaide et al. [1], provides greater penetration through the RPE and allows accurate in vivo deep choroidal imaging and measurement [2]. Changes in choroidal thickness (CT) have been found to correlate with several factors and systemic conditions such as smoking, changes in arterial pressure, hemodialysis, obstructive sleep apnea syndrome, and systemic sclerosis [3–7].

According to the World Health Organization (WHO), the overall global prevalence of iron-deficiency anemia is 25 %, with rates of 12.7 %, 30.2 %, and 41.8 % among adult men, women of reproductive age, and pregnant women, respectively [8]. Infants have the highest

* Correspondence: erhanyumusak@yahoo.com
[1]Department of Ophthalmology, Kırıkkale University School of Medicine, Kırıkkale, Turkey
[5]Kirikkale University Medical Faculty Hospital District Tahsin Duru Akdeniz Caddesi No: 14, Yahsihan/Kırıkkale 71450, Turkey
Full list of author information is available at the end of the article

prevalence of iron-deficiency anemia, followed by pregnant women and women of reproductive age. In women of reproductive age, the risk of iron-deficiency anemia may accompany a range of important causes of morbidity and mortality [9, 10]. These conditions are the most important cause of menorrhagia in patients with iron-deficiency anemia [11, 12].

In this study, we investigated the potential significance of macular thickness and CT in the eyes of patients with iron-deficiency anemia, the most common form of anemia. We also considered the possibility that such changes might serve as an early indicator of underlying hematological disease. Using semi-automated choroidal segmentation software, we measured changes in CT in the eyes of women of reproductive age with iron-deficiency anemia in comparison with a control group.

Methods

This prospective clinical study was conducted between 2014 and 2015 in accordance with the tenets of the Declaration of Helsinki. The trial protocol was approved by the Local Ethical Committee of the Kırıkkale University. Trial registration was requested on October 12, 2015 (decision no:01/04). All patients and control subjects voluntarily participated in the study and signed an informed consent form prepared according to the ethical protocol.

The patient group consisted of patients with a diagnosis of iron-deficiency anemia who were followed by the Hematology Clinic, whereas the control group consisted of healthy adult women of reproductive age. This study included only adult women of reproductive age to avoid the effects of gender, age, and hormonal status. The exclusion criteria were a previously diagnosed systemic or chronic disease or condition (e.g., hypertension, smoking, ocular surgery) in one or both eyes, an axial length >24 ± 1.0 mm, and a refractive measurement exceeding 2.0 diopters.

Patients with a previous diagnosis of iron-deficiency anemia were selected randomly for inclusion in the patient group. The study included 96 eyes from 96 patients followed in this manner, and only the patients right eyes were evaluated to avoid intra-individual bias. In the control group, 60 eyes from 60 patients were also evaluated and fully assessed. Each patient was subjected individually to visual acuity, slit-lamp biomicroscopy, intraocular pressure, and fundus examinations.

CT and macular thickness measurement was performed on an EDI-OCT scanning system (OCT Advance Nidek RS-3000; Nidek Co. Ltd., Gamagori, Japan). In all patients, the central macular thickness (FT) was measured in the right eye prior to evaluation. Patients subsequently underwent EDI-OCT scanning. Technicians then manually drew the choroid and sclera boundaries with assistance from software programs (Fig. 1). These boundaries limited the Bruch membrane between the subfoveal points (FCT) to 500 or 1500 microns in the nasal (N_{500}, N_{1500}) and 500 or 1500 microns in the temporal regions (T_{500}, T_{1500}) for CT measurements (Fig. 2). Choroid and sclera demarcation was performed independently by two experienced technicians. The averages of the obtained values were used.

SSPS statistical software (SPSS for Windows, version 22.0; SPSS, Inc., Chicago, IL, USA) was used for the statistical analysis. The results of the descriptive analysis are presented as numbers, percentages, means, medians, and standard deviations. The paired t test and chi-square test were used to compare variables between the patient and control groups, and Pearson's correlation coefficient was used to evaluate correlations. A multiple linear regression analysis (forward) was used to determine confounding factors among the variables. A P value < 0.05 was considered statistically significant.

Results

The anemia group consisted of 96 female patients of reproductive age. The mean age was 34.08 ± 10.39 years (range: 18–49 years). The control group included 60 patients with a mean age of 32.2 9 ± 8.28 years (range: 17–49 years). The groups did not differ significantly with respect to age (P =0.232). Patients with anemia had a mean hemoglobin level of 9.59 ± 1.18 (range: 6.90–11). The mean duration of anemia was 4.18 ± 3.51 years (range: 1–15 years).

Forty-nine patients with a mean age of 33.86 ± 10.21 years were in the follicular phase of the menstrual cycle. Forty-six patients with a mean age of 34.32 ± 10.68 years were in the luteal phase. There were no significant differences between the patients in each phase with respect to age, hemoglobin level (10.09 ± 1.32 vs. 10.687 ± 1.55), and CT ($P = 0.8$, $P = 0.7$, and P > 0.05, respectively; (Table 1).

No statistically significant difference was observed between the groups with respect to FT (P > 0.05). When all measured CT points were compared, the anemia group had significantly lower values than the control group (Table 2).

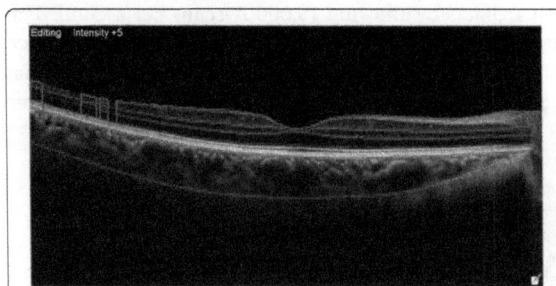

Fig. 1 Choroid boundaries were manually drawn by a technician with software assistance

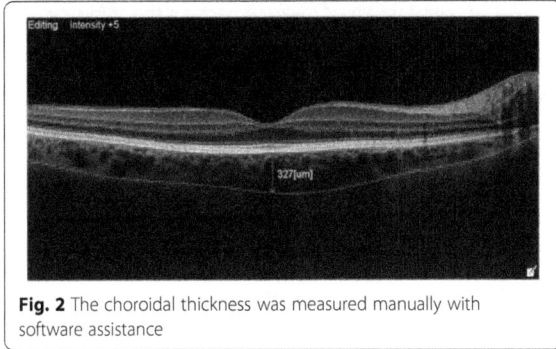

Fig. 2 The choroidal thickness was measured manually with software assistance

In the patient group, no significant association was observed between the duration of anemia and the CT ($P > 0.05$). However, significant correlations were observed between some CT points and the hemoglobin values (temporal–500 micron, $r = -0.287$, $P = 0.001$; nasal–500 microns, $r = -0.287$, $P = 0.005$; nasal–1500 microns, $r = -0.245$, $P = 0.016$; temporal–1500 microns, $r = -0.280$, $P = 0.06$). Moreover, a statistically significant negative correlation was observed between age and CT ($P < 0.05$).

We next assessed the independent effects of age and hemoglobin level on changes in CT through a multiple linear regression analysis. Only age independently affected the FCT ($p = 0.004$), whereas both age and the hemoglobin independently affected the N_{500}, N_{1500}, T_{500}, and T_{1500} values. In other words, no overlap was observed between these factors; each CT point was affected independently by the hemoglobin level and age, with no potential confounding effect ($P < 0.05$ for all; Table 3).

Discussion

The choroid covers the outer retina and is among the most vascularized tissues in the body. This tissue supplies oxygen and nutrition to and provides temperature regulation for the retina. With respect to the retina, the choroid assumes the important roles of growth factor secretion and removal of retinal residues [13]. Both the structure and function

of the choroidal tissue are essential factors ensuring a normal and functional retina. An abnormal choroidal blood volume, impaired photoreceptor function, and/or even a loss of blood flow can lead to injury [14]. The choroid features both sympathetic and parasympathetic innervation to regulate the choroidal blood flow, which is controlled by an autoregulatory mechanism [15].

The CT may be affected by age, axial length, and refractive errors [16, 17]. Diurnal changes in CT have also been reported [18]. The choroid is affected by changes in blood pressure and intraocular pressure through an autoregulatory mechanism [19]. Because the choroid features a rich vascular structure, these changes greatly affect the autoregulation of CT [20]. For example, Tanabe et al. demonstrated a significant relationship between the choroidal vessel diameter and CT [21]. Similarly, Vance et al. found that phoshodiesterase-5 inhibitors such as sildenafil citrate, which promotes smooth muscle relaxation, can lead to an increased CT [22].

In the current study, we found observed a significant reduction in CT in the patient group. In a review of the literature on this subject, we did not identify any previous research that would allow a direct comparison. Karaca et al. collected choroidal measurements at three points in their study of patients with obstructive sleep apnea syndrome and found no significant differences relative to control group measurements [6]. Pekel et al. evaluated choroidal changes in patients who had undergone cardiopulmonary bypass and also failed to detect any significant changes [4]. In addition, Ngo et al. presented a case report of high altitude-induced retinopathy in a patient with significantly increased CT [23].

Hematological diseases affect millions of patients worldwide and are a significant cause of both morbidity and mortality. Anemia consists of a group of hematologic disorders characterized by a decrease in the number of red blood cells and/or hemoglobin level. Factors such as hypoxia, venous stasis, vasospasm, and increased vascular permeability have been proposed in the pathogenesis of anemic retinopathy [24–26].

Table 1 Comparison of patients in two different phases of menstrual cycle (t-test) (LP = Luteal Phase, FP = Follicular phase; std.dev: standart deviation; FCT: choroidal thickness at fovea; N_{500}, choroidal thickness at 500 µm nasal to the fovea; N_{1500}, choroidal thickness at 1500 µm nasal to the fovea; T_{500}, choroidal thickness at 500 µm temporal to the fovea; T_{1500}, choroidal thickness at 1500 µm temporal to the fovea; FT: central macular thickness)

	N	Age	Hbvalue	FT	FCT	N_{500}	N_{1500}	T_{500}	T_{1500}
Mean FP	49	33.86	10.09	224.55	335.06	325.10	319.33	327.80	304.39
LP	47	34.32	10.34	226.66	324.47	318.51	315.04	310.47	288.06
Std. Dev. FP		10.21	1.33	19.23	63.42	81.71	81.71	88.59	92.29
LP		10.68	1.35	20.45	59.47	81.90	78.75	82.39	77.14
P		0.249	0.001 (with control groups)	0253	0.581	0.433	0.643	0.700	0.554

Table 2 The numbers, mean, median ages, minimum, maximum values and choroidal thickness measurements of the study and control groups at baseline. FCT, choroidal thickness at fovea; N500, choroidal thickness at 500 μm nasal to the fovea; N1500, choroidal thickness at 1500 μm nasal to the fovea; T500, choroidal thickness at 500 μm temporal to the fovea; T1500, choroidal thickness at 1500 μm temporal to the fovea; FT: central macular thickness. (t-test)

		Age	Hb value	FT	FCT	N500	N1500	T500	T1500
Anemia	N	96	96	96	96	96	96	96	96
	Mean	34.08	10.21	225.58	329.88	321.88	317.23	319.31	296.40
	Median	34.50	10.65	220.00	326.50	315.00	319.00	321.00	294.00
	Std. Deviation	10.396	1.342	19.760	61.431	81,445	79.810	85.607	85.168
	Minimum	18	7	199	201	121	109	88	79
	Maximum	49	12	291	481	567	575	537	500
Control	N	60	60	60	60	60	60	60	60
	Mean	32.29	14.42	222.45	349.94	347.39	333.74	346.45	326.58
	Median	34.00	14.00	219.00	352.00	344.00	323.00	352.00	315.00
	Std. Deviation	8.283	0.95	13.513	59.064	56.718	55.549	63.100	66.157
	Minimum	17	13	200	217	247	231	231	205
	Maximum	49	16	256	442	508	458	525	474
	P	0.254	0.000	0.276	0.043	0.032	0.157	0.033	0.019

Therefore, we hypothesize that because the choroid is the most vascular area of the eye, the above factors also affect choroidal tissues in patients with iron-deficiency anemia.

In our study, we observed a significant correlation between hemoglobin levels and CT. Moreover, we observed an inverse correlation between age and CT. Ding et al. reported similar results with respect to CT in a study of areas outside the subfoveal wet area in subjects younger than 60 years of age but failed to detect a correlation between age and subfoveal CT [27].

In the Beijing Eye Study, 3468 individuals were examined longitudinally, and several parameters related to the subfoveal CT was assessed [28]. That study observed direct links between age or the degree of myopia and CT. However, the potential associations or lack thereof between blood pressure, ocular perfusion, smoking, and alcohol consumption with diabetes mellitus and arterial hypertension remain controversial. However, that study relied only on single-point measurements. Notably, choroidal volume measurements risk being subject to false information [29].

In our study, we did not observe any significant differences between the two menstrual cycle phases. Because the menstrual cycle has a short duration, it is possible that we were unable observe a hormonal effect, or that the hormonal status does not affect CT. We did observe significant but moderate or weak correlations between the hemoglobin levels and the CT values at some measured points. However, the previously observed inverse correlation between age and CT might have affected this correlation [27]. The patients ranged in age from 17 to 49 years. No significant difference was observed between the duration of anemia duration and CT. This suggests that changes in CT do not progress during the course of anemia.

Table 3 Multiple linear regression analysis between choroidal thickness, age and hemoglobine values

		Beta(β)	P
N_{500}	Hb	−0.290	0.003
	Age	−0.269	0.006
N_{1500}	Hb	−0.249	0.009
	Age	−0.364	0.000
T_{500}	Hb	−0.342	0.000
	Age	−0.289	0.002
T_{1500}	Hb	−0.283	0.003
	age	−0.319	0.001
FCT	Hb	-	-
	Age	−0.291	0.004

FCT choroidal thickness at fovea; N_{500} choroidal thickness at 500 μm nasal to the fovea; N_{1500} choroidal thickness at 1500 μm nasal to the fovea; T_{500} choroidal thickness at 500 μm temporal to the fovea; T_{1500} choroidal thickness at 1500 μm temporal to the fovea; Hb Hemoglobin

Conclusion

Increasing attention is being paid to information about the choroidal structure and function. We think that as future studies of patients with anemia reveal the possible effects of this condition on choroidal tissue, the observation of decreased CT at all measured points in patients with iron-deficiency anemia might suggest the inclusion of this value as a clinical measurement in this patient population.

Abbreviations

EDI-OCT: enhanced-depth imaging optical coherence tomography; CT: choroidal thickness; FCT: choroidal thickness at fovea; N_{500}: choroidal thickness at 500 μm nasal to the fovea; N_{1500}: Choroidal thickness at 1500 μm nasal to the fovea; T_{500}: choroidal thickness at 500 μm temporal to the fovea; T_{1500}: choroidal thickness at 1500 μm temporal to the fovea; FT: foveal thickness (Central macular thickness); LP: luteal Phase; FP: follicular phase; RPE: retinal pigment epithelium; WHO: World Health Organization; Hb: hemoglobin.

Competing interest

The authors declare no competing interests.

Authors' contributions

EY is the first author of this article. Study design: EY, AC, SY. Ethical form preparation and application: AC. Data collection and entry: EY, HD. Contributions of reagents/materials/analytical tools: EY, AC, SY, CDY. Manuscript preparation and analytical data interpretation: EY. Manuscript writing: EY. Manuscript review: KO, EY. All authors read and approved the final manuscript.

Acknowledgements

This study was not supported by any funding project.
In this study, trial registration was requested on January 12, 2015. The trial protocol was approved by the Local Ethical Committee of the Kırıkkale University (decision no:01/04).

Author details

[1]Department of Ophthalmology, Kırıkkale University School of Medicine, Kırıkkale, Turkey. [2]Department of Internal Medicine, Kırıkkale University School of Medicine, Kırıkkale, Turkey. [3]Department of Medical Oncology, Kırıkkale University School of Medicine, Kırıkkale, Turkey. [4]Department of Obstetrics and Gynecology, Kırıkkale University School of Medicine, Kırıkkale, Turkey. [5]Kırıkkale University Medical Faculty Hospital District Tahsin Duru Akdeniz Caddesi No: 14, Yahsihan/Kırıkkale 71450, Turkey.

References

1. Spaide RF, Koizumi H, Pozzoni MC. Enhanced depth imaging spectral domain optical coherence tomography. Am J Ophthalmol. 2009;147:644–52.
2. Margolis R, Spaide RF. A pilot study of enhanced depth imaging optical coherence tomography of the choroid in normal eyes. Am J Ophthalmol. 2009;147:811–5.
3. Jung JW, Chin HS, Lee DH, Yoon MH, Kim NR. Changes in subfovealchoroidal thickness and choroidal extravascular density by spectral domain optical coherence tomography after haemodialysis: A pilot study. Br J Ophthalmol. 2014;98(2):207–12.
4. Pekel G, Alur I, Alihanoglu YI, Yagci R, Emrecan B. Choroidal changes after cardiopulmonary bypass. Perfusion. 2014;29:560–6.
5. Ingegnoli F, Gualtierotti R, Pierro L, Del Turco C, Miserocchi E, Schioppo T, et al. Choroidal impairment and macular thinning in patients with systemic sclerosis: The acute study. Microvasc Res. 2015;97:31–6.
6. Karaca EE, Ekici F, Yalçın NG, Çiftçi TU, Özdek Ş. Macular choroidal thickness measurements in patients with obstructive apnea syndrome. Sleep Breath. 2015;19:335–41.
7. Sizmaz S, Küçükerdönmez C, Pinarci EY, Karalezli A, Canan H, Yilmaz G. The effect of smoking on choroidal thickness measured by optical coherence tomography. Br J Ophthalmol. 2013;97:601–4.
8. McLean E, Cogswell M, Egli I, Wojdyla D, de Benoist B. Worldwide prevalence of anaemia, WHO Vitamin and Mineral Nutrition Information System, 1993–2005. Public Health Nutr. 2009;12(4):444–54.
9. Balarajan Y, Ramakrishnan U, Özaltin E, Shankar AH, Subramanian SV. Anaemia in low-income and middle-income countries. Lancet. 2011;378:2123–35.
10. Kassebaum NJ, Jasrasaria R, Naghavi M, Wulf SK, Johns N, Lozano R, et al. A systematic analysis of global anaemia burden between 1990 and 2010. Blood. 2014;123:615–24.
11. Milman N, Clausen J, Byg KE. Iron status in 268 Danish women aged 18–30 years: Influence of menstruation, contraceptive method, and iron supplementation. Ann Hematol. 1998;77:13–9.
12. Beard JL. Iron requirements in adolescent females. J Nutr. 2000;130(2S Suppl):440S–2S.
13. Parver LM. Temperature modulating action of choroidal blood flow. Eye. 1991;5:181–5.
14. Cao J, McLeod S, Merges CA, Lutty GA. Choriocapillaris degeneration and related pathologic changes in human diabetic eyes. Arch Ophthalmol. 1998;116:589–97.
15. Nickla DL, Wallman J. The multifunctional choroid. ProgRetin Eye Res. 2010;29:144–68.
16. Ikuno Y, Kawaguchi K, Nouchi T, Yasuno Y. Choroidal thickness in healthy Japanese subjects. Invest Ophthalmol Vis Sci. 2010;51:2173–6.
17. Agawa T, Miura M, Ikuno Y, Makita S, Fabritius T, Iwasaki T, et al. Choroidal thickness measurement in healthy Japanese subjects by three-dimensional high-penetration optical coherence tomography. Graefes Arch ClinExpOphthalmol. 2011;249(10):1485–92.
18. Brown JS, Flitcroft DI, Ying GS, Francis EL, Schmid GF, Quinn GE, et al. In vivo human choroidal thickness measurements: Evidence for diurnal fluctuations. Invest Ophthalmol Vis Sci. 2009;50:5–12.
19. Reiner A, Li C, Del Mar N, Fitzgerald ME. Choroidal blood flow compensation in rats for arterial blood pressure decreases is neuronal nitric oxide-dependent but compensation for arterial blood pressure increases is not. Exp Eye Res. 2010;90:734–41.
20. Kiel JW. Choroidal myogenic autoregulation and intraocular pressure. Exp Eye Res. 1994;58:529–43.
21. Tanabe H, Ito Y, Iguchi Y, Ozawa S, Ishikawa K, Terasaki H. Correlation between cross-sectional shape of choroidal veins and choroidal thickness. Jpn J Ophthalmol. 2011;55:614–9.
22. Vance SK, Imamura Y, Freund KB. The effects of sildenafil citrate on choroidal thickness as determined by enhanced depth imaging optical coherence tomography. Retina. 2011;31:332–5.
23. Ngo WK, Tan CS. Choroidal thickness in high-altitude sickness. Indian J Ophthalmol. 2014;62:1106–7.
24. Carraro MC, Rossetti L, Gerli GC. Prevalence of retinopathy in patients with anemia or thrombocytopenia. Eur J Haematol. 2001;67(4):238–44.
25. Aisen ML, Bacon BR, Goodman AM, Chester EM. Retinal abnormalities associated with anemia. Arch Ophthalmol. 1983;101(7):1049–52.
26. Ranil PK, Raman R, Rachepalli SR, Pal SS, Kulothungan V, Lakshmipathy P, et al. Anemia and diabetic retinopathy in type 2 diabetes mellitus. J Assoc Physicians India. 2010;58:91–4.
27. Ding X, Li J, Zeng J, Ma W, Liu R, Li T, et al. Choroidal thickness in healthy Chinese subjects. Invest Ophthalmol Vis Sci. 2011;52:9555–60.
28. Wei WB, Xu L, Jonas JB, Shao L, Du KF, Wang S, et al. Subfoveal choroidal thickness: The Beijing Eye Study. Ophthalmology. 2013;120:175–80.
29. Sanchez-Cano A, Orduna E, Segura F, Lopez C, Cuenca N, Abecia E, et al. Choroidal thickness and volume in healthy young white adults and the relationships between the mand axial length, ammetropy and sex. Am J Ophthalmol. 2014;158(3):574–83.

Oxidative stress and premature senescence in corneal endothelium following penetrating keratoplasty in an animal model

Xiaowen Zhao[1], Ye Wang[1,2*], Yao Wang[1], Suxia Li[1] and Peng Chen[1]

Abstract

Background: The purpose of this study was to address the question of how the premature senescence process may affect corneal endothelium after penetrating keratoplasty, because the quality of donor corneal endothelial cells is important for corneal transplant success.

Methods: The cell senescence and induced oxidative stress in corneal endothelium were assessed using a normal-risk orthotopic mice corneal transplantation model. Senescence associated beta-galactosidase (SA-beta-Gal) staining was used to evaluate premature senescence in the endothelium of corneal allografts. Oxidative Stress and Antioxidant Defense RT^2-PCR Arrays and *in vitro* experimental model using H_2O_2 treatment were used to investigate the possible mechanism.

Results: SA-beta-Gal positivity was observed obviously in mice corneal endothelium of allogenic group and the levels of p16^{INK4a} message and protein increased in endothelium of allogenic group compared to syngenic group. By PCR array, an oxidant-antioxidant imbalance was found in the endothelium of corneal allograft after PKP. The results from mice model were validated using human endothelium samples of corneal allograft after PKP. We also developed an *in vitro* experimental model using H_2O_2 treatment to simulate a state of oxidative stress in cultured human corneal endothelial cells (HCECs) and found that elevated ROS levels, the up-regulation of CDK inhibitors and ROS-mediated p16^{INK4A} up-regulation in HCECs occur via the ASK1-p38 MAPK pathway.

Conclusions: Our results demonstrate the presence of oxidative stress and premature senescence in the endothelium of corneal allografts following PKP.

Keywords: Oxidative stress, Premature senescence, Corneal endothelium, Penetrating keratoplasty

Background

Human corneal endothelial cells (HCECs) form a monolayer with limited regenerative potential, and these cells maintain stromal dehydration via an ion pump mechanism [1]. For the past 50 years, penetrating keratoplasty (PKP) has been the standard treatment for corneal endothelial specific dysfunctional diseases [2]. Rather than replacing the entire cornea, endothelial keratoplasty (EK) replaces the patient's endothelium with a transplanted disc of posterior stroma/Descemets/endothelium (DSEK) or Descemets/endothelium (DMEK) [3]. This relatively new procedure has revolutionized treatment of disorders of the endothelium. Additionally, lamellar keratoplasty (LKP) replaces only the diseased Bowman's layer and the anterior, or upper part of the corneal stroma with donor material. The quality of donor corneal endothelial cells is very important for corneal transplant success. It was reported that the status of donor endothelial cells may be a necessary condition for graft transparency and long-term survival [4, 5]. Endothelial cell loss can lead to corneal opacity over

* Correspondence: wye112002@126.com
[1]State Key Laboratory Cultivation Base, Shandong Provincial Key Laboratory of Ophthalmology, Shandong Eye Institute, Shandong Academy of medical Sciences, No. 5 Yanerdao Rd, Qingdao 266071, China
[2]Current affiliation: Central Laboratory of the Second Affiliated Hospital, Medical College of Qingdao University, Qingdao 266042, China

time after PKP and is substantial 5 years postkeratoplasty [6]. However, there is currently little understanding of the mechanisms of the accelerated postoperative loss of endothelial cells.

DNA breaks and oxidative lesions caused by environmental insults, genetic defects, or endogenous processes belong to certain types of DNA damage. One of the critical effects of oxidative stress caused by reactive oxygen species is the induction of cellular senescence [7, 8]. Numerous studies have reported that premature senescence is closely related to organ transplant [9–12], such as renal transplantation [13]. Cellular senescence is a state of irreversible growth arrest. It can be triggered by many kinds of oncogenic or stressful stimuli including telomere shortening, the epigenetic derepression of the *INK4a/ARF* locus [8, 14]. Studies with clinical outcome of HCECs showed the exhibition signs of oxidative DNA damage and that oxidative stress affects the proliferative capacity of HCECs [15, 16]. These authors also observed that, with respect to the senescence of corneal endothelial cells, age-related relative proliferative capacity and senescence characteristics are not due to replicative senescence caused by critically short telomeres *in vitro* [17].

Studies have indicated that protein kinase activities are redox-sensitive because key cysteine residues in these proteins can undergo post-translational modifications by oxidants [18]. Several signal transduction pathways have been implicated in cell senescence and cell death, including p38 MAPK pathway. Moreover, apoptosis signal-regulating kinase 1 (ASK1) is a key element in the mechanism of stress-induced cell senescence [19]. It was reported that stress-activated ASK1 accelerates endothelial cell senescence in patients with diabetes [20] and that the inhibition of the ASK1-p38 MAPK pathway could be useful for preventing vascular ageing and for treating neurodegenerative and cardiac diseases [18, 21]. However, whether ASK1-p38 MAPK pathway underlying the cell premature senescence in pathogenesis of corneal endothelium after PKP are not well understood.

In this study, we assessed premature senescence and induced oxidative stress in corneal endothelium using a normal-risk orthotopic mice corneal transplantation model. Then, using an oxidative stress and antioxidant defense PCR array, an oxidant-antioxidant imbalance was found to be involved in the endothelium of corneal allograft after PKP. Next, we validated our results from the mice model using human endothelium samples of corneal allograft after PKP. We also developed an *in vitro* experimental model using H_2O_2 treatment to simulate a state of oxidative stress in cultured HCECs and found that elevated ROS levels, the up-regulation of CDK inhibitors and ROS-mediated p16^{INK4A} up-regulation in HCECs occur via the ASK1-p38 MAPK pathway.

Methods

Animals and the normal-risk orthotopic corneal transplantation

The study was approved by the Institutional Animal Care Committee of Shandong Eye Institute, and all of the procedures were performed according to the Association for Research and Vision in Ophthalmology (ARVO) Statement for the Use of Animals in Ophthalmic and Vision Research. Six- to eight-week-old adult BALB/c (H-2d) mice and C57BL/6 (H-2b) mice, weighing 18 to 20 g, were obtained from the Institute of Zoology Chinese Academy of Sciences. The mice were divided into two groups, syngenic groups and allogenic, each containing 20 mice. The corneal transplantations were performed as previously described [22]. Male C57BL/6 mice were used as donors, and same-aged male BALB/c mice were used as recipients. The outcomes of the procedure were compared between syngeneic grafts for which male BALB/c mice were used as both the donors and recipients. Immunosuppressive drugs were not used, either topically or systemically. Only the right eye of each mouse was used for the corneal transplantation; the left eye was undisturbed.

The corneal grafts were collected 4.5 months postgrafting, and the corneal endothelium samples were separated from the grafts. For the PCR Array analysis (SABiosciences Corp., Frederick, MD), the samples were pooled into 6 groups (SP1, SP2, SP3, AP1, AP2, and AP3). Each group comprised three corneal endothelium samples. For the Western blot analyses, the samples were pooled into 6 groups (SW1, SW2, SW3, AW1, AW2, and AW3). Each group comprised two corneal endothelium samples.

Clinical evaluation of grafted mouse corneas, dual staining of corneal endothelium with trypan blue and alizarin red S, and immunohistochemistry

The mouse corneal grafts were examined once per week for two weeks with a slit-lamp biomicroscope (Haag-Streit model BQ-900, Switzerland). Graft opacity was scored using a scale of one to five, as previously described [22]. The corneal grafts were considered to be failures after receiving two successive scores of 3. All of the examinations were performed by two blinded observers. The corneal endothelium was examined by dual staining of the corneal endothelium with trypan blue and alizarin red S (Sigma-Aldrich, Shanghai, China) [23]. For the immunohistochemical analysis of 8-hydroxydeoxyguanosine (8-OHdG) (AB5830; Millipore, Bedford, MA), the corneal samples were fixed in cold methanol and the samples were subjected to staining using the EliVision™ plus kit (Maxim Corp, Fuzhou, China), according to the manufacturer's protocol, and observed using a Fluorescence E800 microscope (Nikon, Tokyo, Japan).

Real time PCR-based array analysis

Total RNA of mouse corneal endothelium was isolated using NucleoSpin RNA II System (Macherey-Nagel, Düren, Germany) according to the manufacturer's instructions. The first-strand cDNA was synthesized from equal amounts of total RNA (1 μg/μl) using a PrimeScript® 1st Strand cDNA Synthesis Kit (TaKaRa, Dalian, China). The real-time PCR array and data analyses were performed using a RT^2 Profiler™ PCR Array Mouse Oxidative Stress and Antioxidant Defense PCR Array (PAMM-065A, SABiosciences Corp., Frederick, MD).

Patient tissue sample collection

After obtaining approval from the Shandong Eye Institute ethics committee and according to the tenets of the Declaration of Helsinki, between December 2005 and December 2010, 15 fresh dysfunctional corneal buttons (7.25 to 8 mm diameter) were collected prospectively from patients with failed corneal transplants. After further sample preparation, five samples were selected for analysis as shown in Table 1. The prospectively enrolled patients from which dysfunctional corneal buttons were obtained provided written informed consent.

Sex-matched normal human cornea samples from organ donors were provided by the International Federation of Eye Banks at the Eye Bank of Shandong, China (Qingdao, China) and were used as controls. Three samples were used for the SA-β-Gal staining (age 21, 25, and 19 years) and four samples were used for the gene expression profiling (age 21, 27, 30 and 31 years). Another five samples (three for 22 years old and two for 25 years old) were used to the HECEs culture. Corneal rims, residual parts dissected from donor corneas by a circular trephine in penetrating keratoplasty, were immediately collected for this study as shown in Table 2. All samples were maintained in corneal storage medium (Optisol; Chiron Ophthalmics, Inc., Irvine, CA) at 4 °C until immediately before the experiment.

RNA extraction and gene expression profiling study

Total RNA was isolated using the NucleoSpin RNA II System (Macherey-Nagel, Duren, Germany), and first-strand cDNA was synthesized using a MMLV Reverse

Transcriptase 1st-Strand cDNA Synthesis Kit (Epicentre Biotechnologies, Madison, WI) according to the manufacturer's protocol. The gene expression profiling study, including labeling, hybridization, scanning, normalization, and data analysis, was performed by KangChen Bio-tech (Shanghai, China) using a Human Genome Oligo Microarray (4x44K, Agilent Technologies, Palo Alto, CA).

Human corneal endothelial cells (HCECs) culture and treatment

Five corneal rims samples from normal donor corneas (three for 22 years old and two for 25 years old) were used to the HCECs culture and cell culture was performed by Wuhan PriCells Biomedical Technology Co., Ltd. (Wuhan, China) according to described protocols [8]. Briefly, Descemet's membrane with intact endothelium was carefully dissected in small strips and then incubated in OptiMEM-I supplemented with 10 % FBS overnight to stabilize the cells before culture. After centrifugation, the strips were incubated in 0.02 % EDTA solution at 37 °C for 1 hour and cells were resuspended in culture medium containing OptiMEM-I, 8 % FBS, 5 ng/mL EGF, 20 ng/mL NGF, 100 g/mL pituitary extract, 20 g/mL ascorbic acid, 200 mg/L calcium chloride, 0.08 % chondroitin sulfate, 50 g/mL gentamicin, and antibiotic/antimycotic solution diluted 1/100. Cultures were then incubated at 37 °C in a 5 % carbon dioxide, humidified atmosphere.

The cultured HCECs were then subjected to various H_2O_2 concentrations (0 to 100 μM) for variable time periods (0 minutes, 1 hours, 2 hours and 6 hours) at 37 °C. The cells with no H_2O_2 treatment were used as controls. In addition, HCECs were also treated with SB203580 (10 μM) (Cell Signaling Technology, Inc., Danvers, MA) and the cells with no SB203580 treatment were used as controls.

Senescence-associated β-galactosidase (SA-β-Gal) activity staining

Following the methods of previous reports [24, 25], human corneal whole mounts were fixed with 4 % formaldehyde (with the endothelial cell side up). The tissues were then incubated at 37 °C overnight using a

Table 1 The information of all the patients

Patient No.	Age/Gender	Affected Eye	History of Ocular Diseases	Time^a(years)	Experiment
1	41/M	OS	Keratoplasty for corneal opacity	5	SA-β-Gal staining
2	35/M	OS	Keratoplasty for corneal opacity	8.5	SA-β-Gal staining
3	62/M	OD	Keratoplastyfor bullous keratopathy	7	gene expression profiling
4	62/M	OD	Keratoplasty for corneal opacity	7	gene expression profiling
5	21/M	OS	Ocular trauma	7	gene expression profiling

F = female; M = male
^{a}years between the first and the second corneal transplantation

Table 2 Donor Information

Age (y)	Hoursª	Daysᵇ	Cause of Death	Experiment	Samples
19	4	1	Motor vehicle accident	SA-β-Gal staining	whole cornea
21	5	2	Cardiac arrest	SA-β-Gal staining	whole cornea
25	4	2	Traumatic injury	SA-β-Gal staining	whole cornea
21	6	2	Motor vehicle accident	gene expression profiling	whole corneal endothelium
27	7	1	Motor vehicle accident	gene expression profiling	whole corneal endothelium
30	6	1	Motor vehicle accident	gene expression profiling	whole corneal endothelium
31	5	2	Motor vehicle accident	gene expression profiling	whole corneal endothelium
22	4	2	Cardiac arrest	HECEs culture	corneal rims
22	1	1	Cardiac arrest	HECEs culture	corneal rims
22	2	1	Motor vehicle accident	HECEs culture	corneal rims
25	2	1	Cardiac arrest	HECEs culture	corneal rims
25	2	1	Motor vehicle accident	HECEs culture	corneal rims

ªNumber of hours between death and corneal preservation
ᵇNumber of days of corneal preservation in corneal storage medium at 4 °C

senescence β-galactosidase staining kit (Beyotime Institute of Biotechnology, Shanghai, China) according to the manufacturer's instructions. The staining was visualized and captured using a microscope that was equipped with a digital camera (Eclipse e800; Nikon).

Immunofluorescent staining

For the immunofluorescent staining, mice corneal tissues were placed with the endothelium side up and fixed with 4 % PFA solution. Then, the samples were incubated overnight at 4 °C with the primary antibodies (p-ASK1 and p-p38). After washing with PBS, the samples were incubated for 1 h with FITC conjugated secondary antibody (1:100; Santa Cruz). The stained cells were counterstained with DAPI and viewed under an Eclipse TE2000-U microscope (Nikon, Tokyo, Japan).

Statistical analysis

All results are expressed as the means ± SDs. The statistical analyses were performed using SPSS 15.0 software (SPSS, Chicago, IL). For the PCR Array and gene expression profiling study, an independent-Samples t-test was performed comparing the two different groups using the Kolmogorov–Smirnov test. For the analysis of the PCR and Western blot results, a One-Way analysis of variance (ANOVA) was performed to compare the groups using the Student–Newman–Keuls test and the Least Significant Difference procedure. P- values of less than 0.05 were considered to be statistically significant.

Information on the Real time PCR, Intracellular reactive oxygen species (ROS) measurement and the detection of mitochondrial ROS, Western blot analysis, and gene expression profiling studies available in the Additional file 1: Materials and Methods.

Results

Premature senescence in the endothelia of corneal allografts following PKP

We assessed premature senescence of endothelia using a normal-risk orthotopic mice corneal transplantation model for three times (totally 60 mice). We collected 8, 11, and 10 corneal grafts for these three times. For each time, four corneal grafts from each of the two groups were used for the detection of staining. That is, one corneal graft was separated into three pieces, and one pieces were used for the staining of the corneal endothelium with trypan blue and alizarin red S. The others were used for staining of SA-β-Gal and immunohistochemical analysis of 8-OHdG.

The results of the clinical evaluation of mouse corneal graft and corneal endothelium are shown in Fig. 1a and e. The original hexagonal structure of endothelial cells was maintained in the syngeneic group (Fig. 1b). The endothelial cell borders of the corneal grafts from the allogeneic group were opaque, and polykaryocytes were observed in corneal endothelium of the allogeneic group (Fig. 1f). SA-β-Gal-positive cells were observed in endothelium of the corneal grafts in allogeneic group (Fig. 1g), whereas SA-β-Gal-positive cells were not observed in endothelium of the corneal grafts in syngeneic group (Fig. 1c). Higher 8-OHdG expression was observed in the nuclei compared to the cytoplasm of the corneal endothelial cells. The percentage 8-OHdG expression was higher in the corneal graft nuclei of allogeneic group (Fig. 1d) than that of syngeneic group (Fig. 1h).

We next compared the expression of p16^INK4A, p21^WAF1/CIP1 and p53 proteins in the endothelium of corneal grafts by western blot analysis (Fig. 2). A significant up-regulation of p16^INK4A, p21^WAF1/CIP1, and p53

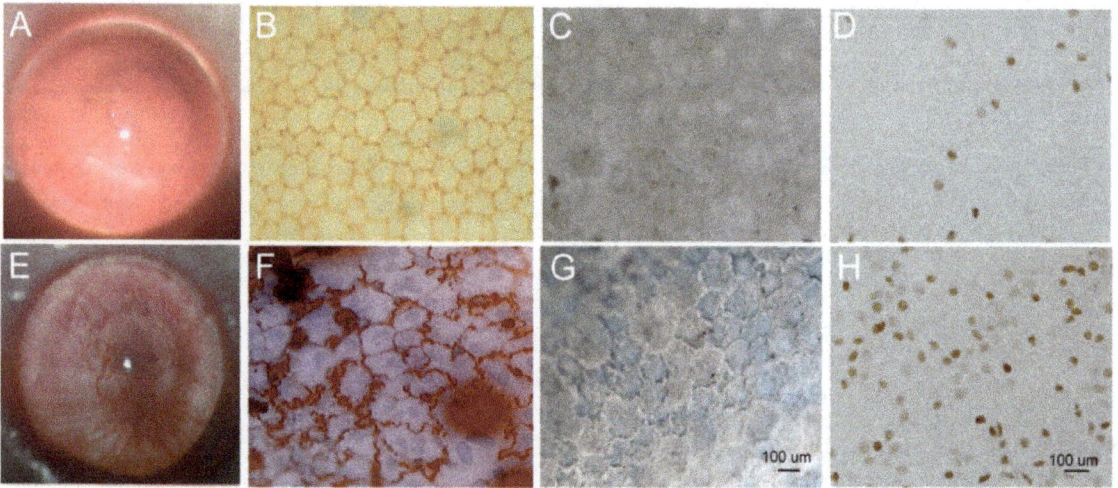

Fig. 1 Premature senescence in mice endothelium of corneal dysfunctional allografts after PKP **a** Clinical evaluation of mouse corneal graft in syngeneic group (after 4.5 months post grafting); **b** Evaluation of endothelium of corneal graft in syngeneic group (*n* = 4); **c** Representative results of SA-β-Gal staining on corneal endothelium in syngeneic group; **d** Representative results of 8-hydroxydeoxyguanosine (8-OHdG) staining on corneal endothelium in syngenic group; **e** Clinical evaluation of mouse corneal graft in allogenic group (after 4.5 months post grafting); **f** Evaluation of endothelium of corneal graft in allogenic group; **g** Representative results of SA-β-Gal staining on corneal endotheliumin in allogenic group; **h** Representative results of 8-OHdG staining on corneal endothelium in allogenic group. Rejection of corneal grafts was observed in allogenic group as opacification of the cornea and new vessel in growth, compared with corneal grafts in syngeneic group **e**. In syngeneic group, the original hexagonal structure was maintained **b** compared with corneal grafts in allogenic group **f**. The endothelial cell borders of corneal grafts in allogeneic group were not clear, and polykaryocytes were observed in corneal endothelium of allogeneic group **f**. Compared with corneal grafts in allogeneic group **g**, SA-β-Gal positive cells were not observed on corneal endotheliumin in syngeneic group **c**. This revealed that dysfunctional corneal allografts exhibited characteristics of premature endothelial senescence. Compared with corneal grafts in syngenic group **d**, the strength and numbers of positive cells of 8-OHdG staining were less than that in allogenic group **h**

protein expression was observed in the corneal endothelium of allogeneic grafts compared with syngeneic grafts.

Then, the Mouse Oxidative Stress and Antioxidant Defense RT^2-PCR Arrays were used to investigate the oxidant-antioxidant imbalance in the endothelium of corneal allografts after PKP. As indicated, a more than two fold change in expression, with $p < 0.05$, was considered to be statistically significant. Of the 84 genes assayed, 27 transcripts (32 %) were down-regulated; of these, 17 were expressed at more than two fold lower levels and 11 (13 %) were more highly expressed, as is shown in the three-dimensional profile (Fig. 3a) and the scatter plot (Fig. 3b). Of the genes that were expressed at lower levels, statistical significance was noted for 23 antioxidant genes

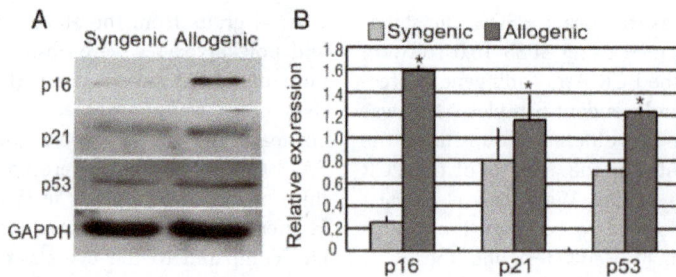

Fig. 2 Up-regulated expression of p16[INK4A], p21[Cip1] and p53 proteins in mice endothelium of dysfunctional corneal allografts Expression of cell senescence related proteins, p16[INK4A], p21[Cip1/CDKN1A] and p53 in mice endothelium of dysfunctional corneal allografts. Changes in protein expression as determined by Western blot. **a** data from the gels; **b** normalization to GAPDH. For each sample, the relative abundance of the protein of interest is determined by calculating the ratio of the intensity of the signal for the protein of interest to that of the normalization control GAPDH. Band densities determined by ImageJ software and compared with syngenic group. Expression of p16[INK4A], p21[Cip1/CDKN1A] and p53 were higher in the corneal endothelium of allogenic group than in the syngenic group (*t*-test, *P* < 0.05, n = 3). Significant differences between the corneal endothelium tissue in syngenic and allogenic groups are indicated by an asterisk (**P* < 0.05)

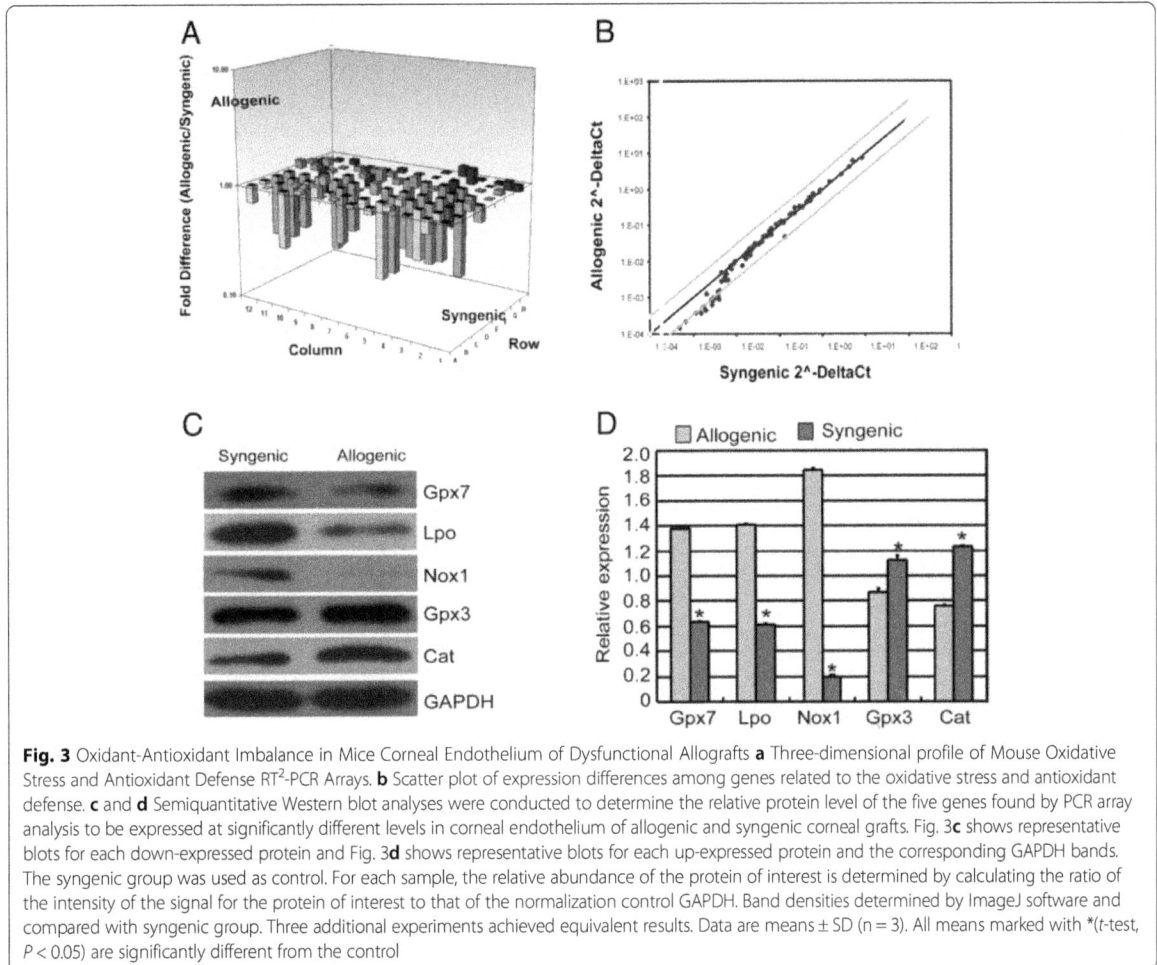

Fig. 3 Oxidant-Antioxidant Imbalance in Mice Corneal Endothelium of Dysfunctional Allografts **a** Three-dimensional profile of Mouse Oxidative Stress and Antioxidant Defense RT²-PCR Arrays. **b** Scatter plot of expression differences among genes related to the oxidative stress and antioxidant defense. **c** and **d** Semiquantitative Western blot analyses were conducted to determine the relative protein level of the five genes found by PCR array analysis to be expressed at significantly different levels in corneal endothelium of allogenic and syngenic corneal grafts. Fig. 3**c** shows representative blots for each down-expressed protein and Fig. 3**d** shows representative blots for each up-expressed protein and the corresponding GAPDH bands. The syngenic group was used as control. For each sample, the relative abundance of the protein of interest is determined by calculating the ratio of the intensity of the signal for the protein of interest to that of the normalization control GAPDH. Band densities determined by ImageJ software and compared with syngenic group. Three additional experiments achieved equivalent results. Data are means ± SD (n = 3). All means marked with *(t-test, $P < 0.05$) are significantly different from the control

(Table 3). The information for the more highly expressed genes is given in Table 4. The genes encoding Glutathione peroxidase 7 (Gpx7), Lactoperoxidase (Lpo) and NADPH oxidase 1 (Nox1) were expressed at 4.48-fold, 4.32-fold and 4.14-fold lower levels, respectively, in allogenic corneal endothelium compared with syngenic corneal endothelium.

In the endothelium of allogenic corneal samples, Gpx7, Lpo, and Nox1 were expressed at 2.22-fold, 2.38-fold and 9.10-fold lower levels, respectively, relative to the endothelium in syngenic corneal samples by Western blot analyses (Fig. 3). In the endothelium of allogenic corneal samples, Gpx3 and Cat were expressed at 1.17-fold and 1.58-fold higher levels, respectively, than in the endothelium in the syngenic corneal samples. Then, we showed the results of the ROS accumulation and activation of ASK1/p38 signal pathway in mouse model in Fig. 4. The elevated ROS levels may be the results of the oxidant-antioxidant imbalance.

Representative results of SA-β-Gal staining on human corneal allografts and in normal human corneal endothelium were shown in Fig. 5-a and b. Compared with normal human corneal endothelium, more SA-β-Gal positive cells were observed on corneal endothelium in corneal allograft after PKP. These results were consistent with that in the mice model. The result of gene expression profiling was shown as the scatterplot in Fig. 5-c. The scatterplot is a visualization that is useful for assessing the variation between endothelium in corneal allografts (Y-axis) and in normal human corneal endothelium (X-axis). Microarray-based GO analysis of differentially expressed genes on endothelium between corneal allograft after PKP and normal human corneal endothelium was shown in Fig. 5-d (the most significantly down-regulated genes) and Fig. 5-e (the most significantly up-regulated genes). The three GO classifications, molecular function (MF), biological process (BP), and cellular component (CC), were evaluated separately and the significant terms of all ontologies are shown.

Table 3 Genes down-regulated in endothelium of mice dysfunctional corneal allografts relative to syngenic control as detected by PCR array

Gene description	Symbol	Fold regulation	P
Antioxidant			
Glutathione Peroxidases (Gpx)			
Glutathione peroxidase 5	Gpx5	−3.18	0.1479
Glutathione peroxidase 6	Gpx6	−3.05	0.0021
Glutathione peroxidase 7	Gpx7	−4.48	0.0017
Peroxiredoxins (TPx)			
Peroxiredoxin 4	Prdx4	−1.22	0.0478
Other Peroxidases			
Lactoperoxidase	Lpo	−4.32	0.0007
Prostaglandin-endoperoxide synthase 2	Ptgs2	−1.43	0.0011
Recombination activating gene 2	Rag2	−3.00	0.0058
Thyroid peroxidase	Tpo	−2.64	0.0016
Other Antioxidants			
Nucleoredoxin	Nxn	−1.19	0.0105
ROS Metabolism			
Superoxide Metabolism			
Cytochrome b-245, alpha polypeptide	Cyba	−1.43	0.0122
Neutrophil cytosolic factor 2	Ncf2	−1.87	0.0045
NADPH oxidase 1	Nox1	−4.14	0.0052
NADPH oxidase 4	Nox4	−1.58	0.022
NADPH oxidase activator 1	Noxa1	−3.11	0.1457
NADPH oxidase organizer 1	Noxo1	−1.63	0.0349
RecQ protein-like 4	Recq14	−1.83	0.0016
Other genes involved in ROS Metabolism			
Interleukin 19	Il19	−3.37	0.0001
Interleukin 22	Il22	−3.41	0.0008
Oxidative stress responsive genes			
Dual oxidase 1	Duox1	−2.65	1.80E-05
Eosinophil peroxidase	Epx	−4.46	2.00E-04
Myeloperoxidase	Mpo	−3.49	0.0041
Membrane protein, palmitoylated 4 (MAGUK p55 subfamily member 4)	Mpp4	−3.11	0.0043
Nudix (nucleoside diphosphate linked moiety X)-type motif 15	Nudt15	−1.18	0.0106
Uncoupling protein 3 (mitochondrial, proton carrier)	Ucp3	−1.58	0.0088
Oxygen transporters			
Hemoglobin, theta 1A	Hbq1a	−3.13	0.0511
Myoglobin	Mb	−3.44	0.0604
Xin actin-binding repeat containing 1	Xirp1	−3.13	0.0003

Table 4 Genes up-regulated in endothelium of mice dysfunctional corneal allografts relative to syngenic control as detected by PCR array

Gene description	Symbol	Fold regulation	P
Antioxidant			
Glutathione Peroxidases (Gpx)			
Glutathione peroxidase 3	Gpx3	1.17	0.0118
Other Peroxidases			
Glutathione reductase	Gsr	1.25	0.0079
Catalase	Cat	1.24	0.0033
Adenomatosis polyposis coli	Apc	1.11	0.0144
Peroxiredoxin 6, pseudogene 1	Prdx6-ps1	1.17	0.0051
Tropomodulin 1	Tmod1	1.37	0.0004
ROS Metabolism			
Superoxide Metabolism			
Stearoyl-Coenzyme A desaturase 1	Scd1	1.09	0.0385
Oxidative stress responsive genes			
Isocitrate dehydrogenase 1 (NADP+), soluble	Idh1	1.19	0.0016
Protein phosphatase 1, regulatory (inhibitor) subunit 15b	Ppp1r15b	1.22	0.0048
Peroxiredoxin 2	Prdx2	1.29	0.0114
Oxygen transporters			
Solute carrier family 38, member 1	Slc38a1	1.11	0.0462

treatment to simulate a state of oxidative stress. Primary culture of human corneal endothelial cells with generic function associated markers such as Na$^+$K$^+$ATPase and ZO-1 as well as PRDX6 were characterized. Intracellular ROS and mitochondria ROS accumulation were compared. ROS generation was observed in HCECs 60 minutes following treatment with 100 µM H$_2$O$_2$ (Fig. 6a-i and 6a -ii). The data indicate that intracellular ROS levels are much higher in HCECs following H$_2$O$_2$ treatment than in untreated cells. SA-β-Gal positivity was also observed in HCECs after 60 minutes of treatment with 100 µM H$_2$O$_2$ (Fig. 6a-iii and 6a-iv). To determine whether ROS production is enhanced in the mitochondria of HCECs following H$_2$O$_2$ treatment, the localization of MitoTracker Green FM with MitoSOX red was performed. As revealed by the localization of Mito Tracker Green (Fig. 6b-ii and 6a-v), H$_2$O$_2$ treated cells exhibited red fluorescence in mitochondria, indicating increased mitochondrial ROS production (Fig. 6b-iv) compared with the control HCECs (Fig. 6b-i).

Inhibitors of cyclin-dependent kinases (CDKs) are considered to play critical roles in cell cycle arrest and

Oxidative stress, elevated ROS levels, the up-regulation of CDK inhibitors and ROS-mediated p16 [INK4A] up-regulation in HCECs occur via the ASK1-p38 MAPK pathway

Given that the oxidant-antioxidant imbalance was involved in endothelium of corneal allografts, we developed an *in vitro* experimental model using H$_2$O$_2$

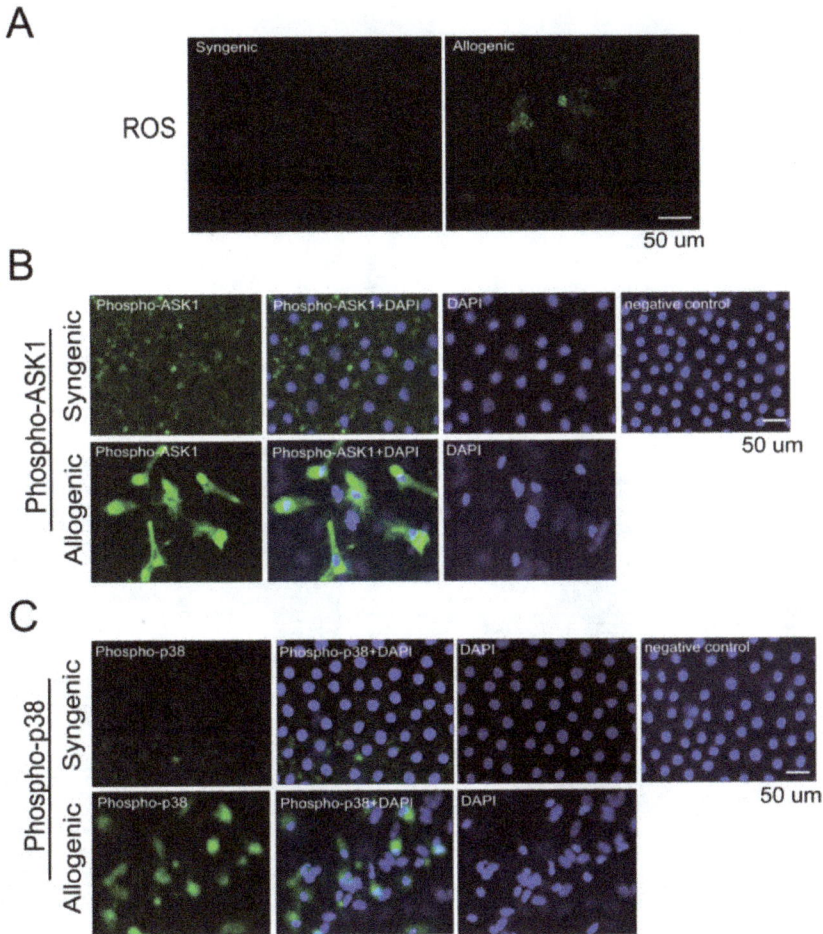

Fig. 4 ROS accumulation and activation of ASK1/p38 signal pathway in Mice Corneal Endothelium of Dysfunctional Allografts **a** Representative results of ROS staining on corneal endothelium in syngenic group and allogenic group; **b** Up-regulation of phospho-ASK1 on corneal endothelium in syngenic group and allogenic group by immunofluorescence detection; **c** Up-regulation of phospho-p38 on corneal endothelium in syngenic group and allogenic group by immunofluorescence detection. Samples of corneal endothelium in syngenic group were used as the control group. 2 corneal grafts from each of the two groups were used for the detection of staining. That is, one corneal graft was separated into two pieces, and one piece was used for the staining of phospho-ASK1. The other was used for staining of phospho-p38

premature senescence [8, 26]. We therefore investigated the effects of ROS on the levels of CDK inhibitors in HCECs, including $p16^{INK4A}$, $p21^{cip1}$, and $p27^{kip1}$. At 2 hours after 100 μM H_2O_2 treatment, a brief up-regulation of $p16^{INK4A}$, $p21^{cip1}$, and $p27^{kip1}$ mRNA was observed in HCECs (Fig. 6c). We also detected the protein expression levels of $p16^{INK4A}$, $p21^{cip1}$, and $p27^{kip1}$ by western blot analysis, as is shown in Fig. 6d. When the HCECs were exposed to 100 μM H_2O_2, the levels of $p16^{INK4A}$, $p21^{cip1}$, and $p27^{kip1}$ protein expression were elevated, and this up-regulation persisted from 2 to 6 hours post-H_2O_2 treatment.

To address whether H_2O_2-induced HCECs senescence is related to the activity of ASK1-p38 MAPK pathway,

the protein levels of ASK1 or phosphorylated ASK1 was measured by Western blot analysis. p38 MAPK activation was then compared between the H_2O_2-treated and untreated HCECs *in vitro*. Fig. 7a presents representative the results of the Western blot studies. The phosphorylation levels of ASK1 and p38 MAPK significantly increased in HCECs following H_2O_2 treatment. We also used siRNA that specifically silences ASK1 and SB203580, a widely used p38 inhibitor, to investigate the molecular mechanisms that underlie H_2O_2-induced endothelial cell senescence in cultured HCECs. By Western blotting analysis, we found that the expression of ASK1 was down-regulated after transfection with ASK1-siRNA and ASK1-siRNA also decreased the activation of

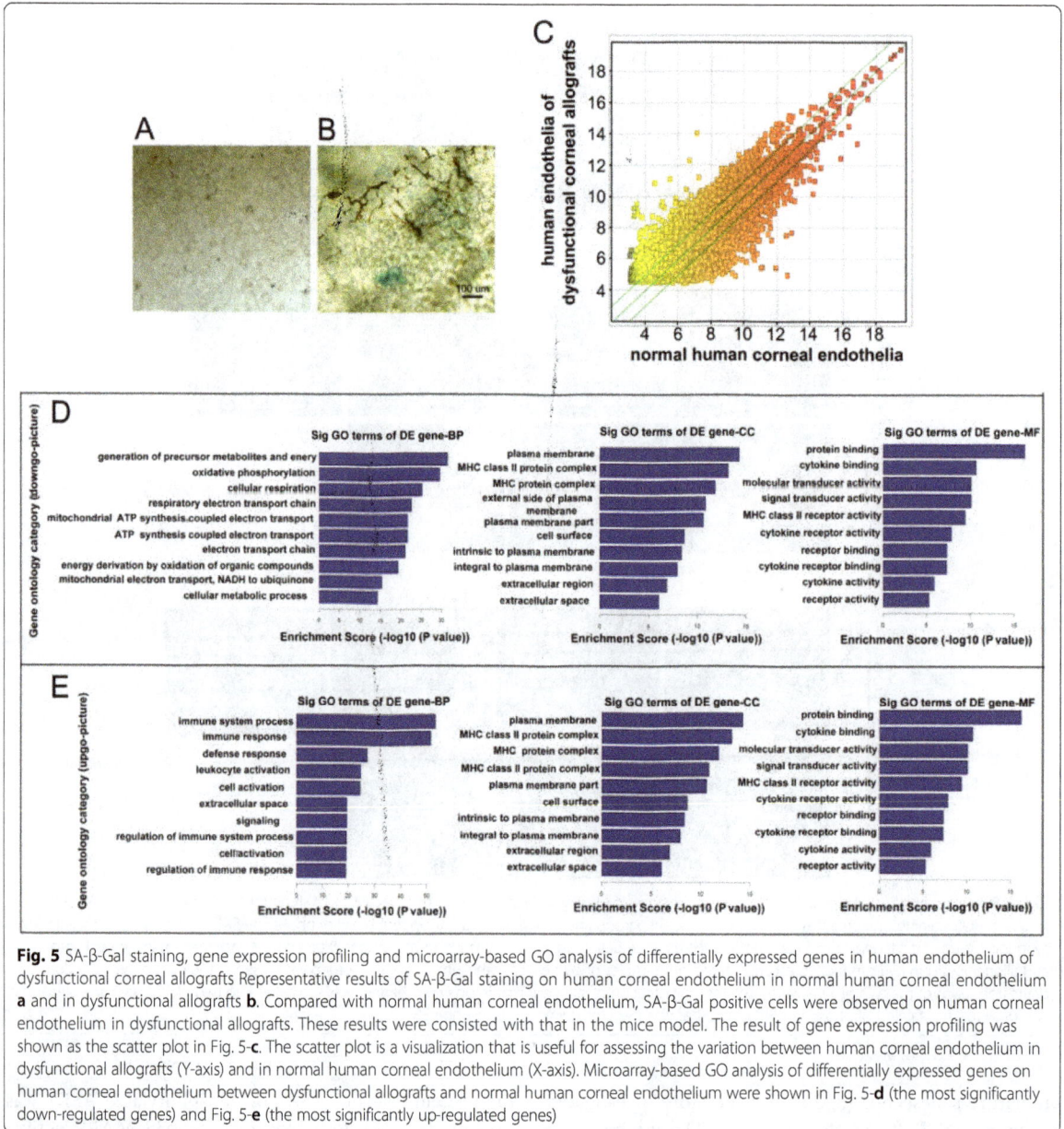

Fig. 5 SA-β-Gal staining, gene expression profiling and microarray-based GO analysis of differentially expressed genes in human endothelium of dysfunctional corneal allografts Representative results of SA-β-Gal staining on human corneal endothelium in normal human corneal endothelium **a** and in dysfunctional allografts **b**. Compared with normal human corneal endothelium, SA-β-Gal positive cells were observed on human corneal endothelium in dysfunctional allografts. These results were consisted with that in the mice model. The result of gene expression profiling was shown as the scatter plot in Fig. 5-**c**. The scatter plot is a visualization that is useful for assessing the variation between human corneal endothelium in dysfunctional allografts (Y-axis) and in normal human corneal endothelium (X-axis). Microarray-based GO analysis of differentially expressed genes on human corneal endothelium between dysfunctional allografts and normal human corneal endothelium were shown in Fig. 5-**d** (the most significantly down-regulated genes) and Fig. 5-**e** (the most significantly up-regulated genes)

MAKP in HCECs (Fig. 7b). By the pharmacological inhibitor SB203580, the expression of p38 was down-regulated in HCECs treated with H_2O_2 (Fig. 7c).

To address whether p38 signaling is required for senescence in response to ROS accumulation in HCECs, we showed the data of the effect of SB203580 on cell senescence in Fig. 8. We found that the ROS levels and the strength of SA-β-Gal staining were decreased after SB203580 treatment (Fig. 8-a and 8-b). We also detected the expression of cell senescence related proteins, including p16^{INK4A}, p27^{kip1} and p53. As shown in Fig. 8-c,

the expression of the three proteins was down-regulated after treatment with SB203580 in HCECs, compared with no treatment of SB203580. These results imply that the ASK1-p38 MAPK pathway may be involved in ROS-induced CECs senescence.

Discussion

In this study, we report a studying on penetrating keratoplasty and in particular the potential mechanisms behind post-operative failure (for example, corneal opacity and the role of the endothelium). We use a

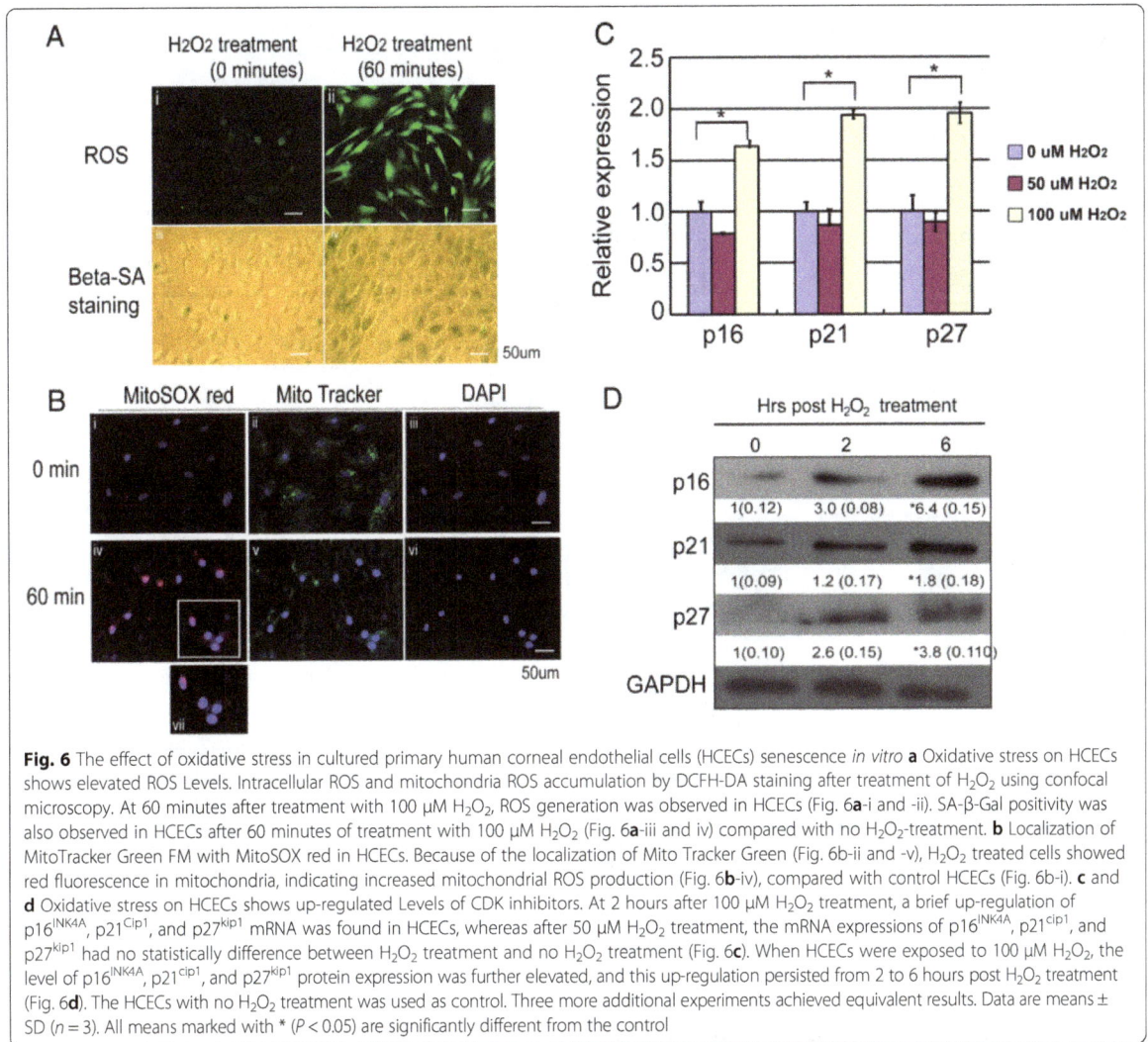

Fig. 6 The effect of oxidative stress in cultured primary human corneal endothelial cells (HCECs) senescence *in vitro* **a** Oxidative stress on HCECs shows elevated ROS Levels. Intracellular ROS and mitochondria ROS accumulation by DCFH-DA staining after treatment of H_2O_2 using confocal microscopy. At 60 minutes after treatment with 100 μM H_2O_2, ROS generation was observed in HCECs (Fig. 6a-i and -ii). SA-β-Gal positivity was also observed in HCECs after 60 minutes of treatment with 100 μM H_2O_2 (Fig. 6a-iii and iv) compared with no H_2O_2-treatment. **b** Localization of MitoTracker Green FM with MitoSOX red in HCECs. Because of the localization of Mito Tracker Green (Fig. 6b-ii and -v), H_2O_2 treated cells showed red fluorescence in mitochondria, indicating increased mitochondrial ROS production (Fig. 6b-iv), compared with control HCECs (Fig. 6b-i). **c** and **d** Oxidative stress on HCECs shows up-regulated Levels of CDK inhibitors. At 2 hours after 100 μM H_2O_2 treatment, a brief up-regulation of p16^{INK4A}, p21^{Cip1}, and p27^{kip1} mRNA was found in HCECs, whereas after 50 μM H_2O_2 treatment, the mRNA expressions of p16^{INK4A}, p21^{cip1}, and p27^{kip1} had no statistically difference between H_2O_2 treatment and no H_2O_2 treatment (Fig. 6c). When HCECs were exposed to 100 μM H_2O_2, the level of p16^{INK4A}, p21^{cip1}, and p27^{kip1} protein expression was further elevated, and this up-regulation persisted from 2 to 6 hours post H_2O_2 treatment (Fig. 6d). The HCECs with no H_2O_2 treatment was used as control. Three more additional experiments achieved equivalent results. Data are means ± SD ($n = 3$). All means marked with * ($P < 0.05$) are significantly different from the control

combination of descriptive data from human PKP samples, together with a mouse model (syngeneic versus allogeneic corneal transplantations) and some cell work *in vitro* with human HCECs treated with peroxide.

In the context of PKP, premature senescence is important clinically not only because aging alters corneal function but also because old corneas perform poorly when transplanted. The endothelium is a major determinant of graft survival. Since stress might accelerate ageing changes, it will be instructive to understand the mechanisms of premature senescence in HECEs. HCECs are arrested in the G1 phase of the cell cycle and given the correct culture medium, HCECs can be grown for many population doublings in culture [27]. We previously reported an age-related increase in p16^{INK4A} expression in normal HCECs *in vivo* [28] and in the senescence accelerated mouse (SAM), indicating that the increased expression of p16^{INK4A} is an age-dependent phenomenon in the corneal endothelium [29]. We also observed that the high expression of p16^{INK4A} and low expression of Bmi1 are associated with cellular senescence of HCECs [30]. Other groups also investigate the characterisation of cellular senescence mechanisms in HCECs [27]. The above studies reported the common aging phenotype and molecular mechansims of normal HCECs.

The accumulation of SA-β-Gal is suggested to be a specific marker of cell senescence [31, 32] and 8-OHdG is the most frequently detected and studied biomarker of ROS for cancer, atherosclerosis and diabetes [33]. In the present study, we found the elevated level of 8-OHdG, suggesting the existence of ROS in corneal endothelium after PKP. Furthermore, the expressions of p16^{INK4a}, p21$^{WAF1/CIP1}$ and p53 proteins in corneal endothelium

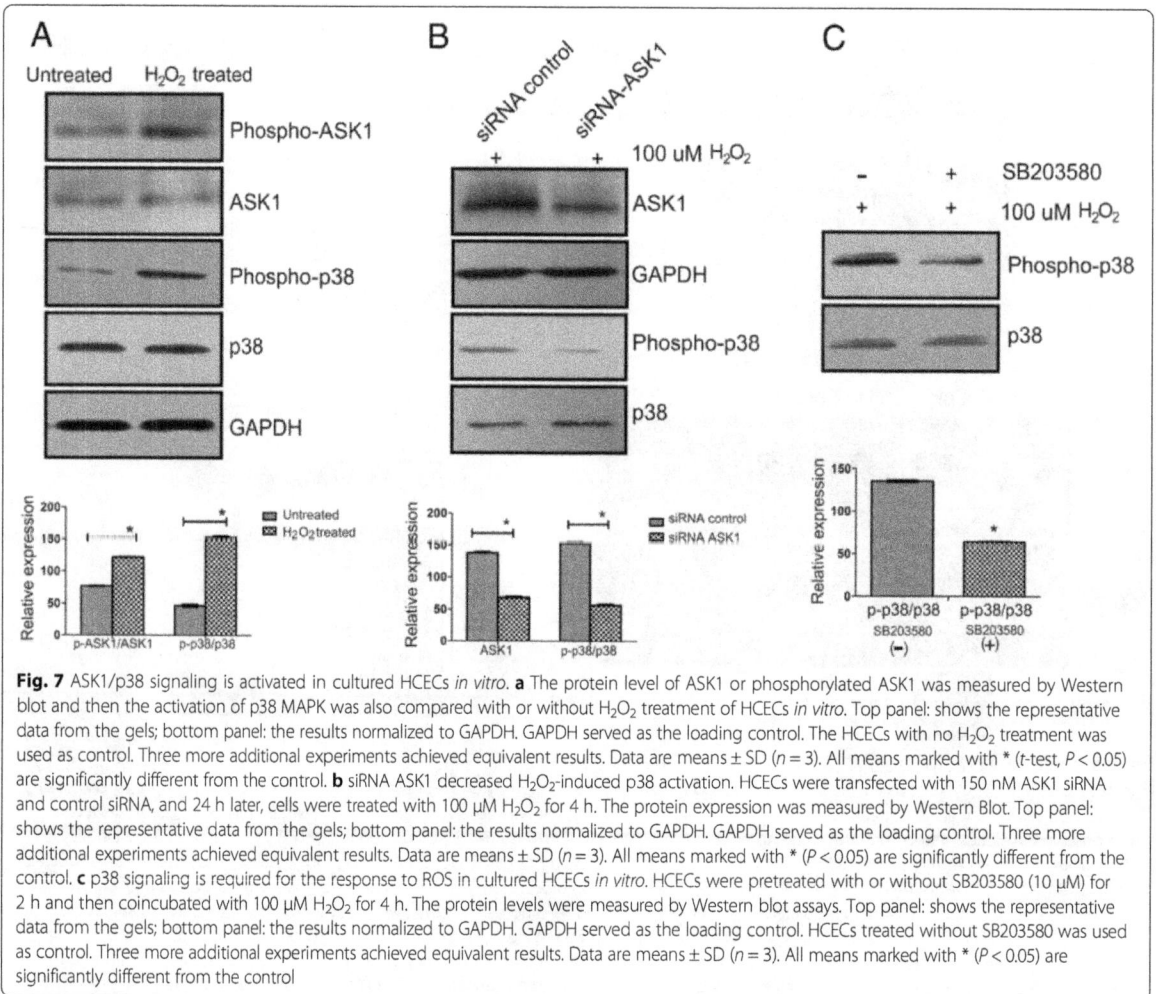

Fig. 7 ASK1/p38 signaling is activated in cultured HCECs in vitro. **a** The protein level of ASK1 or phosphorylated ASK1 was measured by Western blot and then the activation of p38 MAPK was also compared with or without H_2O_2 treatment of HCECs in vitro. Top panel: shows the representative data from the gels; bottom panel: the results normalized to GAPDH. GAPDH served as the loading control. The HCECs with no H_2O_2 treatment was used as control. Three more additional experiments achieved equivalent results. Data are means ± SD (n = 3). All means marked with * (t-test, P < 0.05) are significantly different from the control. **b** siRNA ASK1 decreased H_2O_2-induced p38 activation. HCECs were transfected with 150 nM ASK1 siRNA and control siRNA, and 24 h later, cells were treated with 100 μM H_2O_2 for 4 h. The protein expression was measured by Western Blot. Top panel: shows the representative data from the gels; bottom panel: the results normalized to GAPDH. GAPDH served as the loading control. Three more additional experiments achieved equivalent results. Data are means ± SD (n = 3). All means marked with * (P < 0.05) are significantly different from the control. **c** p38 signaling is required for the response to ROS in cultured HCECs in vitro. HCECs were pretreated with or without SB203580 (10 μM) for 2 h and then coincubated with 100 μM H_2O_2 for 4 h. The protein levels were measured by Western blot assays. Top panel: shows the representative data from the gels; bottom panel: the results normalized to GAPDH. GAPDH served as the loading control. HCECs treated without SB203580 was used as control. Three more additional experiments achieved equivalent results. Data are means ± SD (n = 3). All means marked with * (P < 0.05) are significantly different from the control

of allogeneic grafts were correlated with the accumulation of SA-β-Gal and 8-OHdG, and their expressions were consistent with their induction as a function of cell aging.

ROS play a role in cellular functions including signal transduction at normal concentrations [34]. But an imbalance between generation of ROS and capacity of antioxidants to neutralize ROS can result in disruption of cellular redox status, leading to oxidative stress [35]. Several studies have suggested that low doses of H_2O_2 promote cell proliferation, whereas high levels of ROS can induce DNA damage and trigger cell aging, eventually causing cells to enter senescence prematurely [36, 37]. Thus, we developed an in vitro experimental model using treatment of H_2O_2 to simulate cells in a state of oxidative stress. In this study, the dose of H_2O_2 that is being used was 100 μM. Low concentrations of H_2O_2 (less than 10 μM) were found to stimulate cell proliferation in fibroblasts [38]. Whereas intermediate

concentrations of H_2O_2 (10 ~ 150 μM) caused cell growth arrest and senescence [4, 39].

For PKP, the cumulative burden of injury may exhaust the ability of corneal endothelial cells to repair and remodel to maintain tissue integrity. PKP may represent a final common pathway that greatly accelerated by the special stresses on the transplant, such as aging, nonimmune injury, and rejection. This is more a result of endothelial deterioration for cornea. In our study, the data suggest a ROS/p38 driver of senescence in corneal syngeneic transplants. The reasons for such transplant generate ROS and rigger senescence may be age-related diseases before the transplant, peri-transplant injury or rejection. This is a key question both to understand the significance of our results and also to start to understand why some PKP cases fail. To test this properly would require a quite complex mouse interventional study (p38 inhibition during transplantation), we do attempt a cell line model system to test the causality. Using 100 μM

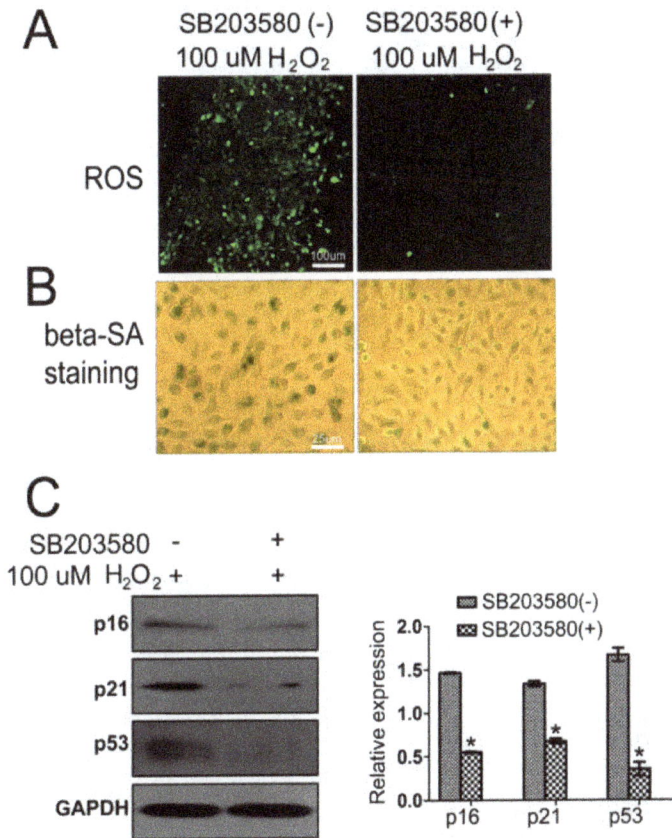

Fig. 8 ASK1/p38 signaling is required for the response to ROS in cultured HCECs *in vitro*. **a** The level of ROS was measured and compared with or without SB203580 treatment of HCECs under H$_2$O$_2$ induced oxidative stress conditions *in vitro*. Bar = 100 μm. The HCECs with no SB203580 treatment was used as control. Three more additional experiments achieved equivalent results. **b** SA-beta-Gal staining was performed and compared with or without SB203580 treatment of HCECs under H$_2$O$_2$ induced oxidative stress conditions *in vitro*. Bar = 25 μm. The HCECs with no SB203580 treatment was used as control. Three more additional experiments achieved equivalent results. **c** The protein level of p16, p21 and p53 was measured by Western blot and compared with or without SB203580 treatment of HCECs *in vitro*. Left panel: shows the representative data from the gels; right panel: the results normalized to GAPDH. GAPDH served as the loading control. The HCECs with no SB203580 treatment was used as control. Three more additional experiments achieved equivalent results. Data are means ± SD ($n = 3$). All means marked with *($P < 0.05$) are significantly different from the control

peroxide we induce senescence in HCECs, and interestingly show that both ROS markers and SA-β-Gal elevation can be suppressed using a p38 small molecule inhibitor (Fig. 8). Although there are some obvious concerns regarding the very high peroxide levels we use, these interventional studies do give initial support for the model we suggest.

Conclusions

In conclusion, our observations indicate an elevation of markers of ROS (both directly and via looking at oxidative defence gene expression), and markers of senescence (SA-β-Gal and proteins such as p16^{INK4a}/p21$^{WAF1/CIP1}$/p53 that are associated with senescence). We also show evidence for activation of the p38MAPK and ASK1 pathway in this situation. These observational data would be consistent with a pathway of ROS > p38/ASK1 > senescence. This in turn suggests a SIPS process taking place in the corneal syngeneic transplants. Our results will give new insights into the molecular pathogenesis of corneal allograft dysfunction, providing future targets for therapeutic intervention.

Abbreviations
HCEC: Human corneal endothelial cells; LKP: Lamellar keratoplasty; PKP: Penetrating keratoplasty; ROS: Reactive oxygen species; SIPS: Stress-induced premature senescence.

Competing interests

The authors declare no conflict of interest.

Author's contributions

YW (Ye Wang) participated in the conception and design of the study and the critical revision of the manuscript for important intellectual content. XZ and SL contributed the animal model for the study. YW (Yao Wang) and PC contributed the cell culture and treatment for the study. XZ performed the data collection and analysis. YW (Ye Wang) interpreted the data and produced the draft of the manuscript. YW (Ye Wang) obtained funding for the study. All authors read and approved the final version of the manuscript.

Acknowledgements

This work was supported by the National Natural Science Foundation of China (81370990,81300742 and 30901637), the Shandong Province Natural Science Foundation (BS2012YY030 and BS2013YY013) and the Shandong Provincial Excellent Innovation Team Program.

References

1. Laule A, Cable MK, Hoffman CE, Hanna C. Endothelial cell population changes of human cornea during life. Arch Ophthalmol. 1978;96(11):2031–5.
2. Bourne WM, Hodge DO, Nelson LR. Corneal endothelium five years after transplantation. Am J Ophthalmol. 1994;118(2):185–96.
3. Prokhorenko VI, Nagy AM, Waschuk SA, Brown LS, Birge RR, Miller RJ. Coherent control of retinal isomerization in bacteriorhodopsin. Science. 2006;313(5791):1257–61.
4. Hori J, Streilein JW. Dynamics of donor cell persistence and recipient cell replacement in orthotopic corneal allografts in mice. Invest Ophthalmol Vis Sci. 2001;42(8):1820–8.
5. [[Lagali L, 2010 #132], Lagali N, Stenevi U, Claesson M, Fagerholm P, Hanson C, et al. Swedish Society of Corneal S: Donor and recipient endothelial cell population of the transplanted human cornea: a two-dimensional imaging study. Invest Ophthalmol Vis Sci. 2010;51(4):1898–904.
6. Lass JH, Gal RL, Dontchev M, Beck RW, Kollman C, Dunn SP, et al. Donor age and corneal endothelial cell loss 5 years after successful corneal transplantation. Specular microscopy ancillary study results. Ophthalmology. 2008;115(4):627–32. e628.
7. Campisi J. Senescent cells, tumor suppression, and organismal aging: good citizens, bad neighbors. Cell. 2005;120(4):513–22.
8. Collado M, Blasco MA, Serrano M. Cellular senescence in cancer and aging. Cell. 2007;130(2):223–33.
9. Koppelstaetter C, Schratzberger G, Perco P, Hofer J, Mark W, Ollinger R, et al. Markers of cellular senescence in zero hour biopsies predict outcome in renal transplantation. Aging Cell. 2008;7(4):491–7.
10. McGlynn LM, Stevenson K, Lamb K, Zino S, Brown M, Prina A, et al. Cellular senescence in pretransplant renal biopsies predicts postoperative organ function. Aging Cell. 2009;8(1):45–51.
11. Hubbard WJ, Dashti N. Aging and transplantation - a topic for biomedicine or bioethics? Aging Dis. 2012;2(2):181–5.
12. Melk A, Schmidt BM, Braun H, Vongwiwatana A, Urmson J, Zhu LF, et al. Effects of donor age and cell senescence on kidney allograft survival. Am J Transplant. 2009;9(1):114–23.
13. Joosten SA, van Ham V, Nolan CE, Borrias MC, Jardine AG, Shiels PG, et al. Telomere shortening and cellular senescence in a model of chronic renal allograft rejection. Am J Pathol. 2003;162(4):1305–12.
14. Herbig U, Ferreira M, Condel L, Carey D, Sedivy JM. Cellular senescence in aging primates. Science. 2006;311(5765):1257.
15. Joyce NC, Zhu CC, Harris DL. Relationship among oxidative stress, DNA damage, and proliferative capacity in human corneal endothelium. Invest Ophthalmol Vis Sci. 2009;50(5):2116–22.
16. Joyce NC, Harris DL, Zhu CC. Age-related gene response of human corneal endothelium to oxidative stress and DNA damage. Invest Ophthalmol Vis Sci. 2011;52(3):1641–9.
17. Konomi K, Joyce NC. Age and topographical comparison of telomere lengths in human corneal endothelial cells. Mol Vis. 2007;13:1251–8.
18. Schroeter H, Boyd C, Spencer JP, Williams RJ, Cadenas E, Rice-Evans C. MAPK signaling in neurodegeneration: influences of flavonoids and of nitric oxide. Neurobiol Aging. 2002;23(5):861–80.
19. Ichijo H, Nishida E, Irie K, ten Dijke P, Saitoh M, Moriguchi T, et al. Induction of apoptosis by ASK1, a mammalian MAPKKK that activates SAPK/JNK and p38 signaling pathways. Science. 1997;275(5296):90–4.
20. Yokoi T, Fukuo K, Yasuda O, Hotta M, Miyazaki J, Takemura Y, et al. Apoptosis signal-regulating kinase 1 mediates cellular senescence induced by high glucose in endothelial cells. Diabetes. 2006;55(6):1660–5.
21. Soga M, Matsuzawa A, Ichijo H. Oxidative Stress-Induced Diseases via the ASK1 Signaling Pathway. Int J Cell Biol. 2012;2012:439587.
22. Cursiefen C, Cao J, Chen L, Liu Y, Maruyama K, Jackson D, et al. Inhibition of hemangiogenesis and lymphangiogenesis after normal-risk corneal transplantation by neutralizing VEGF promotes graft survival. Invest Ophthalmol Vis Sci. 2004;45(8):2666–73.
23. Taylor MJ, Hunt CJ. Dual staining of corneal endothelium with trypan blue and alizarin red S: importance of pH for the dye-lake reaction. Br J Ophthalmol. 1981;65(12):815–9.
24. Mimura T, Joyce NC. Replication competence and senescence in central and peripheral human corneal endothelium. Invest Ophthalmol Vis Sci. 2006;47(4):1387–96.
25. Mishima K, Handa JT, Aotaki-Keen A, Lutty GA, Morse LS, Hjelmeland LM. Senescence-associated beta-galactosidase histochemistry for the primate eye. Invest Ophthalmol Vis Sci. 1999;40(7):1590–3.
26. Serrano M, Hannon GJ, Beach D. A new regulatory motif in cell-cycle control causing specific inhibition of cyclin D/CDK4. Nature. 1993;366(6456):704–7.
27. Sheerin AN, Smith SK, Jennert-Burston K, Brook AJ, Allen MC, Ibrahim B, et al. Characterization of cellular senescence mechanisms in human corneal endothelial cells. Aging Cell. 2012;11(2):234–40.
28. Song Z, Wang Y, Xie L, Zang X, Yin H. Expression of senescence-related genes in human corneal endothelial cells. Mol Vis. 2008;14:161–70.
29. Xiao X, Wang Y, Gong H, Chen P, Xie L. Molecular evidence of senescence in corneal endothelial cells of senescence-accelerated mice. Mol Vis. 2009;15:747–61.
30. Wang Y, Zang X, Chen P. High expression of p16INK4a and low expression of Bmi1 are associated with endothelial cellular senescence in the human cornea. Mol Vis. 2012;18:803–15.
31. Bodnar AG, Ouellette M, Frolkis M, Holt SE, Chiu CP, Morin GB, et al. Extension of life-span by introduction of telomerase into normal human cells. Science. 1998;279(5349):349–52.
32. Sigal SH, Rajvanshi P, Gorla GR, Sokhi RP, Saxena R, Gebhard Jr DR, et al. Partial hepatectomy-induced polyploidy attenuates hepatocyte replication and activates cell aging events. Am J Physiol. 1999;276(5 Pt 1):G1260–72.
33. Wu LL, Chiou CC, Chang PY, Wu JT. Urinary 8-OHdG: a marker of oxidative stress to DNA and a risk factor for cancer, atherosclerosis and diabetics. Clin Chim Acta. 2004;339(1–2):1–9.
34. Kamsler A, Daily D, Hochman A, Stern N, Shiloh Y, Rotman G, et al. Increased oxidative stress in ataxia telangiectasia evidenced by alterations in redox state of brains from Atm-deficient mice. Cancer Res. 2001;61(5):1849–54.
35. Rhee SG. Cell signaling. H2O2, a necessary evil for cell signaling. Science. 2006;312(5782):1882–3.
36. Bennett MR. Reactive oxygen species and death: oxidative DNA damage in atherosclerosis. Circ Res. 2001;88(7):648–50.
37. Cooke MS, Evans MD, Dizdaroglu M, Lunec J. Oxidative DNA damage: mechanisms, mutation, and disease. FASEB J. 2003;17(10):1195–214.
38. Kim BY, Han MJ, Chung AS. Effects of reactive oxygen species on proliferation of Chinese hamster lung fibroblast (V79) cells. Free Radic Biol Med. 2001;30(6):686–98.
39. Taniyama Y, Griendling KK. Reactive oxygen species in the vasculature: molecular and cellular mechanisms. Hypertension. 2003;42(6):1075–81.

Efficacy of intravitreal ranibizumab combined with Ahmed glaucoma valve implantation for the treatment of neovascular glaucoma

Min Tang[1], Yang Fu[1], Ying Wang[2], Zhi Zheng[2], Ying Fan[2], Xiaodong Sun[2] and Xun Xu[1*]

Abstract

Background: Neovascular glaucoma is a refractive glaucoma. Recently, anti-VEGF factors have been used alone or in combination for the treatment of neovascular glaucoma. However, the medium- and long-term efficacy of such drugs remains to be evaluated. This study was to determine the efficacy of intravitreal ranibizumab combined with Ahmed glaucoma valve implantation for the treatment of neovascular glaucoma.

Methods: In this prospective non-randomized study, 43 neovascular glaucoma patients (43 eyes) were assigned to receive either 0.5 mg intravitreal ranibizumab for three to 14 days before Ahmed glaucoma valve implantation (injection group, $n = 21$) or Ahmed glaucoma valve implantation alone (control group, $n = 22$). The patients were followed up for six to 12 months. Differences in surgical success rate, intraocular pressure, best corrected visual acuity, anti-glaucoma medications and postoperative complications were compared between the two groups. Surgical success was defined as IOP $> = 6$ mm Hg and $< = 21$ mm Hg, with or without the use of anti-glaucoma medications, and without severe complications or reoperation.

Results: Of the 43 patients, 40 completed the 6-month follow-up and 37 completed the 1-year follow-up. Success rate was 73.7 % vs. 71.4 % at six months and 72.2 % vs. 68.4 % at 12 months in the injection group and the control group respectively. No significant difference was noted between the two groups (six months: $P = 0.87$, 12 months: $P = 1.00$). There were no significant differences in the two groups with respect to intraocular pressure, best corrected visual acuity, anti-glaucoma medications or postoperative complications at six months or 12 months.

Conclusions: Single intravitreal ranibizumab (0.5 mg) before surgery has no significant effect on the medium- or long-term outcomes of neovascular glaucoma treated with Ahmed glaucoma valve implantation.

Trial registration: Chinese Clinical Trial Registry (ChiCTR-OOC-14005709, Trial registration date: 2014-12-01)

Keyword: Ahmed glaucoma valve, Ranibizumab, Neovascular glaucoma

* Correspondence: tmsmile@sina.com.cn
We regard Min Tang and Yang Fu as co-first authors.
[1]Department of Ophthalmology, Shanghai General Hospital of Nanjing Medical University, No.100 Haining Road, Hongkou District, Shanghai 200080, China
Full list of author information is available at the end of the article

Background

Neovascular glaucoma (NVG) is a medical condition in which neovascularization involving the iris and the anterior chamber angle is accompanied by the formation of a fibrovascular membrane that results in secondary angle closure and obstructs the aqueous outflow. The main causes include diabetic retinopathy (DR), retinal vein occlusion (RVO), retinal artery occlusion (RAO) and ocular ischemic syndrome [1]. Ahmed glaucoma valve (AGV) implantation is an effective treatment for NVG, but the procedure is associated with poor outcomes [2]. A study found that vascular endothelial growth factor (VEGF) is a key factor causing NVG, as demonstrated by significantly higher VEGF levels in the aqueous humor of NVG patients [3]. VEGF levels in the aqueous humor are known to play a significant role in determining the outcomes of NVG patients after AGV implantation [4].

Because of their role in inhibiting intraocular neovascularization and mitigating damage to the blood ocular barrier due to leakage from new vessels, anti-VEGF factors have been used alone or in combination for the treatment of NVG. However, currently available evidence remains insufficient to confirm the effectiveness of such drugs. Ranibizumab (Lucentis) is now used in the treatment of age-related macular degeneration and macular edema as an anti-VEGF factor [5, 6], but it remains unclear whether ranibizumab will affect the efficacy of AGV implantation for NVG patients.

This prospective study was designed to compare the difference in efficacy at a follow-up of six to 12 months in NVG patients with or without a single intravitreal injection of ranibizumab (IVR) before AGV implantation.

Methods

This study was a prospective, non-randomized, open-label, controlled study. This study enrolled patients admitted to the Department of Ophthalmology of Shanghai General Hospital from December 2012 to March 2014. Inclusion criteria were: 1) NVG patients (NVG was diagnosed by the presence of active neovascularization in the iris and/or angle, high intraocular pressure (IOP > 21 mm Hg, 1 mm Hg = 0.133 kPa, Goldmann applanation tonometer) and underlying ischemic retinal diseases); 2) IOP > 21 mm Hg, with or without anti-glaucoma medications or panretinal photocoagulation (PRP) before; 3) 18 to 85 years old; 4) patients who chose IVR before AGV implantation or AGV implantation only should complete a follow-up of six to 12 months. Exclusion criteria were: 1) patients combined with other types of glaucoma or other serious eye diseases; 2) patients who had received glaucoma surgery or other intraocular surgery in either eye; 3) patients who had received intravitreal injection in either eye within three months before surgery; 4) patients who failed to complete

the scheduled follow-ups for various reasons; 5) IOP measurements were made inaccurate for various reasons; 6) IOP decreased (<= 21 mm Hg) after IVR and/or PRP; 7) cataract surgery or vitreous surgery was needed during the primary surgery; 8) surgery or intravitreal injection was required for both eyes; and 9) pregnant patients or patients combined with other serious uncontrolled medical diseases. This study was approved by the Ethics Committee of Shanghai General Hospital (registration number: 2012 K061), and it was registered with the Chinese Clinical Trial Registry (registration number: ChiCTR-OOC-14005709). All patients signed an informed consent before participation in this study.

Grouping method: NVG patients through preliminary screening would be educated about IVR on its effect, side-effect, risks, price and so on, then they chose to accept IVR before AGV implantation (injection group) or AGV implantation only (control group) at the discretion of themselves and signed an informed consent.

Endpoints were: 1) completion of the scheduled follow-up over the 6-month or 12-month period; 2) failure to be followed up as scheduled, being lost to follow up, undergoing intraocular surgery including cyclophotocoagulation during the follow-up period, or receiving intravitreal injection during the follow-up period (collectively referred to as dropouts).

We tried to do PRP for patients before IVR or AGV implantation if possible, and evaluated again whether they needed IVR or AGV implantation. As to those who could not accept PRP due to very high IOP or corneal edema pre-surgery, we applied this therapy just after surgery (usually 1 or 2 weeks later). Patients would not be enrolled if their IOPs were controlled by PRP before AGV implantation (IOP < = 21 mm Hg).

IVR was performed three to 14 days prior to AGV implantation. Under topical anesthesia, a needle was introduced through the conjunctival surface 3.8 mm from the corneal limbus in the affected eye for intravitreal injection of 0.5 mg/0.05 mL ranibizumab (Lucentis, 10 mg/mL; Novartis, Basel, Switzerland). The puncture site was pressed with a cotton swab for 5 to 10 s after the needle was withdrawn. IOP and light perception were examined. Sometimes anterior chamber paracentesis was performed in patients with higher IOP. All patients were observed more than three days. After that, AGV implantation would be performed, once the IOPs of patients reached 40 mm Hg during time, or it would be done two weeks after IVR. Otherwise, Patients would not be enrolled by the study if their IOPs were controlled just by IVR (IOP < = 21 mm Hg).

AGV implantation was performed under peribulbar anesthesia, a fornix-based conjunctival flap superior and temporal to the affected eye was prepared until the equator and a mitomycin C-soaked (0.4 mg/mL) cotton swab was applied to the area for two to five minutes before rinsing thoroughly with saline. An AGV (Model FP7) drainage plate was fixed with 6–0 suture on the surface of the sclera, with its anterior border 8 to 10 mm from the limbus. A 27G needle was introduced into the interlamellar space of the sclera 5 mm behind the limbus and pushed forward until into the anterior chamber, where viscoelastic agent was injected while the needle was being withdrawn slowly. A drainage tube was implanted into the anterior chamber two to three mm deep through the needle tract, and was mildly ligated with 8–0 absorbable suture (6 to 7 mm behind the limbus) before the conjunctival flap was tightly stitched. A small amount of aqueous humor was drained through a clear corneal if necessary incision to bring intraocular pressure slightly higher than normal IOP. All the procedures were completed by the authors.

Levofloxacin eye drops were applied at short intervals before surgery. Tobramycin and dexamethasone ophthalmic solution was applied postoperatively once every two hours for a total of three days, followed by four times a day for two weeks. Tropicamide or atropine was administered for two weeks for pupil dilation treatment where appropriate. Some patients received panretinal photocoagulation within one month after surgery. Anti-glaucoma medications were administered in light of IOP during follow-up.

The mean of three consecutive outpatient IOP measurements just before surgery was used as the baseline IOP. Patients were followed up on schedule (1–3d, 2w ± 1d, 1m ± 3d, 3m ± 5d, 6m ± 7d, 12m ± 14d) after surgery. Best corrected visual acuity (BCVA) and IOP were determined and slit-lamp microscopy with a preset lens was performed as a routine. Other tests including gonioscopy, ultrasound biomicroscopy, perimetry and retinal nerve fiber layer scan were conducted in selected patients where appropriate. IOP, surgical success rate, BCVA, anti-glaucoma medications and postoperative complications were used as major outcome measures at each follow-up time interval. Surgical success was defined as IOP > = 6 mm Hg and < = 21 mm Hg, with or without the use of anti-glaucoma medications, and without severe complications or reoperation [7]. Surgical failure was defined as IOP persistently < 6 mm Hg or > 21 mm Hg for more than two weeks, or loss of light perception, or the occurrence of any serious complication including endophthalmitis, corneal decompensation, malignant glaucoma, severe choroidal detachment (>180°), severe choroidal hemorrhage (>180°), retinal detachment, ocular atrophy, or displacement, withdrawal or exposure of drainage tube, or necessity of reoperation for other reasons.

Statistical analysis was performed using statistical package SAS9.13. Differences in gender and diagnoses at baseline and postoperative complications, and dropout rates during follow-up were compared between the two groups using chi-square, corrected chi-square test or Fisher's exact probability test. Differences in age, IOP, BCVA, and medications at baseline and IOP decline, BCVA, and medications during follow-up were compared using the t test. Difference in success rates throughout follow-up was compared using the Log-Rank test. P value < 0.05 was considered statistically significant.

Results

A total of 43 patients (43 eyes) were enrolled. The patients were divided into the injection group ($n = 21$), who received AGV implantation three to 14 days (average 8.6 ± 2.2 days) subsequent to IVR, and the control group ($n = 22$), who received AGV implantation alone. The baseline information of the two groups is presented in Table 1. There were no significant differences in baseline measures between the two groups.

Of the 43 patients, 40 completed the 6-month follow-up and 37 completed the 1-year follow-up. In particular, in the injection group two patients received intraocular surgery (at three months and six months) and one patient was lost to follow up (at 12 months). In the control group two patients received intraocular surgery (at six months and 12 months) and one patient were lost to follow up (at 12 months). The dropout rates were not significantly different between the two groups (six months: $P = 0.52$; 12 months: $P = 0.95$).

The mean IOPs at various time points throughout follow-up decreased significantly from baseline in both groups (ANOVA, $\alpha = 0.05$). IOP rose gradually in both groups with the passage of time. IOPs at various time points throughout follow-up were not significantly different between the two groups (Table 2). The success rates declined gradually in both groups with the passage of time. Success rates at various time points throughout follow-up (Table 3) were not significantly different between the two groups ($P = 0.84$, Fig. 1).

The two groups showed different patterns of BCVA changes after surgery. In the injection group, BCVA improved significantly and peaked for one to three months before declining sharply to levels comparable to that of the control group. In the control group, BCVA increased slightly, peaked at one month, and then gradually declined. Inter-group statistical analysis showed significant differences only at three-month follow-up (Table 4). BCVAs in both groups fell back to the baseline at six months or 12 months.

The number of anti-glaucoma medications used at various time points throughout follow-up in both groups declined significantly from baseline (ANOVA, $\alpha = 0.05$). And the number of medications increased gradually in both groups with the passage of time. There was no

Table 1 Characteristics of patients with NVG

	Injection Group	Control Group	P
Total Patients	21	22	
Gender			0.45
Male	10	13	
Female	11	9	
Age	60.1 ± 13.8 (32–81)	58.6 ± 17.3 (28–81)	0.76
Diagnosis			0.90
CRVO	8	7	
BRVO	2	2	
DR	11	13	
Baseline IOP (mm Hg)	46.4 ± 13.3 (24.5–76.0)	45.0 ± 14.9 (23.5–78.5)	0.74
Prior intravitreal injection	0	0	
NVI/NVA Degree			0.90
NVI only	3	2	
NVI&NVA (Open-angle)	5	4	
NVI&NVA (partial Closed-angle)	2	3	
NVI&NVA (Closed-angle)	11	13	
PRP before			0.55
none	12	9	
Incomplete	6	8	
complete	3	5	
BCVA (LogMAR)	1.1 ± 0.4 (0.3–1.6)	1.2 ± 0.4 (0.4–1.6)	0.65
Pre-medications	2.5 ± 0.5 (2–3)	2.6 ± 0.5 (2–3)	0.66

Note: The difference in gender was compared between the two groups using the chi-square test, the difference in NVI/NVA degree was compared using two-tailed Fisher's exact test, and the differences in diagnosis and PRP before were compared using the corrected chi-square test. Differences in age, IOP, BCVA and anti-glaucoma medications were compared using the t test

significant difference at various time points between the two groups (Table 5).

Of the 21 patients in the injection group, anterior uveitis developed in seven patients one day after surgery, but was resolved with topical steroid drops within two weeks; proliferative membrane formed in the pupil in one patient and was removed using YAG laser. Nine

patients experienced mild hyphema, which resolved itself within two weeks. Two patients developed mild vitreous hemorrhage, which resolved itself within a month. Two patients experienced transient ocular hypertension (> = 30 mm Hg) and mild corneal edema one day after surgery due to excessive viscoelastic residues, which were alleviated after eyeball massage. Blood clots developed in the drainage tube in three patients, but resolved themselves in two and were cured by YAG laser at day 3 after surgery. The lens of the eye turned cloudy rapidly in one patient within days after surgery, who underwent cataract surgery two months after surgery and withdrew from this study. Of the 23 patients in the control group, 10 patients developed postoperative anterior uveitis, which was revolved within two weeks after topical steroid drops. Nine patients experienced mild hyphema, which resolved itself within two weeks. Five patients developed mild vitreous hemorrhage, which resolved itself within a month. Four patients experienced transient ocular hypertension (including two combined with corneal edema), which were alleviated after eyeball massage. Blood clots developed in the drainage tube in four patients, but resolved themselves. One patient developed conjunctival retraction at three months which did not cause drainage tube exposure and therefore was left unattended. Mild choroidal hemorrhage in local areas developed in one patient one day after surgery as revealed by B ultrasonography (less than 90°) and resolved itself gradually within two months. No serious complications such as malignant glaucoma, sustained low IOP, endophthalmitis, lose of light perception, and retinal detachment occurred in either of the two groups (Table 6).

Discussion

Patients with early NVG have an open angle and normal or slightly elevated IOP. Aggressive treatment with glaucoma medications and laser therapy can bring the disease under control in some of these patients. However, as the disease progresses, the angle is gradually closed and IOP often continues to rise, leading to a poor response to medications or laser, and surgery is usually

Table 2 IOP (mm Hg) in both groups

	Pre-surgery	2 weeks	1 month	3 months	6 months	12 months
Injection Group IOP (mean ± SD)	46.4 ± 13.3	14.5 ± 4.4	16.9 ± 4.2	18.1 ± 3.8	20.5 ± 4.5	21.1 ± 4.2
(Minimum - Maximum)	(24.5–76.0)	(6.5–24.0)	(9.0–26.0)	(10.0–24.0)	(14.0–28.0)	(15.5–28.0)
Control Group IOP (mean ± SD)	45.0 ± 14.9	15.6 ± 5.6	17.1 ± 5.3	19.4 ± 5.0	20.2 ± 3.9	22.1 ± 4.7
(Minimum - Maximum)	(23.5–78.5)	(6.0–27.5)	(8.0–28.0)	(12.0–31.5)	(14.5–27.0)	(12.0–30.0)
P	0.74	0.51	0.85	0.35	0.83	0.53

Note: IOPs before surgery and at two weeks, one month, three months, six months and 12 months after surgery were determined using an applanation tonometer (mean of 9 am and 4 pm measurements). Differences in IOPs at various time points throughout follow-up were compared between the two groups using the t test

Table 3 Success rates of the two groups

	2 weeks	1 month	3 months	6 months	12 months
Injection Group	95.2 %	90.5 %	80.0 %	73.7 %	72.2 %
(Successful subjects/total subjects)	(20/21)	(19/21)	(16/20)	(14/19)	(13/18)
Control Group	90.9 %	81.8 %	77.3 %	71.4 %	68.4 %
(Successful subjects/total subjects)	(20/22)	(18/22)	(17/22)	(15/21)	(13/19)
P	0.57	0.41	0.83	0.87	1.00

Note: Success was defined as IOP $\geq$ 6 mm Hg and $\leq$ 21 mm Hg, with or without the use of anti-glaucoma medications, and without severe complications or reoperation. The differences in the success rates were compared between the two groups using the corrected chi-square test (two weeks, one month, and three months) and chi-square test (six months) and two-tailed Fisher's exact test (12 months)

required. AGV implantation is an effective method for the treatment of NVG, especially for patients with angle closure; however, NVG is associated with unfavorable outcomes [2]. In this study, success was achieved in 71.4 % of the 22 patients in the control group at six months and 68.4 % at 12 months. Some clinical studies using the same surgical procedure have reached similar results. For instance, Yalvac IS et al. [8] performed AGV implantation alone in 38 patients with NVG and achieved success in 63.2 % of the patients at one year. Shen CC et al. [9] reported a success rate of 70 % and 60 % at one year and two years, respectively. In a retrospective study, Netland PA et al. [2] reported a success rate of 73.1 % at one year, 61.9 % at two years, and only 20.6 % at five years, and considered NVG a high risk factor of AGV implantation failure.

The course of NVG depends on the occurrence and development of new vessels in the iris and the anterior chamber angle. Anti-VEGF factors can inhibit intraocular neovascularization, promote atrophy, and mitigate damage to the blood-ocular barrier as a result of leakage from new vessels. A study shows that ranibizumab can lower IOP and alleviate rubeosis in patients with NVG [10]. Therefore, anti-VEGF factors have been used alone or in combination for the treatment of NVG. However, currently available clinical evidence is inconclusive to establish the effectiveness of such drugs, especially in the medium- and long-term [11, 12]. Our study examined

the efficacy of AGV implantation with or without a single preoperative injection of 0.5 mg ranibizumab in patients with NVG. After a follow-up period of six months to one year, the results showed that there was no significant difference between the two groups in terms of IOP control, success rate, or anti-glaucoma medications.

Currently available studies on glaucoma treatment have reported the use of anti-VEGF factors under the conjunctiva [13] and in the anterior chamber [7] and vitreous cavity [14–16], and even reported that topical eye drops containing ranibizumab (2 mg/mL) after filtering surgery can reduce the formation of bleb scarring [17]. However, there are large discrepancies in the conclusions reached by a number of small-scale clinical studies on NVG. Elmekawey H et al. [7] injected 0.5 mg ranibizumab into the anterior chamber in 13 patients once and two patients twice, and performed trabeculectomy at four weeks when the new vessels resolved on the surface of the iris. Success was achieved in 93.3 % of the patients at six months. Lüke J et al. [10] used repeated intravitreal injections of ranibizumab for the treatment of iris neovascularization (2.3 times/year) and neovascular glaucoma (3.6 times/year), in combination with traditional therapies such as laser photocoagulation, cryotherapy, and vitrectomy. This treatment approach improved rubeosis and angle closure and achieved effective control of IOP. However, in a retrospective study, Ma KT et al. [18] analyzed the outcomes of NVG patients

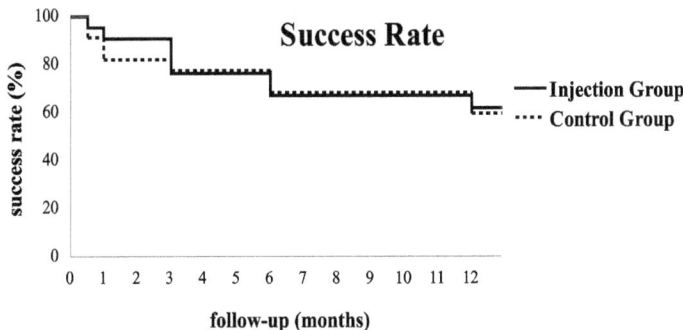

Fig. 1 Success rates in both groups. Note: Difference in success rate throughout follow-up was compared between the two groups using the Log-Rank test ($P = 0.84$)

Table 4 Best corrected visual acuities in both groups

		Pre-surgery	2 weeks	1 month	3 months	6 months	12 months
Injection Group	No.	27.4 ± 20.0	29.3 ± 16.0	39.2 ± 16.6	38.7 ± 16.0	29.7 ± 14.4	24.3 ± 11.1
	LogMAR	1.1 ± 0.4	1.1 ± 0.3	0.9 ± 0.3	0.9 ± 0.3	1.1 ± 0.3	1.2 ± 0.2
Control Group	No.	24.2 ± 19.5	28.7 ± 15.0	30.6 ± 15.6	28.0 ± 14.7	26.4 ± 13.6	22.1 ± 13.9
	LogMAR	1.2 ± 0.4	1.1 ± 0.3	1.1 ± 0.3	1.1 ± 0.3	1.2 ± 0.3	1.2 ± 0.3
P		0.65	0.81	0.086	0.045	0.39	0.60

Note: Best corrected visual acuities (BCVAs) were determined by ETDRS digital letters before surgery, and two weeks, one month, three months, six months and 12 months after surgery. The differences in BCVAs at various time points throughout follow-up were compared between the two groups using the t test

who received AGV implantation combined intraoperative vitreous injection of 1.25 mg bevacizumab, and found that its one-year success rate did not differ significantly from AGV implantation alone. As our point of view, the possible reasons for the discrepancies of the above studies may include different usages of anti-VEGF factors (especially single or repeated injections) and baseline differences in patients.

Intravitreal injection of anti-VEGF factors can help reduce macular edema and improve vision in patients with RVO and DR [19–21]. Our data showed that early postoperative BCVA improved from baseline in the two groups, because IOP was brought under control and corneal edema was alleviated in most patients. However, with the extension of the follow-up period, BCVA gradually declined, which may be caused by retinal deterioration and worsened cataracts. In comparison, postoperative BCVA improved more notably and this improvement lasted longer in patients administered with ranibizumab (about three months). The average BCVA in the injection group at three months was higher than that in the control group, which is positive for the quality of life and compliance of patients. Nevertheless, the beneficial effect from ranibizumab disappeared thereafter and BCVA started to move closer between the two groups, with no significant difference in medium- and long-term vision outcomes between the two groups. Collectively, our results suggest that single IVR before surgery can only enhance vision in the early period after surgery.

We observed that ranibizumab alleviated rubeosis in patients and this effect started to appear two to three days after administration as measured by slit lamp examination. However, there was no marked difference in the incidence of postoperative complications between the two groups. Early postoperative complications after

AGV implantation surgery for NVG included hyphema, choroidal detachment, vitreous hemorrhage, and obstruction of drainage valves. The occurrence of these complications was associated with a number of factors such as the severity of neovascularization of the iris and the anterior chamber angle, the severity of underlying diseases, the level of baseline IOP, and changes in perioperative IOP (especially during surgery). For this reason, we sought to achieve success in our first attempt when preparing a scleral tunnel to avoid sharp IOP decline as a result of repeated puncture of the anterior chamber. Meanwhile an appropriate amount of viscoelastic was injected into the anterior chamber to bring IOP slightly higher than normal levels. The drainage tube was partially ligated using absorbable suture. These measures contribute to the maintenance of anterior chamber and IOP during surgery and within a short period after surgery. Therefore, no serious complications occurred in early postoperative periods in both groups, which, therefore, rendered the role of ranibizumab less significant. Nakatake S et al. [22] studied a group of NVG patients who had received trabeculectomy and also found that the use of bevacizumab injections had no notable effect on the incidence of preoperative complications such as hyphema and choroidal detachment. However, as ranibizumab was applied for a short time, our study failed to establish a correlation between ranibizumab and medium- and long-term complications after AGV implantation, such as drainage valve exposure or fiber encapsulation.

As a non-randomized study, anti-VEGF treatment was assigned at the discretion of the subjects, and the sample size was relative small, so bias would be inevitable between groups. To some extent, our study demonstrates that single IVR before AGV implantation has no

Table 5 Glaucoma medications usage in both groups

	Pre-surgery	2 weeks	1 month	3 months	6 months	12 months
Injection Group	2.5 ± 0.5	0.2 ± 0.4	0.6 ± 0.6	0.7 ± 0.6	1.0 ± 0.7	1.1 ± 0.8
Control Group	2.6 ± 0.5	0.2 ± 0.4	0.7 ± 0.7	0.7 ± 0.7	1.1 ± 0.8	1.3 ± 0.9
P	0.66	0.94	0.59	0.93	0.71	0.47

Note: The differences in the number of glaucoma medications used at various time points throughout follow-up were compared between the two groups using the t test

Table 6 Postoperative complications in both groups

	Injection Group	Control Group	P
Anterior uveitis	7 (33.3 %)	10 (47.6 %)	0.42
Worsened corneal edema	2 (9.5 %)	2 (9.1 %)	0.96
Hyphema	9 (42.9 %)	9 (40.9 %)	0.90
Vitreous hemorrhage	2 (9.5 %)	5 (22.7 %)	0.23
Transient ocular hypertension	2 (9.5 %)	4 (18.2 %)	0.41
Malignant glaucoma	0	0	
Sustained low IOP	0	0	
Drainage tube obstruction/displacement/exposure	3 (14.3 %)	4 (18.2 %)	0.73
Lens opacity	1 (4.8 %)	0	
Choroidal hemorrhage/detachment	0	1 (4.5 %)	
Retinal detachment	0	0	
Conjunctival retraction/rupture	0	1 (4.5 %)	
Endophthalmitis	0	0	
Loss of light perception	0	0	
Total	12 (57.1 %)	14 (63.6 %)	0.66

Note: The differences in postoperative complications were compared between the two groups using the chi-square or corrected chi-square test

significant effect on the medium- and long-term outcomes of NVG patients. As these drugs act in a very time-dependant manner, it is necessary to carry out repeated injections to control the progression of the disease according to changes in rubeosis, IOP, BCVA or the fundus during follow-up. Further studies are needed to explore how to choose and evaluate clinical indicators used to determine the timing of repeated administration. However, we presume that the use of anti-VEGF factors as needed may signal the direction of single or combined treatment modalities for NVG in the future.

Conclusions
Single intravitreal ranibizumab (0.5 mg) before surgery has no significant effect on the medium- or long-term outcomes of neovascular glaucoma treated with Ahmed glaucoma valve implantation.

Abbreviations
AGV: Ahmed glaucoma valve; BCVA: best corrected visual acuity; DR: diabetic retinopathy; IOP: intraocular pressure; IVR: intravitreal injection of ranibizumab; NVA: neovascularization of the angle; NVG: neovascular glaucoma; NVI: neovascularization of the iris; PRP: panretinal photocoagulation; RAO: retinal artery occlusion; RVO: retinal vein occlusion; VEGF: vascular endothelial growth factor.

Competing interests
The authors declare that they have no competing interests.

Authors' contributions
MT participated in the conception and design of the study, performed the IVR and AGV implantations and drafted the manuscript. YFu participated in the collection and analyses of the data and revised the manuscript. YW, ZZ, YFa and XS collected the data. XX conceived the study and revised the manuscript. All authors read and approved the final manuscript.

Acknowledgments
This study was supported by National Natural Science Foundation of China (81170862). We thank Medjaden Editorial Office for medical writing services in this manuscript.

Author details
[1]Department of Ophthalmology, Shanghai General Hospital of Nanjing Medical University, No.100 Haining Road, Hongkou District, Shanghai 200080, China. [2]Department of Ophthalmology, Shanghai General Hospital, Shanghai Jiao Tong University, School of Medicine, Shanghai 200080, China.

References
1. Vasudev D, Blair MP, Galasso J, Kapur R, Vajaranant T. Intravitreal bevacizumab for neovascular glaucoma. J Ocul Pharmacol Ther. 2009;25: 453–8.
2. Netland PA. The Ahmed glaucoma valve in neovascular glaucoma (An AOS Thesis). Trans Am Ophthalmol Soc. 2009;107:325–42.
3. Lim TM, Bae SH, Cho YJ, Lee JH, Kim HK, Sohn YH. Concentration of Vascular Endothelial Growth Factor after Intracameral Bevacizumab Injection in Eyes With Neovascular Glaucoma. Korean J Ophthalmol. 2009;23(3):188–92.
4. Kim YG, Hong S, Lee CS, Kang SY, Seong GJ, Ma KT, et al. Level of vascular endothelial growth factor in aqueous humor and surgical results of ahmed glaucoma valve implantation in patients with neovascular glaucoma. J Glaucoma. 2009;18(6):443–7.
5. Kaiser PK, Do DV. Ranibizumab for the treatment of neovascular AMD. Int J Clin Pract. 2007;61(3):501–9.
6. Rotsos TG, Moschos MM. Cystoid macular edema. Clin Ophthalmol. 2008; 2(4):919–30.
7. Elmekawey H, Khafagy A. Intracameral ranibizumab and subsequent mitomycin C augmented trabeculectomy in neovascular glaucoma. J Glaucoma. 2014;23(7):437–40.
8. Yalvac IS, Eksioglu U, Satana B, Duman S. Long-term results of Ahmed glaucoma valve and Molteno implant in neovascular glaucoma. Eye(Lond). 2007;21(1):65–70.
9. Shen CC, Salim S, Du H, Netland PA. Trabeculectomy versus Ahmed Glaucoma Valve implantation in neovascular glaucoma. Clin Ophthalmol. 2011;5:281–6.
10. Lüke J, Nassar K, Lüke M, Grisanti S. Ranibizumab as adjuvant in the treatment of rubeosis iridis and neovascular glaucoma-results from a prospective interventional case series. Graefes Arch Clin Exp Ophthalmol. 2013;251(10):2403–13.
11. Laplace O. Surgical session: neovascular glaucoma and anti-vascular endothelial growth factor treatment. J Fr Ophtalmol. 2009;32(3):230–5.
12. Park SC, Su D, Tello C. Anti-VEGF therapy for the treatment of glaucoma: a focus on ranibizumab and bevacizumab. Expert Opin Biol Ther. 2012;12(12): 1641–7.
13. Liarakos VS, Papaconstantinou D, Vergados I, Douvali M, Theodossiadis PG. The effect of subconjunctival ranibizumab on corneal and anterior segment neovascularization: study on an animal model. Eur J Ophthalmol. 2014;24(3): 299–308.
14. Desai RU, Singh K, Lin SC. Intravitreal ranibizumab as an adjunct for Ahmed valve surgery in open-angle glaucoma: a pilot study. Clin Experiment Ophthalmol. 2013;41(2):155–8.
15. Li Z, Zhou M, Wang W, Huang W, Chen S, Li X, et al. A prospective comparative study on neovascular glaucoma and non-neovascular refractory glaucoma following Ahmed glaucoma valve implantation. Chin Med J(Engl). 2014;127(8):1417–22.
16. Mathew R, Barton K. Anti-vascular endothelial growth factor therapy in glaucoma filtration surgery. Am J Ophthalmol. 2011;152(1):10–5.
17. Bochmann F, Kaufmann C, Becht CN, Guber I, Kaiser M, Bachmann LM, et al. Influence of topical anti-VEGF (Ranibizumab) on the outcome of filtration surgery for glaucoma - Study Protocol. BMC Ophthalmol. 2011;17(11):1–9.
18. Ma KT, Yang JY, Kim JH, Kim NR, Hong S, Lee ES, et al. Surgical results of Ahmed valve implantation with intraoperative bevacizumab injection in patients with neovascular glaucoma. J Glaucoma. 2012;21(5):331–6.

19. Kwong TQ, Mohamed M. Anti-vascular endothelial growth factor therapies in ophthalmology: current use, controversies and the future. Br J Clin Pharmacol. 2014;78(4):699–706.

20. Terai N, Haustein M, Siegel A, Stodtmeister R, Pillunat LE, Sandner D. Diameter of retinal vessels in patients with diabetic macular edema is not altered by intravitreal ranibizumab (lucentis). Retina. 2014;34(7):1466–72.

21. Couturier A, Dupas B, Guyomard JL, Massin P. Surgical outcomes of florid diabetic retinopathy treated with antivascular endothelial growth factor. Ratina. 2014;34(10):1952–9.

22. Nakatake S, Yoshida S, Nakao S, Arita R, Yasuda M, Kita T, et al. Hyphema is a risk factor for failure of trabeculectomy in neovascular glaucoma: a retrospective analysis. BMC Ophthalmol. 2014;14:55.

Dietary profile of patients with Stargardt's disease and Retinitis Pigmentosa: is there a role for a nutritional approach?

Francesco Sofi[1,2,3], Andrea Sodi[4*], Fabrizio Franco[4], Vittoria Murro[4], Dania Biagini[2], Alba Miele[4], Giacomo Abbruzzese[4], Dario Pasquale Mucciolo[1], Gianni Virgili[1,3], Ugo Menchini[4], Alessandro Casini[1,2] and Stanislao Rizzo[4]

Abstract

Background: Stargardt's disease (STGD) and Retinitis Pigmentosa (RP) are inherited retinal degenerations that may be affected, in opposite way, by diet.

Methods: Dietary profile was assessed in 24 patients with STGD and in 56 patients with RP. We documented in only 6 out of 24 (25 %) STGD patients a daily intake of vitamin A within the recommended range while 14/24 (58.3 %) reported a high daily intake and 4/24 (16.7 %) showed a low daily intake. With regard to RP, 4/56 (7.1 %) reported to be within the recommended range, 37/56 (66.1 %) reported high daily intake and 15/56 (26.8 %) showed low daily intake of vitamin A.

Results: Interestingly, STGD patients with low vitamin A intake (<600 μg RAE/day) showed significantly better visual acuity with respect to those introducing higher intake of vitamin A.

Conclusion: The present study suggests insuitable nutrient intakes among patients with STGD and RP, especially for daily intake of vitamin A. The results may be used to provide tailored nutritional interventions in these patients.

Keywords: Stargardt's disease, Retinitis Pigmentosa, Vitamin A, Diet

Background

Vitamin A plays a crucial role in the biochemistry of visual signal cascade and the maintenance of an optimal vitamin A status has been considered relevant for a normal retinal physiology [1, 2].

Stargardt's Disease (STGD) and Retinitis Pigmentosa (RP) are genetic-based relevant ocular diseases that may be affected, in opposite way, by vitamin A intake and other nutrients [3–5].

In an animal model of STGD vitamin A supplementation has been shown to accelerate the accumulation of toxic by-products, being prevented by a reduction of its serum levels with possible implications for the treatment [6]. Moreover, in such patients a supplementation with

lutein, a retinal carotenoid, increases macula pigment density but it seems not to be associated with changes in central vision over a 6 months-follow up period [7]. Conversely, RP patients seems to get beneficial effects from a supplementation with vitamin A, since it has been associated with an improved preservation of cone electroretinogram amplitudes and has been proposed as a treatment to slow the progression of the disease [8]. Moreover, for RP patients assuming vitamin A therapy addition of the polyunsaturated fatty acid docosahexaenoic acid has been showed to slow the course of the disease over the first two years of supplementation [9–11]. Similarly, an increased dietary intake of lutein, a retinal carotenoid, seems to slow visual function loss in RP adult patients assuming vitamin A [12]. In the light of all these clinical observations, nutritional indications and/or supplementations for patients suffering from these retinal dystrophies are usually given but, to the

* Correspondence: asodi@tin.it
Guarantor of the paper: F. Sofi
[4]Department of Surgery and Translational Medicine, Eye Clinic, University of Florence, Florence, Italy
Full list of author information is available at the end of the article

best of our knowledge, no data on dietary habits of these patients are presently available.

The purpose of this study was to evaluate the dietary habits and nutritional intake of vitamin A in patients with STGD and RP, in order to suggest tailored dietary modifications in such diseases.

Methods

Study population

The study populations comprised 24 patients with a STGD [12 M, 12 F; median age: 34 years (range: 13–64)] and 56 patients with RP [23 M, 33 F; median age: 45 years (range: 14–85)] referring to the Eye Clinic of the University of Florence, Italy for clinical evaluation. For patients under 18 years of age, the informed consent was obtained from their parents.

The criteria for STGD phenotype included the following: appearance in the first or second decade of life; bilateral progressive central vision loss; macular atrophy/dystrophy; normal calibre of retinal vessels; absence of pigmented bone spicules; and normal or mildly abnormal full-field electroretinogram. Flecks at the posterior pole and dark choroid at fluorescein angiography were present in most of the cases but their absence was not considered an exclusion criterion. All the patients carried bi-allelic mutations of the ABCA4 gene [13, 14]. The clinical diagnosis of RP was based on the history of night blindness, typical retinal pigmentary changes, attenuated retinal vessels, reduced or absent electroretinogram response and progressive peripheral visual field loss. For these patients the molecular analysis could not be performed.

Figure 1 illustrates a typical STGD while Fig. 2 shows the fundus appearance of a classic RP.

All the patients included in the study were clinically evaluated by means of a standard ophthalmologic examination, electroretinography (Electrophysiological Diagnostic

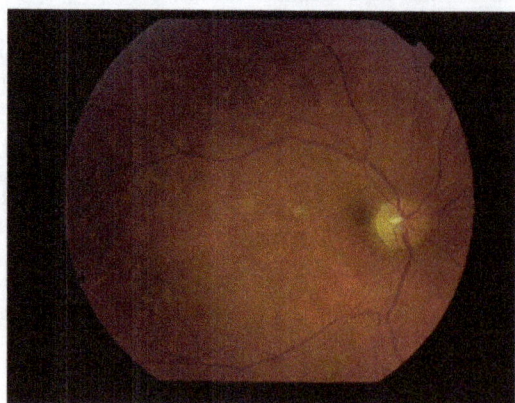

Fig. 1 STGD: macular atrophy and flecks at the posterior pole

Unit Retimax, Roland Consult, Brandenburg, Germany) performed according to the existing ISCEV Guidelines, OCT scan (Topcon 3D OCT-1000, Topcon Medical Systems Inc, Oakland, NJ, USA) and automated visual field examination (Humprey Automated Perimeter, Carl Zeiss, Dublin, CA, USA). Fluorescein angiography (Zeiss Retinograph with Image Processing Software Visupac, Carl Zeiss, Dublin, CA, USA) was obtained in 15 STGD patients either to refine the diagnosis or to investigate the possible presence of dark choroid.

In both groups age of onset of the visual symptoms and visual acuity at the time of the dietary analysis were considered as possible markers of disease severity. The study adhered to the tenets of the Declaration of Helsinki and was approved by the AOU Careggi Ethics Committee. Each patient gave written informed consent.

Dietary analysis

Trained dieticians collected data in order to assess the habitual consumption of 109 food items, with the aid of software specific for the analysis of food habits and the estimation of nutrient and caloric intake (WinFood, release 1.5; Medimatica, Martinsicuro, Te, Italy). For each specific food item a commonly used portion size was specified and subjects were asked how often they had consumed that unit (never, daily, weekly, monthly) on average during the past year. Emphasis was paid to ensure that the answers were related to a yearlong dietary pattern and not to last few months, especially in terms of seasonal changes of diet. Nutrient intakes were presented for comparison with the dietary reference intakes (RDI) for males and females aged 18–59 years [15].

Statistical analysis

Statistical analysis was performed by using the SPSS (Statistical Package for Social Sciences Inc., Chicago, IL, USA) software for Macintosh (Version 19.0). Values are expressed as mean ± standard deviation (SD) or median and range, as appropriate. Chi-square test was used to test for proportions. T-test was used for comparisons between single groups for normally distributed parameters and Mann–Whitney test was used for comparison of age between groups. A p-value <0.05 was considered to indicate statistical significance.

Results

Clinical characteristics

The median age at onset of symptoms was 20.5 years (range: 8–39) for STGD and 30 years (range: 2–72) for RP, with the median duration of the disease of 11.5 years (range: 0–39) and 14 years (range: 0–53) for STGD and RP, respectively.

At the moment of the dietary analysis Snellen equivalent visual acuity was 3.8 ± 3.1 in the right eye and 3.8 ±

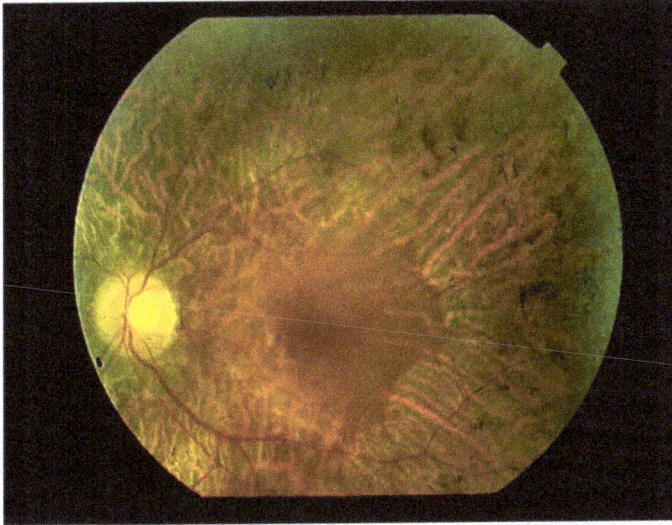

Fig. 2 RP: Pale optic disc, attenuated retinal vessels, midperipheral dystrophy of the retinal pigment epithelium with typical pigmentary changes

3.2 in the left eye for STGD as compared to 5.4 ± 3.8 in the right eye and 5.1 ± 3.7 in the left eye for RP patients.

Dietary profile

Dietary pattern of the study population is described in Tables 1 and 2, for STGD and RP respectively. Macronutrient distributions were not significantly different between males and females for both groups of patients. By comparing the dietary patterns with the dietary reference intakes reported by the Italian Society of Human Nutrition (Italian Society of Human Nutrition, [15]) in order to prevent the major chronic diseases we can observe some divergences from the recommendations. Indeed, in both males and females the study populations showed a slightly increased contribution of total fat from the diet, with a considerably low contribution from polyunsaturated fats. In addition, a low intake of fibre is showed in both genders of the two groups of patients as well as a high intake of cholesterol was demonstrated in all the patients.

As considering minerals and vitamins, both groups of patients reported insufficient intake of some minerals and vitamins, as showed by low intake of calcium, magnesium, potassium, vitamin B6, folic acid and vitamin D.

In Table 3, prevalence of patients following recommendations for a healthy diet is reported. Notably, a high proportion of patients consume a hyperlipidic diet with a contribution from total fat >30 % of the total energy in 19/24 (79.2 %) STGD and 45/56 (80.4 %) RP patients. More importantly, almost the total number of patients enrolled in the study showed an insufficient intake for polyunsaturated fats, and a high proportion of the patients reported a high intake of cholesterol

from the diet. Similarly, almost the totality of the patients did not reach current recommendations for fibre intake.

Vitamin A and other nutrients

With regard to vitamin A intake, only 6 out of 24 STGD patients (25 %) reported a daily intake of vitamin A that follows the recommendations for a healthy diet (Table 3 and Fig. 3). Contrarily to what suggested for patients with such disease, interestingly, in 14/24 (58.3 %) a high intake of vitamin A from the diet was reported. In this group of patients the average intake of dietary vitamin A was 1329.8 µg RAE/day (SD: 828.4) with a range of 706.3–3863.2 µg RAE/day, and one patient exceeded the upper toxicity level (3000 µg RAE/day). Looking at the clinical characteristics, it came evident that such patient presented with a very low visual acuity (right eye: 1.0; left eye: 1.2) and an early age of onset of the disease (19 years). Similarly, as far as RP is concerned, only 4 out of 56 patients (7.1 %) reported to meet the current recommendations for daily intake of vitamin A from the diet. Even in this group of patients, contrarily to what usually recommended by physicians, a relatively high proportion of patients, i.e., 15/56 (26.8 %) reported to consume a low intake of vitamin A (<600 µg RAE/day) (Fig. 3).

Interestingly, STGD patients with low vitamin A intake (<600 µg RAE/day) showed significantly better visual acuity (right eye: 6.8 ± 3.4; left eye: 7.0 ± 3.8 vs. 3.2 ± 2.8 and 3.2 ± 2.7; p = 0.04) with respect to those introducing higher intake of vitamin A (>700 µg RAE/day). On the other hand, RP patients with high vitamin A intake (>700 µg RAE/day) showed a higher, albeit not

Table 1 Dietary profile and nutrient intake in patients with Stargardt's Disease

	Males (n = 12)		Females (n = 12)	
	Mean (SD)	DRI	Mean (SD)	DRI
Energy, kcal	2249.9 (309.4)	2200	1773 (338.2)	1800
% of energy from carbohydrates	51.3 (4.4)	45–60 %	52.4 (7.9)	45–60 %
% of energy from protein	15.6 (1.8)	15–20 %	15.8 (2)	15–20 %
% of energy from fats	33.2 (5)	<30 %	34.8 (7.3)	<30 %
% of energy from saturated fats	8.7 (2.3)	<10 %	9.8 (3)	< 10 %
% of energy from monounsaturated fats	15.3 (2.7)	15–20 %	14.9 (4.7)	15–20 %
% of energy from polyunsaturated fats	3.4 (0.6)	5–10 %	3.5 (0.9)	5–10 %
EPA, mg	230 (130)	>250	120 (70)	>250
DHA, mg	290 (70)		130 (90)	
Cholesterol, mg	286.7 (104.8)	<200	209.5 (56.9)	<200
Dietary fibre, g	18.5 (4.3)	25	16.3 (4.6)	25
Calcium, mg	707.3 (250.6)	1000	615.9 (220.8)	1000
Magnesium, mg	146.4 (32.1)	240	130.9 (26.3)	240
Potassium, mg	2394.8 (767.1)	3900	2225.3 (495.5)	3900
Sodium, mg	1462.3 (606)	1500	1476.2 (832.2)	1500
Iron, mg	10.2 (1.7)	10	13.5 (2.3)	18
Vitamin A, μg RAE	1277.9 (962.8)	700	729.4 (258.8)	600
Thiamin, mg	1.23 (0.25)	1.2	1.19 (0.32)	1.1
Riboflavin, mg	1.56 (0.47)	1.6	1.16 (0.32)	1.3
Niacin, mg	16.9 (2.4)	18	13.9 (2.9)	18
Vitamin B6, mg	1.14 (0.43)	1.3	1.17 (0.53)	1.3
Folic acid, mg	193.2 (100.3)	400	201.5 (80.9)	400
Vitamin C, mg	161.7 (103.6)	105	136.2 (73.8)	85
Vitamin D, μg	3.41 (1.71)	15	2.33 (1.65)	15
Vitamin E, mg	11.1 (3.5)	15	7.92 (3.7)	15

The dietary reference intakes (DRI) are presented using adequate intake and population reference intake for males and females aged 18–59 years according to the Dietary Reference Values of the Italian Society of Human Nutrition [15]
EPA eicosapentaenoic acid, *DHA* docosahexaenoic acid, *RAE* retinol activity equivalent

significant, age of onset of the disease (30.8 ± 5.7 years) vs. those reporting low vitamin A intake (25.5 ± 9.0 years).

Finally, intake of EPA and DHA from diet was also evaluated. Among STGD patients, 10 out of 24 (41.7 %) patients reported not to reach the recommendations for these relevant nutrients (>250 mg/day). A similar result has been reported in the RP group since 17 out of 56 (30.4 %) patients showed not to reach the current recommendations for the introduction of EPA + DHA with the diet.

Discussion

Over the last years, some nutrients like vitamin A, docosahexaenoic acid, and lutein have been proposed to influence the clinical course of the two most common retinal dystrophies, STGD and RP [8, 9, 12]. In fact in STGD vitamin A cannot be properly metabolized because of ABCA4 protein impairment and gives origin to toxic byproducts which are the main components of lipofuscin [2, 6]. On the other side in most RP patients genetic abnormalities prevent the appropriate processing of vitamin A in phototransduction and visual cycle [2, 4, 5, 16]. Indeed, in opposite ways, both STGD and RP may be significantly influenced by dietary intake of these nutrients.

In STGD, experimental studies in animal models suggested that a reduction of vitamin A dietary intake, and their resulting circulating levels, might arrest the accumulation of retinal toxic metabolites, so ameliorating the clinical course of the disease [17]. However, a low vitamin A diet has never been proposed and evaluation of dietary profiles of these patients has never been conducted. Conversely, in RP, nutritional supplementation with vitamin A associated with docosahexaenoic acid or lutein has been already evaluated in clinical trials [8, 10, 12],

Table 2 Dietary profile and nutrient intake in patients with Retinitis Pigmentosa

	Males (n = 23)		Females (n = 33)	
	Mean (SD)	DRI	Mean (SD)	DRI
Energy, kcal	1994.9 (436.4)	2200	1830 (362.1)	1800
% of energy from carbohydrates	47.9 (7.9)	45–60 %	49.6 (6.2)	45–60 %
% of energy from protein	16.7 (2.6)	15–20 %	17.7 (2.8)	15–20 %
% of energy from fats	34.6 (6.2)	<30 %	34.1 (5.6)	<30 %
% of energy from saturated fats	9.3 (2.8)	< 10 %	9.3 (2.3)	< 10 %
% of energy from monounsaturated fats	15.6 (3.6)	15–20 %	15 (3.7)	15–20 %
% of energy from polyunsaturated fats	3.6 (1)	5–10 %	3.4 (0.9)	5–10 %
EPA, mg	180 (130)	>250	230 (60)	>250
DHA, mg	190 (150)		280 (60)	
Cholesterol, mg	284.4 (113.9)	<200	266.3 (87.6)	<200
Dietary fibre, g	15.5 (4.5)	25	15.9 (4.3)	25
Calcium, mg	596.9 (198.8)	1000	662.5 (213.9)	1000
Magnesium, mg	138.8 (50.4)	240	139.6 (33.6)	240
Potassium, mg	2432.8 (511.5)	3900	2423.9 (552.5)	3900
Sodium, mg	1626.8 (563.1)	1500	1357.8 (443.1)	1500
Iron, mg	11.7 (3.7)	10	10.9 (2.8)	18
Vitamin A, µg RAE	1332.9 (205.7)	700	1368.9 (498.7)	600
Thiamin, mg	1.07 (0.35)	1.2	1.05 (0.21)	1.1
Riboflavin, mg	1.56 (0.47)	1.6	1.16 (0.32)	1.3
Niacin, mg	17.3 (5.4)	18	15.4 (4.9)	18
Vitamin B6, mg	1.26 (0.43)	1.3	1.33 (0.39)	1.3
Folic acid, mg	203.9 (80.4)	400	221.2 (66.8)	400
Vitamin C, mg	112.1 (60.6)	105	136.3 (50.5)	85
Vitamin D, µg	3.83 (2.76)	15	4.44 (2.24)	15
Vitamin E, mg	9.7 (3.6)	15	9.2 (3.1)	15

The dietary reference intakes (DRI) are presented using adequate intake and population reference intake for males and females aged 18–59 years according to the Dietary Reference Values of the Italian Society of Human Nutrition [15]
EPA eicosapentaenoic acid, *DHA* docosahexaenoic acid, *RAE* retinol activity equivalent

Table 3 Prevalence of men and women following the dietary reference intake (DRI) for selected nutrients

	Stargardt's disease		Retinitis pigmentosa	
	Males (n = 12)	Females (n = 12)	Males (n = 23)	Females (n = 33)
Carbohydrates (45–60 % TE), n (%)	11 (91.7)	7 (58.3)	13 (56.5)	23 (69.7)
Protein (15–20 % TE), n (%)	7 (58.3)	7 (58.3)	14 (60.9)	22 (66.7)
Fats (<30 % TE), n (%)	2 (16.7)	3 (25)	5 (21.7)	6 (18.7)
SFA (<10 % of total fats), n (%)	8 (66.7)	7 (58.3)	15 (65.2)	19 (57.6)
MUFA (15–20 % of total fats), n (%)	8 (66.7)	5 (41.7)	10 (43.5)	15 (45.5)
PUFA (5–10 % of total fats), n (%)	0 (0)	0 (0)	1 (4.3)	0 (0)
Cholesterol (<200 mg), n (%)	3 (25)	6 (50)	5 (21.7)	8 (24.2)
Dietary fibre (>25 g), n (%)	0 (0)	0 (0)	0 (0)	1 (3)
Vitamin A (600–700 µg RAE), n (%)	1 (8.3)	5 (41.7)	2 (8.7)	2 (6.1)
EPA + DHA (>250 mg), n (%)	10 (83.3)	4 (33.3)	15 (65.2)	24 (72.7)

DRIs for the selected macronutrient or nutrient are reported in brackets
STGD Stargardt's Disease, *PR* pigmentosa retinitis, *TE* total energy, *SFA* saturated fats, *MUFA* monounsaturated fats, *PUFA* polyunstaurated fats, *EPA* eicosapentaenoic acid, *RAE* retinal activity equivalent, *DHA* docosahexaenoic acid

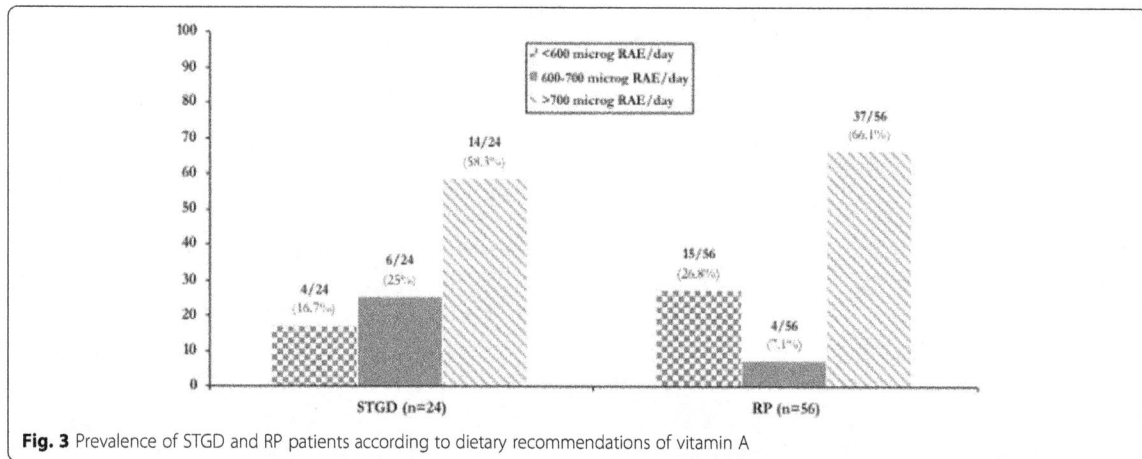

Fig. 3 Prevalence of STGD and RP patients according to dietary recommendations of vitamin A

showing some beneficial effects, even if the efficacy and safety of this approach is still controversial: in fact, the high doses of vitamin A proposed in RP patients have the potential risk of bone and liver damage, and severe birth defects if assumed by pregnant women [18].

In our study we investigated the dietary habits of some patients affected by RP or STGD in order to seek for possible tailored dietary intervention to suggest to these patients. The study population showed some divergences from nutritional recommendations that may be corrected through a nutritional intervention. Indeed, a high proportion of patients consume a hyperlipidic diet with a high assumption of cholesterol and a low intake of polyunsaturated fatty acids and fibre. Interestingly, with regard to vitamin A intake, we reported that the daily intake of vitamin A in STGD patients was higher than what recommended in a relevant portion of the study population. In this group of patients, the high intake of vitamin A was also associated with a worst clinical course of the disease in terms of visual acuity. Conversely, in RP patients vitamin A intake was lower than dietary recommendations in a relevant percentage of RP patients, with a resultant - even if not significant - worst clinical profile in terms of earlier age of onset of the disease. These data, showing a relevant prevalence of insuitable nutrient intakes among our patients with retinal dystrophies, supports the possible influence of diet on the pathogenesis of some inherited retinal degenerations and suggests a nutritional intervention in these patients.

Actually, the dietary pattern of these patients may play a significant role in the clinical course of the disease and may represent a therapeutic approach for disorders presently without effective treatment.

The study has some limitations. First, the small sample size of the study population does not allow us to establish possible relationships between nutrients and different clinical features of the retinal degenerations. On the other

hand, it should be noted that STGD is a relatively rare condition and this is the first study investigating this issue. Second, the nature of the study i.e., cross-sectional design does not give us the opportunity to confirm a causal relationship between nutritional and clinical characteristics of these diseases. Moreover RP and STGD may show a very high phenotypic variability and so the association between nutrients intake and clinical course must be considered not conclusive. Third, circulating levels of vitamin A could not be measured in such patients. The measurements of serum vitamin A levels would have improved the knowledge of the pathophysiological mechanisms at the basis of the onset and of the grade of severity of the disease. Finally the possible influence of multiple lifestyle features (like smoking, drugs assumption, BMI) should be considered in future investigations.

Conclusions

Nevertheless, despite all these limitations, the strength of the present study is that it is the first study that evaluated the dietary profile of patients with retinal dystrophies. The altered intake of many nutrients in the diet of these patients supports the idea that a nutritional intervention can be attempted before giving a prescription with nutritional supplementations. Further studies are requested to evaluate the balance between the possible clinical benefits of a reduced vitamin A intake and the potential ocular (night blindness and xerophthalmia) and systemic (depression, skin problems and others) risk of vitamin A deficiency.

Abbreviations
RAE: retinal activity equivalent; RP: Retinitis Pigmentosa; STGD: Stargardt's disease.

Competing interests
All authors declare that there are no competing interest.

Dietary profile of patients with Stargardt's disease and Retinitis Pigmentosa: is there a role...

33

Authors' contributions

Conception and design: FS, AC, AS. Analysis and interpretation of the data: FS, VM, AM, GA, FF, AS. Drafting of the article: FS, FF, RA, GFG, UM, AC, AS Dietary analysis: FS, AC, DB. Clinical evaluation of patients: AS, VM, AM, GA. Critical revision of the article for important intellectual content: RA, GFG, UM, AC. Final approval of the article: FS, FF, RA, GFG, UM, AC, AS. Statistical expertise: FS.

Financial disclosure

Nothing to declare

Author details

[1]Department of Experimental and Clinical Medicine, University of Florence, Florence, Italy. [2]Agency of Nutrition, University Hospital of Careggi, Florence, Italy. [3]Don Carlo Gnocchi Foundation Italy, Onlus IRCCS, Florence, Italy. [4]Department of Surgery and Translational Medicine, Eye Clinic, University of Florence, Florence, Italy.

References

1. Lien EI, Hammond BR. Nutritional influences on visual development and function. Progr Ret Eye Res. 2011;30:188–203.
2. Palczewski K. Chemistry and Biology of Vision. J Biol Chem. 2012;287:1612–9.
3. Chappelow AV, Traboulsi EI. Stargardt Disease. In: Traboulsi EI, editor. Genetic Diseases of the Eye. Oxford-New York: Oxford University Press; 2012. p. 467–75.
4. Hartong DT, Berson EL, Dryja TP. Retinitis pigmentosa. Lancet. 2006;368: 1795–809.
5. Ferreyra HA, Heckenlively JR. Retinitis Pigmentosa. In: Traboulsi EI, editor. Genetic Diseases of the Eye. Oxford-New York: Oxford University Press; 2012. p. 381–92.
6. Radu RA, Yuan Q, Hu J, Peng JH, Lloyd M, Nusinowitz S, et al. Accelerated accumulation of lipofuscin pigments in the RPE of a mouse model for ABCA4-mediated retinal dystrophies following Vitamin A supplementation. Invest Ophthalmol Vis Sci. 2008;49:3821–9.
7. Aleman TS, Cideciyan AV, Windsor EA, Schwartz SB, Swider M, Chico JD, et al. Macular pigment and lutein supplementation in ABCA4-associated retinal degenerations. Invest Ophthalmol Vis Sci. 2007;48:1319–29.
8. Berson EL, Rosner B, Sandberg MA, Hayes KC, Nicholson BW, Weigel-DiFranco C, et al. A randomized trial of vitamin A and vitamin E supplementation for retinitis pigmentosa. Arch Ophthalmol. 1993;111:761–72.
9. Berson EL, Rosner B, Sandberg MA, Moser A, Brockhurst RJ, Hayes KC, et al. Clinical trial of docosohexanoic acid in patients with Retinitis Pigmentosa receiving vitamin A treatment. Arch Ophthalmol. 2004;122:1297–305.
10. Berson EL, Rosner B, Sandberg MA, Weigel-DiFranco C, Moser A, Brockhurst RJ, et al. Further evaluation of docosohexanoic acid in patients with Retinitis Pigmentosa receiving vitamin A treatment. Arch Ophthalmol. 2004;122: 1306–14.
11. Berson EL, Rosner B, Sandberg MA, Weigel-Di Franco C, Willett W. ω-3 intake and visual acuity in patients with Retinitis Pigmentosa receiving vitamin A. Arch Ophthalmol. 2012;130:707–11.
12. Berson EL, Rosner B, Sandberg MA, Weigel-DiFranco C, Brockhurst RJ, Hayes KC, et al. Clinical trial of lutein in patients with Retinitis Pigmentosa receiving vitamin A. Arch Ophthalmol. 2010;128:403–11.
13. Koenekoop RK. The gene for Stargardt disease, ABCA4, is a major retinal gene: a mini-review. Ophthalmic Genet. 2003;24:75–80.
14. Passerini I, Sodi A, Giambene B, Mariottini A, Menchini U, Torricelli F. Novel mutations of the ABCR gene in Italian patients with Stargardt Disease. Eye. 2010;24:158–64.
15. Italian Society of Human Nutrition. Livelli di Assunzione di Riferimento di Nutrienti ed energia per la popolazione italiana 2012. Available at: http://www.sinu.it/html/pag/larn-2014.asp (accessed on August, 28 2013).
16. Perusek L, Maeda T. Vitamin A derivatives as treatment options for retinal degenerative diseases. Nutrients. 2013;5:2646–66.
17. Radu RA, Han Y, Bui TV, Nusinowitz S, Bok D, Lichter J, et al. Reductions in serum vitamin A arrest accumulation of toxic retinal fluorophores: a potential therapy for treatment of lipofuscin-based retinal diseases. Invest Ophthalmol Vis Sci. 2005;46:4393–401.
18. Massof RW, Fishman GA. How strong is the evidence that nutritional supplements slow the progression of Retinitis Pigmentosa? Arch Ophthalmol. 2010;128:493–5.

5

Neovascular glaucoma: a retrospective review from a tertiary center in China

Na Liao, Chaohong Li, Huilv Jiang, Aiwu Fang, Shengjie Zhou and Qinmei Wang[*]

Abstract

Background: The purpose of this study is to report the prevalence, etiology, treatment and outcomes of neovascular glaucoma (NVG) in a tertiary care ophthalmic center in China.

Methods: Medical records of patients diagnosed as NVG at the Wenzhou Medical University between 2003 and 2014 were reviewed. Success was defined as IOP between 6 and 21 mmHg without topical or systemic glaucoma medications with retention of presenting visual acuity (VA).

Results: NVG was diagnosed in 483 of 8306 (5.8 %) of all glaucoma patients. Etiology is reported for all 310 eyes of 284 patients managed in the department. Interventions depended on insurance as well as personal finances; outcomes are reported for the 149 eyes of 138 patients with complete data that met follow up requirements. Diabetic retinopathy (DR,39.7 %) was the major cause of NVG. Kaplan Meier survival analysis showed a success rate of 84.8 % at 1 year, 47.5 % at 3 years and 21.9 % at 5 years. Major interventions included glaucoma drainage device (GDD) in 103 eyes and trans-scleral cyclophotocoagulation (TSCPC) in 22 eyes. Complications were more common in the GDD group.

Conclusions: NVG comprised 5.8 % of glaucoma patients seen in a tertiary Chinese hospital. DR was identified as the commonest cause and probably reflects the increasing prevalence of diabetes in China. Surgical interventions were partly determined by insurance status and personal finances. GDD was the commonest surgical intervention used and also had the most complications.

Keywords: Neovascular glaucoma, Etiology, Glaucoma drainage device

Background

Neovascular glaucoma (NVG) is a secondary, refractory condition that accounts for 0.7–5.1 % of glaucoma in an Asian population [1, 2]. The condition is secondary to obstruction of the trabecular meshwork by neo-vascular membrane that develops in response to retinal ischemia [3, 4]. Current surgical options for intraocular pressure (IOP) control in NVG comprise augmented trabeculectomy, glaucoma drainage devices (GDD) and cyclophotocoagulation (CPC) while prognostic factors include young age, previous vitrectomy and post-surgery complications [4–6]. Recent prospective data on the management of refractory glaucoma from China reported GDD as safe and effective for some of the conditions but with a relatively poor outcome in

NVG [7]. Late presentation and loss of follow up are additional challenges for the management of NVG in China [8].

There is paucity of data from China relating the causes and management of NVG. The objective of this study is to report the causes, management and outcomes of NVG in a tertiary facility in China.

Methods

The study was approved by the ethics committee of the Wenzhou medical university. As this was a retrospective study with de-identified data informed consent was not required. The records of all patients diagnosed as NVG between June 2003 and March 2014 at the eye hospital of Wenzhou Medical University, Wenzhou, China were reviewed. The diagnosis of NVG was based on an IOP > 21 mmHg on applanation tonometry associated with neo-vascularization of the iris and/or angle of the anterior

* Correspondence: wqm3@mail.eye.ac.cn
School of Optometry and Ophthalmology and Eye Hospital, Wenzhou Medical University, Wenzhou, Zhejiang, China

chamber detected by slit lamp bio-microscopy and gonio-scopy [9]. All patients with NVG treated in our hospital were investigated to determine the cause. Other data extracted from the records included age, gender, affected eye, visual acuity(VA), lens status, IOP, number of glau-coma medications used at presentation and at last visit, types of intervention, history of previous intraocular sur-gery, use of anti-VEGF agents and post operative compli-cations. Etiology of NVG was reported for all patients managed in the hospital. Patients with a follow up of less than 6 months were excluded, as were those without IOP and VA data at the final visit.

All patients received treatment for the underlying cause as well as medical treatment for control of IOP. Surgery was undertaken if further IOP lowering was deemed necessary either for retention of vision or for comfort. The overall management however depended not only on surgeon preference but also on insurance cover as well as capacity to pay. While 95 % of our patients had medical insurance, reimbursement is not uniform and payment for prosthesis like GDD is usual.

Surgery if indicated was undertaken by one of 5 sur-geons. For patients with useful vision, most surgeons preferred GDD as the first surgical option. Trabeculect-omy was offered for such patients if economic factors precluded the use of a GDD, while trans-scleral cyclo-photocoagulation (TSCPC) was generally offered those without useful vision. Endoscopic cyclophotocoagulation (Endo-CPC) was introduced in our hospital in 2006 and was combined with cataract surgery/vitrectomy or used in isolation for refractory NVG in some pseduophakic eyes. Anti-vascular endothelial growth factor (anti-VEGF) became available in the clinic from 2008 and was used on a case-by-case basis determined primarily by insurance cover and affordability.

All GDD surgery was performed using Ahmed im-plants (New World Medical, Inc., Rancho Cucamonga, CA, USA). The surgical technique used for GDD and trabeculectomy were similar to that described in the lit-erature [10, 11]. All trabeculectomies were performed with adjunctive mitomycin C, but the decision to use mitomycin with GDD was made by the individual sur-geon. TSCPC was performed using the G probe with the diode laser (Iridex Corporation, Mountain View, CA, USA); Endo-CPC; was undertaken with the Endo-OPTIKS machine (Endo-OPTIKS, Little Silver, NJ, USA). The tech-nique of TSCPC and Endo-CPC used was similar to that described [12, 13]. For TSCPC, three to four quadrants were treated with the G probe with about 20 spots avoid-ing the 3 and 9 o'clock positions with parameters adjusted to avoid a 'pop'. For Endo-CPC about 200 degrees of ciliary processes were coagulated.

Success was defined as an IOP between 6 and 21 mmHg without topical or systemic glaucoma medications with retention of presenting VA; this visual criteria was applied to patients with a VA of light perception or better [5]. Snellen's VA was converted to the logarithm of the min-imal angle of resolution (LogMAR) for analysis. An im-provement or decrease in visual acuity was defined as a change of two or more lines on the LogMAR scale. Log-MAR values for low vision were defined as follows: count-ing fingers (CF) =2.3; hand motions (HM) =2.6; light perception (LP) =2.9; and no light perception (NLP) =4 [14]. For those with low vision, a difference of one low vision category post-surgery was considered as change. Patients with incomplete data (lack of IOP and VA) and follow up less than 6 months were excluded from the analysis of outcomes.

Statistical analysis

All statistical analyses were performed using SPSS soft-ware version 15.0 (SPSS, Inc., Chicago, IL) and $p < 0.05$ was considered significant. Normality of variables was ascertained using Kolmogorov-Smirnov tests. Continuous normally distributed data were presented as mean ± stand-ard deviation; proportions (%) were used to describe cat-egorical variables while non-normal distribution variables were presented as median (interquartile range). The paired student t-test and Wilcoxon signed-rank test was performed to compare the IOP and mean number of anti-glaucoma medications at presentation and at last visit respectively. Kaplan Meir survival analysis was used to report success rates. Cox's proportional hazards regression model [odds ratio (OR) with 95 % confidence interval (CI)] was used to report the association of poten-tial prognostic factors: age, binocular involvement, lens status, previous intraocular surgery (vitrectomy or cataract surgery), systemic diseases, use anti-VEGF for underlying cause, history of PRP and influence of postoperative complications.

Results

NVG was diagnosed in a total of 483 (5.8 %) of the 8306 glaucoma patients seen during the study period. 199 patients elected to seek care elsewhere while 284 were investigated and managed at the Wenzhou medical uni-versity eye department. Etiology of NVG was established and reported for these 284 patients. After excluding 14 patients lacking IOP or VA data at their last visit and 132 patients with less than 6 months follow up, 149 eyes of 138 patients (85 males and 53 females) were available for reporting interventions and outcomes.

Patient demographics are shown in Table 1. All patients were Han-Chinese. The mean age was 64.2 ± 14.0 years (range, 10–94 years) and the median follow-up 18.5 months (range, 6.07–103.8 months). There were 105 phakic (70.5 %), 11 aphakic (7.4 %) and 33 pseudo-phakic (22.1 %) eyes. The causes of NVG are listed in

Table 1 Demographic Data

Clinical characteristics of eyes with neovascular glaucoma (N = 149)	
Age in years (range)	64.2 ± 14.0 (10–94)
Eyes (%)	
Right	76 (51.0 %)
Left	73 (49.0 %)
Gender (%)	
Male	85 (61.6 %)
Female	53 (38.4 %)
Lens (%)	
Phakic	105 (70.5 %)
Aphakic	11 (7.4 %)
Pseudophakic	33 (22.1 %)
Presenting Vision	
Improvement VA	21 (22.6 %)
Unchanged[a]	34 (36.6 %)
Decrease VA	38 (40.9 %)
Decrease to NLP	16 (17.2 %)
Previous VA = 1	2
Previous VA = CF	1
Previous VA = HM	6
Previous VA = LP	7
IOP at presentation[b]	43.5 ± 10.9
IOP at final follow-up[b]	19.0 ± 11.4
Glaucoma medications	
Median at presentation (IQR)	2 (3)
Median at final follow up (IQR)	0 (1.5)
Median interval of follow up in months (IQR)	18.5 (17.6)
History of intraocular surgery	54 (36.2 %)
Complications	38 (25.5 %)
Enucleation (%)	5 (3.4 %)
Hypotony (%)	8 (5.4 %)

IOP intraocular pressure, VA visual acuity, IQR interquartile range
[a]56 eyes with NLP at presentation were excluded
[b]5 enucleation and 2 phthisis bulbi excluded

Table 2. Diabetic retinopathy (123/310 eyes, 39.7 %) was the commonest followed by CRVO (66/310 eyes, 21.3 %). The primary cause could not be determined in 59 eyes (19.0 %). 26 patients had bilateral NVG; 15 of these patients presented with bilateral NVG while 11 were diagnosed in the fellow eye after 1 to 16 months. 20/26 (76.2 %) cases with bilateral NVG were caused by DR, two were due to bilateral CRVO, one had bilateral uveitis, one was ascribed to bilateral BRVO, one was caused by the ocular ischemia syndrome while the cause in one bilateral case remained unknown.

In eyes with presenting VA of LP or better (93 eyes of 86 patients), VA was retained in 34 eyes (36.6 %),

Table 2 Etiological Factors Associated with NVG

Causes of neovascular glaucoma	Eyes (%)
Retinal ischemic disease	
DR	123 (39.7)
CRVO	66 (21.3)
BRVO	5 (1.6)
CRAO	3 (1.0)
RD	17 (5.5)
Others[a]	9 (2.9)
Ocular ischemia syndrome	7 (2.3)
Uveitis	6 (1.9)
Trauma	13 (4.2)
Surgical causes	3 (1.0)
Radiation	1 (0.3)
Unknown	59 (19.0)

DR diabetic retinopathy, CRVO central retinal vein occlusion, CRAO central retinal artery occlusion, BRVO branch retinal vein occlusion, RD retinal detachment
[a]Including Coat's exudative retinopathy (4), Ischemic optic neuropathy (2), Hypertensive retinopathy (1) and Persistent Hyperplastic Primary Vitreous (1) and Eales' disease (1)

decreased in 38 eyes (40.9 %) and improved in 21 (22.6 %) eyes. Deterioration of vision to NLP occurred in 16/93 (17.2 %) eyes. Two of these 16 eyes had useful VA (LogMAR = 1) prior to surgery. One case was caused by severe DR while the other was caused by BRVO. Both were managed with a GDD; one case developed retinal detachment.

Of the 149 eyes, two developed phthisis bulbi and 5 required enucleation. Excluding these 7 eyes, IOP decreased from a mean (± SD) of 43.5 ± 10.9 to 19.0 ± 11.4 mmHg ($p = 0.000$). The number of glaucoma medications was reduced from 2 (interquartile range =3) to 0 (interquartile range = 1.5) after interventions ($p = 0.000$)

Kaplan-Meier survival analysis is shown in Fig. 1. Success was achieved in 84.8 % at 1 year, 47.5 % at 3 years and 21.9 % at 5 years. Six eyes that required combinations of GDD, TSCPC or trabeculectomy were excluded from this analysis (3 eyes that underwent TSCPC followed by GDD or Trabeculectomy and 3 that required TSCPC following GDD). Of the remaining 143 eyes, 103 eyes underwent GDD, 22 eyes were treated with TSCPC, 7 eyes had trabeculectomy, 3 eyes underwent Endo-CPC and 8 eyes underwent combined surgery. Table 3 details the treatment modalities and their outcomes. Age, lens status, the use of anti-VEGF, postoperative complications, PRP, prior-intraocular surgery did not have a statistically significant influence on outcome (Table 4).

Postoperative complications are summarized in Table 5. Shallow anterior chamber was the commonest complication (12/143, 8.4 %) followed by hypotony (8/143, 5.6 %). Tube-related complications included occlusion/

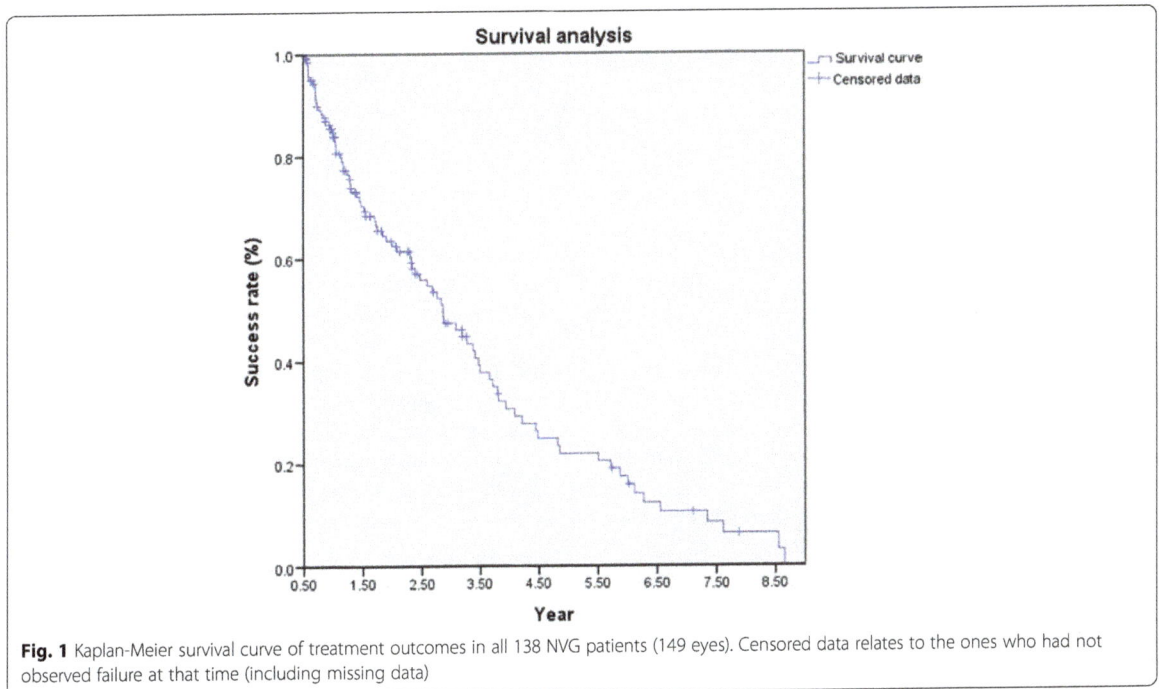

Fig. 1 Kaplan-Meier survival curve of treatment outcomes in all 138 NVG patients (149 eyes). Censored data relates to the ones who had not observed failure at that time (including missing data)

displacement of the tube and occurred in 2 eyes. Most complications occurred in the GDD group.

Discussion

A survey by the Beijing union medical college hospital and WHO in 1996 reported that the prevalence of secondary glaucoma in the population over the age of 50 years was 0.12 % and accounted for 5.9 % of all glaucoma [15]. NVG per se was not reported, but as it is a secondary glaucoma, we can infer that the proportion of NVG in that survey was lower than 5.9 %. NVG was diagnosed in 5.8 % of 8306 glaucoma patients seen in our tertiary hospital. This is similar to the 6.7 % of 1232

Chinese subjects diagnosed as glaucoma in a population based survey in Singapore [16]. Although it cannot really be compared to population-based data, Our data provides the prevalence of NVG in a tertiary eye hospital in China.

DR (39.7 %) followed by CRVO (21.3 %) was the major cause of NVG in this series. While the etiology could only be determined for the 284 patients who elected to continue their care in our center, the pattern is consistent with reports from other countries [17–19]. A recent hospital based report from China provides conflicting results: CRVO (39.2 %) was reported as the commonest cause in 120 NVG eyes [20]. Diabetes, a major cause of NVG has

Table 3 Treatment and results ($N = 143$ eyes)[a]

Treatments[N(%)]	No. cases	Complete success rate	Decreased VA	The percentage of IOP reduction
TB	7 (4.9 %)	4 (57.1 %)	2 (28.6 %)	70.0 %
GDD	103 (72.0 %)	46 (32.2 %)	35 (34.0 %)	54.8 %[b]
TSCPC	22 (15.4 %)	7 (31.8 %)	4 (18.2 %)	66.8 %[c]
Endo-CPC	3 (2.1 %)	0	3 (100 %)	17.2 %[d]
Combined surgery	8 (5.6 %)	4 (50.0 %)	1 (12.5 %)	61.1 %
Vitrectomy & GDD	3	1	0	48.2 %
Cataract & GDD	3	3	0	73.6 %
Cataract & Endo-CPC	2	0	1	60.5 %

TB trabeculectomy, GDD glaucoma drainage devices, TSCPC trans sclera cyclophotocoagulation, Endo-CPC endoscopic cyclophotocoagulation
[a]6 eyes treated with multiple operations excluded
[b]GDD group excludes 1 enucleated eye
[c]TSCPC group excludes 3 enucleated eyes and 1 with phthisis bulbi
[d]Endo-CPC group excludes 1 eye with phthisis

Table 4 Prognostic factors

Parameters	P	Odds ratio	95 % confidence interval
Age	0.85	1.07	0.53–2.16
Binocular	0.34	1.36	0.72–2.56
Lens status	0.99	1.00	0.72–1.39
Prior surgery	0.78	1.10	0.59–2.02
Hypertension	0.34	1.28	0.77–2.11
Diabetes	0.18	0.69	0.40–1.19
Anti-VEGF	0.32	1.79	0.58–5.56
Complications	0.30	0.78	0.48–1.25
PRP	0.43	1.22	0.74–2.01

increased in China over the years and has a current reported prevalence of 23 %, affecting an estimated 92.4 million adults in the mainland [21]. Our data seems to suggest a change in etiology of NVG that is likely linked to the increasing prevalence of diabetes in China. Lack of data and the retrospective nature of the study contributed to our inability to identify the cause in 19 % of cases.

VA results were sobering. Acuity was poor to start with and could only be preserved or improved in 59 % of cases while 41 % worsened, with 16 eyes deteriorating to no light perception. Improvement in vision occurred in 21/93 eyes (90 % due to resolution of corneal edema, hyphema and/or vitreous hemorrhage). GDD was the commonest surgical intervention used and also had the most complications. Interventions in our hospital depend on surgeon preference and experience as well as cover by medical insurance. GDD (103/143, 70.2 %) was the first option for controlling IOP in NVG patients with potential for vision. TSCPC was the second choice (22/143, 15.4 %) and tended to be used in those with a poorer prognosis.

Kaplan-Meier survival analysis showed a 84.8 probability of success at 1 year, 62.6 % at 2 years and 21.9 % at 5 years.

Table 5 Postoperative complications (N = 143 eyes)[a]

Complications	Number (%)	Group with highest incidence
Hyphema	4 (2.8)	GDD (4)
Shallow anterior chamber	12 (8.4)	GDD (10)
Choroidal detachment	2 (1.4)	GDD (2)
Ciliary body detachment	4 (2.8)	GDD (4)
Tube related complications[b]	2 (1.9)	-
Bleb-related complications[c]	3 (2.6)	GDD (3)
Hypotony	8 (5.6)	GDD (4)
Endophthalmitis	0	-

GDD glaucoma drainage devices
[a]6 eyes treated with multiple operations were excluded
[b]103 eyes treated with GDD were analyzed
[c]22 eyes treated with TSCPC, 3 with Endo-CPC and 2 with cataract & Endo-CPC were excluded

Nakatake, etc. found that success rate of primary trabeculectomy (with or without anti-VEGF) prior to surgery was 70.9 % after 1 year, decreasing to 60.8 % in 2 years [6]. A recent report from Japan showed that the success rate was higher (83 % at 3 years) if trabeculectomy was preceded by a preoperative intravitreal injection of Bevacizumab [22]. A publication from Korea reported a success rate of 79 % at 1 year decreasing to less than 60 % at 2 years [23]. As our numbers were small we could not report the outcomes for each intervention separately and our results cannot be easily compared to previous reports. However our findings do reflect the reality of management, outcome and poor follow up even in a tertiary care center China. The high success rate at 1 year could be due to inclusion criteria, exclusion of patients with follow up less than 6 months as well as loss to follow up.

Cox proportional hazards model showed that factors like systemic disease, lens status, complications, anti-VEGF agents, PRP and prior-intraocular surgery did not influence the treatment outcome of NVG, but our numbers are small. While, anti-VEGF agents may be beneficial for the management of NVG reducing the need for glaucoma surgery and decreasing complications in eyes with neovascular glaucoma, the addition of intravitreal bevacizumab did not seem to increase the success rate in previous studies [24, 25]. All cases that required PRP underwent the procedure, but its influence on incidence of NVG is not clear [26, 27]. While PRP eliminates the stimulus for neovascularization it does not affect existing peripheral anterior synechiae (PAS) [28].

The complications encountered following intervention in this study were those usually reported after such interventions. Shallow anterior chamber was the most frequent early complication (8.5 %), while hypotony was the most frequent late complication (5.6 %). The extreme low complication rate could not compare with previous reports from Asian directly [6, 29]. It is very likely that the discrepancy between complication rates in our study and others are related to the poor follow up rates in the current study (i.e. patients with mild complications mostly like lost follow-up) and some data unavailable in this retrospective study. Given the limitations of sample size we too found that larger IOP reductions could be achieved with tube surgery compared to TSCPC but the postoperative complications were higher and included some sight threatening ones [30]. Although we did not encounter any endophthalmitis, phthisis and severe pain requiring enucleation occurred in 5 patients, three of those in the TSCPC group.

The limitations of the study include the retrospective design, exclusion of a large number of cases due to lack of follow up and lack of data as well as the lack of standardized management. The lack of a preferred practice or standardized regime also meant that the numbers for some interventions were too small to conduct any analysis. The fact that the management is affected by insurance status and personal finances made it difficult to create a protocol or standardize procedures, but this as well as poor follow up is the reality in China. This case series does however demonstrate the changing etiology of NVG in China, has the longest follow-up of NVG in an Asian population and reflects the reality of management in China.

Conclusion

Diabetic retinopathy was the commonest detected cause of NVG encountered in a tertiary hospital in China. Cases present late, follow up is poor and management is partly determined by surgeon preference, insurance cover and personal finances. The increasing prevalence of diabetes in China will likely lead to a higher incidence of NVG and other related complications.

Competing interests
The authors declare that they have no competing interests.

Authors' contributions
NL was responsible for, collection of data, analysis and interpretation of results and wrote the first draft of the manuscript. CHL participated in its design and helped to draft the manuscript. HLJ was involved in data collection. AWF and SJZ helped perform the analysis; QMW conceived the study. All authors read and approved the final manuscript.

Acknowledgements
This work was supported in part by the National Science and Technology Ministry (2012BAI08B04); National Natural Science Foundation of China (81300804);the Scientific Research Fund of Wenzhou Medical University (QTJ11022).

References
1. Wong TY, Chong EW, Wong WL, Rosman M, Aung T, Loo JL, et al. Prevalence and causes of low vision and blindness in an urban malay population: the Singapore Malay Eye Study. Arch Ophthalmol. 2008;126(8):1091–9.
2. Narayanaswamy A, Baskaran M, Zheng Y, Lavanya R, Wu R, Wong WL, et al. The prevalence and types of glaucoma in an urban Indian population: the Singapore Indian Eye Study. Invest Ophthalmol Vis Sci. 2013;54(7):4621–7.
3. Brown GC, Magargal LE, Schachat A, Shah H. Neovascular glaucoma. Etiologic considerations. Ophthalmology. 1984;91(4):315–20.
4. Sivak-Callcott JA, O'Day DM, Gass JD, Tsai JC. Evidence-based recommendations for the diagnosis and treatment of neovascular glaucoma. Ophthalmology. 2001;108(10):1767–76. quiz1777, 1800.
5. Takihara Y, Inatani M, Fukushima M, Iwao K, Iwao M, Tanihara H. Trabeculectomy with mitomycin C for neovascular glaucoma: prognostic factors for surgical failure. Am J Ophthalmol. 2009;147(5):912–8. 918 e911.
6. Nakatake S, Yoshida S, Nakao S, Arita R, Yasuda M, Kita T, et al. Hyphema is a risk factor for failure of trabeculectomy in neovascular glaucoma: a retrospective analysis. BMC Ophthalmol. 2014;14:55.
7. Li Z, Zhou M, Wang W, Huang W, Chen S, Li X, et al. A prospective comparative study on neovascular glaucoma and non-neovascular refractory glaucoma following Ahmed glaucoma valve implantation. Chin Med J (Engl). 2014;127(8):1417–22.
8. Zhang X, Zhou M. Neovascular glaucoma: challenges we have to face. Chin Med J (Engl). 2014;127(8):1407–9.
9. Netland PA. The Ahmed glaucoma valve in neovascular glaucoma (An AOS Thesis). Trans Am Ophthalmol Soc. 2009;107:325–42.
10. Oguri A, Takahashi E, Tomita G, Yamamoto T, Jikihara S, Kitazawa Y. Transscleral cyclophotocoagulation with the diode laser for neovascular glaucoma. Ophthalmic Surg Lasers. 1998;29(9):722–7.
11. Takada S, Hoshino Y, Ito H, Masugi Y, Terauchi T, Endo K, et al. Extensive bowel necrosis related to bevacizumab in metastatic rectal cancer patient: a case report and review of literature. Jpn J Clin Oncol. 2015;45(3):286–90.
12. Uram M. Endoscopic cyclophotocoagulation in glaucoma management. Curr Opin Ophthalmol. 1995;6(2):19–29.
13. Zhang SH, Dong FT, Mao J, Bian AL. Factors related to prognosis of refractory glaucoma with diode laser transscleral cyclophotocoagulation treatment. Chin Med Sci J. 2011;26(3):137–40.
14. Sidoti PA, Dunphy TR, Baerveldt G, LaBree L, Minckler DS, Lee PP, et al. Experience with the Baerveldt glaucoma implant in treating neovascular glaucoma. Ophthalmology. 1995;102(7):1107–18.
15. Zhao J, Sui R, Jia L, Ellwein LB. Prevalence of glaucoma and normal intraocular pressure among adults aged 50 years or above in Shunyi county of Beijing. Zhonghua Yan Ke Za Zhi. 2002;38(6):335–9.
16. Foster PJ, Oen FT, Machin D, Ng TP, Devereux JG, Johnson GJ, et al. The prevalence of glaucoma in Chinese residents of Singapore: a cross-sectional population survey of the Tanjong Pagar district. Arch Ophthalmol. 2000;118(8):1105–11.
17. Al-Shamsi HN, Dueker DK, Nowilaty SR, Al-Shahwan SA. Neovascular glaucoma at king khaled eye specialist hospital - etiologic considerations. Middle East Afr J Ophthalmol. 2009;16(1):15–9.
18. Shen CC, Salim S, Du H, Netland PA. Trabeculectomy versus Ahmed Glaucoma Valve implantation in neovascular glaucoma. Clin Ophthalmol. 2011;5:281–6.
19. Woodcock MG, Richards JC, Murray AD. The last 11 years of Molteno implantation at the University of Cape Town. Refining our indications and surgical technique. Eye (Lond). 2008;22(1):18–25.
20. Liu L. Etiology analysis of neovascular glaucoma in 120 cases. Int J Ophthalmol. 2011;11(3):521–3.
21. Yang SH, Dou KF, Song WJ. Prevalence of diabetes among men and women in China. N Engl J Med. 2010;362(25):2425–6. author reply 2426.
22. Kobayashi S, Inoue M, Yamane S, Sakamaki K, Arakawa A, Kadonosono K. Long-term Outcomes After Preoperative Intravitreal Injection of Bevacizumab Before Trabeculectomy for Neovascular Glaucoma. J Glaucoma. 2015 Jan 9. doi:10.1097/IJG.0000000000000211.
23. Lee HY, Park JS, Choy YJ, Lee HJ. Surgical outcomes of different Ahmed Glaucoma Valve implantation methods between scleral graft and scleral flap. Korean J Ophthalmol. 2011;25(5):317–22.
24. Wakabayashi T, Oshima Y, Sakaguchi H, Ikuno Y, Miki A, Gomi F, et al. Intravitreal bevacizumab to treat iris neovascularization and neovascular glaucoma secondary to ischemic retinal diseases in 41 consecutive cases. Ophthalmology. 2008;115(9):1571–80. 1580 e1571-1573.
25. Fong AW, Lee GA, O'Rourke P, Thomas R. Management of neovascular glaucoma with transscleral cyclophotocoagulation with diode laser alone versus combination transscleral cyclophotocoagulation with diode laser and intravitreal bevacizumab. Clin Experiment Ophthalmol. 2011;39(4):318–23.
26. Striga M, Ivanisevic M. Comparison between efficacy of full- and mild-scatter (panretinal) photocoagulation on the course of diabetic rubeosis iridis. Ophthalmologica. 1993;207(3):144–7.
27. Hayreh SS, Klugman MR, Podhajsky P, Servais GE, Perkins ES. Argon laser panretinal photocoagulation in ischemic central retinal vein occlusion. A 10-year prospective study. Graefes Arch Clin Exp Ophthalmol. 1990;228(4):281–96.
28. Ehlers JP, Spirn MJ, Lam A, Sivalingam A, Samuel MA, Tasman W. Combination intravitreal bevacizumab/panretinal photocoagulation versus panretinal photocoagulation alone in the treatment of neovascular glaucoma. Retina. 2008;28(5):696–702.
29. Yildirim N, Yalvac IS, Sahin A, Ozer A, Bozca T. A comparative study between diode laser cyclophotocoagulation and the Ahmed glaucoma valve implant in neovascular glaucoma: a long-term follow-up. J Glaucoma. 2009;18(3):192–6.
30. Bloom PA, Clement CI, King A, Noureddin B, Sharma K, Hitchings RA, et al. A comparison between tube surgery, ND:YAG laser and diode laser cyclophotocoagulation in the management of refractory glaucoma. Biomed Res Int. 2013;2013:371951.

Surgical outcomes of 23-gauge transconjunctival pars plana vitrectomy combined with lensectomy for glaucomatous eyes with extremely shallow anterior chamber and cataract

Zhaotian Zhang[†], Shaochong Zhang[†], Xintong Jiang, Suo Qiu and Yantao Wei[*]

Abstract

Background: Glaucoma combined with an extremely shallow anterior chamber and cataracts remains as a complex condition to deal with. And the emergence of microincision vitrectomy surgery (MIVS) system may provide an ideal option for the treatment of that. We report a clinical study of surgical outcomes of 23-gauge transconjunctival pars plana vitrectomy (PPV) combined with lensectomy in the treatment of glaucomatous eyes with extremely shallow anterior chamber and cataract.

Methods: Prospective, nonrandomized and noncomparative case series study. Consecutive patients with secondary glaucoma, extremely shallow anterior chamber and cataract were recruited to have combined surgeries of 23-gauge transconjunctival pars plana vitrectomy and lensectomy. The main outcomes were best corrected visual acuity (BCVA), intraocular pressure (IOP), anterior chamber depth (ACD), number of anti-glaucoma medications and surgery-associated complications.

Results: Seventeen consecutive patients with secondary glaucoma, extremely shallow anterior chamber and cataract were recruited. The mean follow-up was 21.2 ± 8.8 months. Postoperatively, there was no significant improvement of BCVA ($P = 0.25$). The mean intraocular (IOP) decreased significantly from 43.14 ± 6.53 mmHg to 17.29 ± 1.80 mmHg ($P < 0.001$), and the mean depth of anterior chamber increased significantly from 0.507 ± 0.212 mm to 3.080 ± 0.313 mm ($P < 0.001$). The mean number of anti-glaucoma medications decreased from 4.1 ± 0.8 to 0.6 ± 0.8 ($P < 0.001$). No severe vision-threatening intra- or post-operative complications occurred.

Conclusions: Glaucoma with an extremely shallow anterior chamber and cataract can be managed well with the combined surgeries of 23-gauge pars plana vitrectomy and lensectomy. The surgical procedure is an effective and safe method to resolve the pupillary block and deepen the anterior chamber.

Keywords: 23 gauge, Transconjunctival, Pars plana vitrectomy, Pars plana lensectomy, Glaucoma, Shallow anterior chamber, Cataract

* Correspondence: weiyantao75@126.com
†Equal contributors
State Key Laboratory of Ophthalmology, Zhongshan Ophthalmic Center, Sun Yat-sen University, No.54, South Xianlie Road, Guangzhou 510060, China

Background

Glaucoma combined with an extremely shallow anterior chamber and cataracts is a complex condition often associated with malignant glaucoma, phacomorphic glaucoma, spherophakia or nanophthalmos. In such patients, the primary mechanism is anterior dislocation of lens-iris diaphragm resulted from pupillary or cilliary blockage [1–5]. Elevated intraocular pressure (IOP) and long-lasting contact of the lens-iris diaphragm to the corneal endothelium eventually lead to corneal decompensation and severe impairment of visual function. Therefore, besides control of the IOP, cataract extraction and anterior chamber formation are considered to be necessary [1, 5]. However, the crowded anterior chamber poses several difficulties during phacoemulsification, including poor construction of corneal incision, more endothelial cell loss, iris prolapse, difficult capsulorhexis and high risk of complications [6, 7].

Previous studies have demonstrated the effectiveness of vitrectomy combined with lensectomy or phacoemulsification in the treatment of malignant glaucoma [6, 8]. However, conventional 20-gauge vitrectomy system requires opening of the conjunctiva, which causes extensive conjunctival scarring [9, 10]. With the rapid development of surgical instrumentations, the microincision vitrectomy surgery (MIVS) system provides a promising technique with multiple advantages over the 20-gauge vitrectomy system [11–15]. MIVS system (23-gauge or 25-gauge) may be a feasible alternative to overcome the technical difficulties mentioned above [8–11].

According to the latest literatures, there have been few studies on the use of 23 or 25-gauge MIVS in the severe anterior segment eyes diseases. Therefore we conducted the current study to investigate its potential application in this series of diseases. In the study, we adopted 23-gauge transconjunctival PPV combined with pars plana lensectomy (PPL) in eyes with glaucoma, cataract and extremely shallow anterior chamber. Considering the severe irreversible vision defect induced by glaucoma and possible complications after intraocular lens (IOL) implantation, IOL was not determined to be implanted in any eyes of the patients. The aim of the surgery is to remove the lens and vitreous, create a communication between the anterior chamber and the vitreous cavity, and thereby reform the anterior chamber.

Methods

The study was approved by the Institutional Review Board of Zhongshan Ophthalmic Center affiliated to Sun Yat-sen Univeristy (Guangzhou, China). And it was performed in accordance with the World Medical Association's Declaration of Helsinki. Inclusion criteria for patients included medically uncontrolled IOP, extremely shallow central and peripheral anterior chamber and lens nucleus of grade 2or 3. Exclusion criteria were patients with uncontrolled ocular

infection, significant opacity of the cornea, lens nucleus of grade 4 or harder, severe systemic diseases and those unable to have scheduled follow-ups. The procedures were fully explained to each patient, and written informed consent was obtained from each subject. Written consent of publishing case details was also obtained from each subject. Seventeen eyes of 17 consecutive patients were prospectively recruited from January 2011 to February 2013 at Zhongshan Ophthalmic Center of Sun Yat-sen University.

All eligible patients underwent comprehensive ophthalmologic examinations, including best-corrected visual acuity (BCVA), non-contact tonometry and slit-lamp microscope. The nuclear sclerosis was graded using the Lens Opacity Classification System (LOCS III) [16]. The anterior chamber angle and anterior chamber depth (ACD) were examined by ultrasound biomicroscope (UBM Plus, Model P45; Pardigm Medical Industries, Salt Lake City, UT, USA). The ACD was defined as the distance between the posterior corneal surface and the anterior lens surface. B-scan ultrasonography was performed to determine status of the vitreous and retina. The axial length was also measured by A-scan ultrasound biometry.

One hour before surgery, 20 % mannitol was intravenously administered to all the patients. All surgeries were performed under retrobulbar anesthesia by one experienced ophthalmologist (S.Z) using 23-gauge system (Constellation Vitrectomy System, Alcon Laboratories, USA). Transconjunctival incisions were created about 3.0–3.5 mm from the limbus using trocars at the inferotemporal, superotemporal, and superonasal quadrants. Using the 23-gauge instruments, the anterior vitreous was firstly cut off. And then lensectomy was performed to extract the lens nucleus and cortex. Peripheral lens capsule was preserved for the secondary implantation of posterior IOL. Once there was any nucleus fragment dropping into the vitreous cavity, total vitrectomy was determined to remove the lens fragments and the residual vitreous. By means of the previous steps, the communication between the anterior chamber and the vitreous cavity was constructed. The anterior chamber was accessed through the superior trocar and the pupil, viscoelastic agents were then injected to separate the peripheral iris-corneal adhesion. As mentioned above, we determined that IOL implantation would not a feasible option for the patients, so all the eyes were not implanted with IOL finally. After all the procedures were completed, the cannulas were removed. And the incisions were sealed by a single stich with 7–0 Vicryl sutures if obvious leakage was observed.

Postoperatively, tobramycin, nonsteroidal anti-inflammatory and dexamethasone eye drops were consecutively administered four times daily for 4–6 weeks. Anti-glaucoma eye drops or oral medicine was administered if necessary.

Table 1 The characteristics of 17 patients with secondary glaucoma, extremely shallow anterior chamber and cataract

No	Age	Sex	Eye	Diagnosis	Nucleus density	Prior surgeries	BCVA Pre-	BCVA Post-	IOP (mmHg) Pre-	IOP (mmHg) Post-	No. of glaucoma medication Pre-	No. of glaucoma medication Post-	ACD (mm) Pre-	ACD (mm) Post-	AL (mm)	Follow-up (month)
1	65	F	os	Phaco glaucoma	Mature white	No	HM	HM	49.4	16.5	4	0	0.544	2.869	22.77	18
2	41	F	os	Malig glaucoma	2	Trab+ACF	0.02	0.02	39.5	18.7	4	0	0.317	2.955	21.23	12
3	69	M	os	Malig glaucoma	3	Trab	0.04	0.05	43.2	18.5	5	1	0.405	2.797	22.27	30
4	71	M	os	Phaco glaucoma	Mature white	No	HM	HM	41.7	17.4	5	0	0.220	2.980	24.83	24
5	59	F	os	Malig glaucoma	2	Trab+ACF	HM	FC	42.0	18.9	4	1	0.693	2.750	22.21	30
6	63	F	od	Malig glaucoma	3	Trab+ACF	0.04	0.02	38.5	18.2	3	0	1.050	3.463	22.30	36
7	67	M	os	Malig glaucoma	3	Trab	HM	HM	49.8	17.5	5	2	0.762	2.676	23.85	18
8	68	F	os	Spherphakia, glaucoma	2	No	FC	0.02	35.3	17.3	3	0	0.580	3.581	21.60	24
9	45	F	od	Uveitis, glaucoma	3	LPI	LP	FC	41.4	14.7	4	0	0.261	3.069	23.49	30
10	58	F	od	Malig glaucoma	3	Trab	FC	0.02	50.9	16.2	5	1	0.630	2.750	21.72	18
11	42	F	od	Uveitis, glaucoma	3	LPI	HM	FC	33.6	16.1	4	0	0.378	2.823	21.62	24
12	40	F	od	Malig glaucoma	2	Trab	HM	HM	37.5	15.4	3	0	0.542	2.951	21.94	12
13	62	M	od	Phaco glaucoma	Mature white	No	HM	FC	42.8	20.8	3	1	0.460	3.520	22.31	36
14	57	M	os	Malig glaucoma	2	Trab+ACF	HM	FC	60.3	18.5	5	2	0.635	2.962	21.98	12
15	44	F	od	Spherphakia, glaucoma	2	no	0.02	0.02	39.4	15.7	4	0	0.322	3.551	21.67	9
16	50	F	os	Malig glaucoma	2	Trab+ACF	FC	FC	42.7	14.1	5	1	0.524	3.360	22.10	15
17	57	M	os	Malig glaucoma	3	Trab	HM	FC	45.3	19.5	4	2	0.295	3.298	21.45	12

BCVA best-corrected visual acuity; CF counting fingers; HM hand motion; M male; F female; ACD anterior chamber depth; AL axial length; IOP intraocular pressure; Trab trabeculectomy; LPI laser peripheral iridectomy; ACF anterior chamber reformation; Phaco glaucoma: phacomorphic glaucoma; Malig glaucoma: malignant glaucoma; Pre-: preoperative; Post-: postoperative

Follow up examinations were scheduled at 1 week, 1 month, 3 months, 6 months, and 1 year after the surgery. If necessary, extra revisits were performed. At each postoperative visit, BCVA was assessed with Snellen visual charts, IOP was measured by non-contact tonometry, slit-lamp microscope and ophthalmoscope were performed, and the number of anti-glaucoma medications being used was also recorded. All the postoperative ACD was examined by anterior segment coherence tomography (AS-OCT, VisanteTM; Carl Zeiss Meditec, Dublin, CA, USA). In the aphakic eyes, the ACD was defined as the distance between the posterior corneal surface and the plane of the pupil. Improved VA was defined as improvement of more than one Snellen line, same as within one line and worse as loss of more than one Snellen line.

All Snellen visual acuity values were converted to the logarithm of the minimum angle of resolution (logMAR) for statistical analysis. Visual acuity of light perception (LP) was assigned as 2.9 logMAR, hand movements (HM) as 2.6 logMAR, and counting fingers (CF) as 2.3 logMAR. All data were analyzed using the SPSS 13.0 statistical software (SPSS Inc., Chicago, IL, USA). The Shapiro normality test was performed on all the continuous data. Paired t-test and Wilcoxon matched-pairs signed rank test were used as appropriate. All the continuous data were expressed as mean ± standard deviation (SD). A P value less than 0.05 was considered statistically significant.

Results

There were totally 17 consecutive patients (17 eyes) included in the study, with 10 eyes (58.8 %) diagnosed as malignant glaucoma, three eyes (17.6 %) as phacomorphic glaucoma, two eyes (11.8 %) as glaucoma secondary to spherophakia and two eyes (11.8 %) as glaucoma secondary to uveitis. The mean age of the patients was 56.35 years (range 40–71 years). Previous surgical interventions included trabeculectomy in ten eyes, anterior chamber reformation in five eyes, and laser peripheral iridectomy in two eyes. The lens nucleus density was classified from grade 2 in seven eyes (41.2 %) to grade 3 in seven eyes (41.2 %) and mature white cataract was diagnosed in three eyes (17.6 %). The mean axial length was 22.31 ± 0.94 mm (range 21.23–24.83 mm). The mean postoperative follow-up duration was 21.2 ± 8.8 months (range 9–40 months). The baseline characteristics of all patients were summarized in Table 1. A typical case (Case 9) was demonstrated in Fig. 1.

Preoperatively, the BCVA was 8/200 in two eyes (11.8 %), 4/200 in two eyes (11.8 %), CF in three eyes (17.6 %), HM in nine eyes (52.9 %), and LP in one eye (5.9 %). At the final visit, the BCVA was 10/200 in one eye (5.9 %), 4/200 in five eyes (29.4 %), CF in seven eyes (41.2 %), HM in four eyes (23.5.8 %). The preoperative and postoperative logMAR BCVA had no statistical difference (2.32 ± 0.47 VS 2.28 ± 0.42) (P = 0.25).

The mean IOP was 43.14 ± 6.53 mmHg (range 33.6–60.3 mmHg) preoperatively, which significantly decreased to 21.12 ± 4.76 mmHg (P < 0.001) at 1 day and

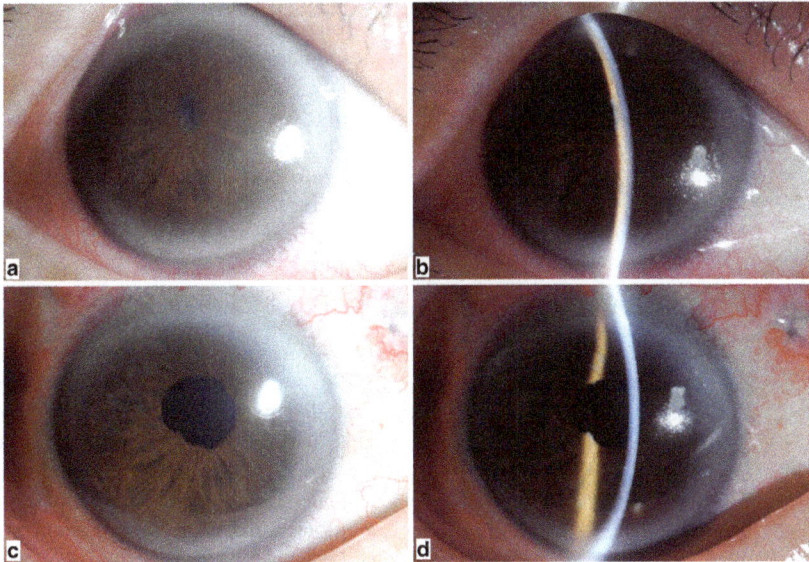

Fig. 1 A 45-year-old man presented with glaucoma secondary to uveitis in his right eye (Case 9). Before surgery: **a** anterior segment photograph shows marked iris atrophy and pupillary occlusion. **b** slit lamp biomicroscopy examination revealed an extremely shallow anterior chamber. The central ACD was 0.261 mm. One week after surgery: **c** The image on the left demonstrates a quiet anterior chamber and a relative normal pupil. **d** The slit lamp photography shows a significantly deep anterior chamber. The central ACD has increased to 3.069 mm at the center after 23-gauge PPV and PPL

20.28 ± 4.85 mmHg ($P < 0.001$) at 7 days postoperatively. One month after the surgery, the mean IOP of 17.45 ± 2.42 mmHg was maintained with/without topical anti-glaucoma medications. However, a slow elevation of IOP was observed in two eyes during the follow-up (Case 9 and Case 11), which underwent glaucoma valve implantation due to the failure of IOP-lowering medications. At the final visit, the mean IOP was 17.29 ± 1.80 mmHg (range 14.4–20.8 mmHg) in 17 eyes. Changes in IOP measurements during the follow-up were shown in Fig. 2.

With regard to anti-glaucoma medications, patients were administered a mean of 4.1 ± 0.8 (range 3–5) medications before surgery. At the last follow-up, anti-glaucoma medications had decreased significantly to 0.6 ± 0.8 (range 0–2) ($P < 0.001$). And nine eyes (52.9 %) maintained the IOP in a normal range without any anti-glaucoma eye drops.

The mean preoperative ACD was 0.507 ± 0.212 mm (range 0.220–1.05 mm). At the final follow-up, the mean ACD was 3.080 ± 0.313 mm (range 2.676–3.581 mm), which was statistically significant compared with the preoperative one ($P < 0.001$).

There were no severe perioperative complications occurred. During the surgery, slight iris hemorrhage occurred in one eye (Case 9) during the separation of iris posterior synechia, but it stopped soon after temporarily rising of irrigation pressure. Peripheral retinal hole was found in one eye, which subsequently received retinal laser photocoagulation. At the end of the surgery, four eyes (23.5 %) required suturing to stop visible leakage at the sclerotomy sites. No postoperative complications such as hypotony, conjunctival leakage, corneal decompensation, endophthalmitis, suprachoroidal hemorrhage, vitreous hemorrhage, choroidial detachment, or retinal detachment were observed. Failure of pre-existing filtering bleb was not found in any eyes.

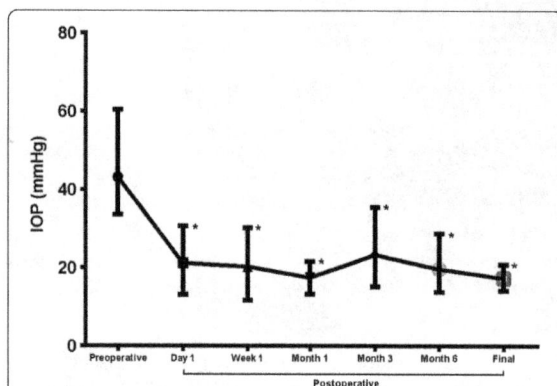

Fig. 2 IOP changes before and after 23-gauge PPV and PPL (* = presence of statistical significance to the preoperative IOP)

Discussion

Although this study enrolled patients with different types of glaucoma, the common features of all were medically uncontrolled IOP (43.14 ± 6.53 mmHg) and extremely shallow anterior chamber (0.507 ± 0.212 mm). In our case series, lens extraction was considered to be the definite treatment to deepen the anterior chamber and relieve pupillary block. However, the crowded anterior chamber disturbs the surgical manipulation of phacoemulsification in such eyes. The peripheral iridocorneal apposition makes it difficult to properly construct a clear corneal incision. The narrow anterior chamber puts the cornea under higher risk of damage by ultrasound waves and/or mechanical contact of the surgical instruments. Additionally, corneal edema and pupillary abnormities are commonly found in this kind of patients, both of which may increase the difficulty of capsulorhexis [6, 7]. Consequently, clear corneal phacoemulsification was considered to be fraught with higher risk of intra- and postoperative complications in our case series.

In such instance, PPV combined with PPL may be a relatively safer manipulation. Using vitrectomy cutter, cataract can be managed with enough working space from vitreous cavity. The lens was extracted by mechanical cutting, which exert less damage to the corneal endothelial cells as compared to ultrasound energy in phacoemulsification. Moreover, there was less need of repeated exchange of instruments, which would reduce IOP fluctuation during the procedure. In the current study, 23-gauge vitrectomy instrumentations were adopted to remove cataract and anterior vitreous through the transconjunctival incision. The main advantage of 23-gauge system is that incision of the conjunctiva is not required, which reduces operating times, minimizes conjunctiva trauma, and decreases postoperative inflammation [12–15]. Considering the rigidity and effectiveness of its instrumentations, 25-gauge system was not used in the present study.

According to our data, the combined surgery was effective in relieving the pupil block and reforming the anterior chamber. Intraoperatively, we observed significant deepening of the anterior chamber and elimination of aqueous blockade in all eyes. At the final revisit, the anterior chamber was maintained well with a mean depth of 3.080 mm. In our case series, the majority of patients (58.8 %) were diagnosed as malignant glaucoma. Previous studies have reported that PPV is an effective treatment to break the cycle of aqueous misdirection. However, several reports showed that the recurrence of malignant glaucoma is more likely in phakic eyes undergone PPV alone (26 ~ 75 %) compared with pseudophakic eyes and those received PPV and PPL (0 ~ 17 %) [8–10]. For these reasons, it is concluded that vitrectomy combined with lens extraction provide therapeutic advantage in phakic eyes with malignant glaucoma. In our surgical procedure with 23-gauge vitrectomy system,

PPV and PPL were performed via the same transconjunctival sclerotomies without the creation of corneal incision. During the mean follow-up of 21.2 months, none of the patients suffered a recurrence of aqueous misdirection.

Although the anterior chamber was effectively deepened in all eyes, the aqueous outflow route was not successfully reconstructed in some cases due to the extensive peripheral anterior synechia or irreversible trabecular injury. Despite an initial normalizing of the IOP with/without anti-glaucoma medications in all patients, we observed a slow increase of IOP in two eyes with initial diagnosis of uveitis. During the follow-up period, implantations of Ahmed valve drainage device (New World Medical, Rancho Cucamonga, CA, USA) were eventually performed in these eyes (Case 9 and Case 11). Un Chul Park et al. reported that the success rate of Ahmed valve implantation in the vitrectomized group was similar to that of the nonvitrectomized group [17]. Nevertheless, conventional 20-gauge vitrectomy has been reported to cause conjunctiva scarring and recession in multiple quadrant, which may induce impairment of the pre-existing filtering bleb or exert challenge to the further glaucoma surgery [18]. In the current study, we found that the conjunctival adhesion caused by 23-gauge trocar was minimal, which didn't disturb the implantation of the drainage device. Moreover, there was no suturing-associated failure of pre-existing filering bleb observed in our cases series. At the end of the follow-up, the mean IOP was 17.29 ± 1.80 mmHg with no need of glaucoma medications in 52.9 % of eyes.

The major complication of MISV is postoperative hypotony (IOP < 5 mmHg) resulted from leaking sclerotomies. As previously reported, the incidence of postoperative hypotony was 2.6 % after 23-gauge vitrectomy and 3.8 to 20 % after 25-gauge MIVS. [19–22] Postoperative hypotony can precipitate the occurrence of delayed subchoroidal hemorrhage, the incidence of which is 10-fold greater than that in the intraoperative period [23, 24]. In the present study, postoperative hypotony was not found in any of the case. The mean IOP was 21.12 ± 4.76 mmHg at 1 day and 20.28 ± 4.85 mmHg at 7 days after the surgery. The meticulous checks for the leaking sclerotomy and appropriate suturing were considered as the main causes of the low incidence of postoperative hypotony in our case series. The rate of sclerotomy suturing in this study was 23 %, which was higher than that reported by the available literatures (1.3–11.2 %) for 23-gauge vitrectomy [20, 25, 26]. The possible explanation was that vitreous base dissection was performed more thoroughly in most cases, which resulted in poorer closure due to the reduced "plugging effect" of remnant vitreous under the sites of sclerotomy. The sclerotomies were sutured by single-needle stitch to minimize the scar formation of corresponding conjunctiva. In our case series, the stable postoperative IOP may explain the

low rate of complications including suprachoroidal hemorrhage, vitreous hemorrhage, choroidial detachment, and retinal detachment.

As described by Liu et al., phacoemulsification-posterior capsulorhexis–anterior vitrectomy– intraocular lens (IOL) implantation was performed in patients with phakic malignant glaucoma, which helped to improve the postoperative visual acuity [27]. Howerver, according to our data, the preoperative visual acuity was quite poor (2.32 ± 0.47) and 88.2 % eyes had BCVA of 20/400 or worse. The main causes of reduced vision in our patients were corneal edema, cataract, and glaucomatous optic nerve damage. Even after removal of lens, no significant increase in the mean BCVA was observed at the end of the follow-up. Owing to the little benefit of visual function achieved from the surgery, the goal of our surgery is to reform the anterior chamber, decrease the IOP and preserve existing vision. Therefore, the IOL was not determined to be implanted in our cases, which might reduce the surgery manipulation and the risks of complications.

Despite the advantages mentioned above, our study also has some limitations. One drawback was that ultrasonic fragmatome is not available in the 23-gauge vitrectomy system. It is almost impossible to manipulate the lens nucleus more than grade 4 using 23-gauge vitrectomy cutter. For this reason, eyes with lens nucleus of grade 4 or harder was considered as contraindication for this microincision technique, and thus not included in this study. This limitation may be resolved by the advancement in surgical instrumentation. More recently, Spierer et al. describe the application of a 20-gauge transconjunctival vitrectomy trocar system, which may offer combined 20-gauge fragmatome and 23-gauge vitrectomy for the management of denser lens nucleus in such eyes [28].

Conclusion

In conclusion, our findings showed that the 23-gauge transconjunctival PPV combined with PPL was relatively safe and effective in the management of patients with glaucoma, extremely shallow anterior chamber and cataract. Definite anterior chamber formation and IOP reduction could be achieved by the combined surgical approach, with preservation of residual vision and decrease of anti-glaucoma medications. The procedure could be considered as a therapeutic option for eyes with poor visual function and no plan of IOL implantation.

Abbreviations
BCVA: best corrected visual acuity; IOP: intraocular pressure; ACD: anterior chamber depth; PPV: pars plana vitrectomy; MIVS: microincision vitrectomy surgery; logMAR: logarithm of the minimum angle of resolution; LP: light perception; HM: hand movements; CF: counting fingers; IOL: intraocular lens; PPL: pars plana lensectomy.

Competing interests

The authors have no financial or proprietary interest in a product, method, or material described herein.

Authors' contributions

Z.Z. and Y.W. were involved with the design of the research. S.Z. performed all the surgeries. X.J. and S.Q. assembled and analyzed the data. All of the authors reviewed the data and participated in the writing of the manuscript. All authors read and approved the final manuscript.

Acknowledgements

Part of this study was supported by a grant from the Innovation Foundation of State Key Laboratory of Ophthalmology (2011C04), a grant from National Natural Science Foundation of China (81170866), and a grant from Provincial Natural Science Foundation of Guangdong (S2011010004979).

References

1. Ruben S, Tsai J, Hitchings R. Malignant glaucoma and its management. Br J Ophthalmol. 1997;81:163–7.
2. Kanamori A, Nakamura M, Matsui N, Tomimori H, Tanase M, Seya R, et al. Goniosynechialysis with lens aspiration and posterior chamber intraocular lens implantation for glaucoma in spherophakia. J Cataract Refract Surg. 2004;30:513–6.
3. Lee JW, Lai JS, Yick DW, Tse RK, et al. Retrospective case series on the long-term visual and intraocular pressure outcomes of phacomorphic glaucoma. Eye. 2010; 24:1675–80.
4. Yalvac IS, Satana B, Ozkan G, Eksioglu U, Duman S. Management of glaucoma in patients with nanophthalmos. Eye. 2008;22:838–43.
5. Quigley HA, Friedman DS, Congdon NG. Possible mechanisms of primary angle-closure and malignant glaucoma. J Glaucoma. 2003;12:167–80.
6. Sharma A, Sii F, Shah P. Vitrectomy-phacoemulsification- vitrectomy for the management of aqueous misdirection syndromes in phakic eyes. Ophthalmology. 2006;113:1968–73.
7. Behndig A. Phacoemulsification in spherophakia with corneal touch. J Cataract Refract Surg. 2002;28:189–91.
8. Chaudhry NA, Flynn Jr HW, Murray TG, Nicholson D, Palmberg PF. Pars plana vitrectomy during cataract surgery for prevention of aqueous misdirection in high-risk fellow eyes. Am J Ophthalmol. 2000;129:387–8.
9. Byrnes GA, Leen MM, Wong TP, Benson WE. Vitrectomy for ciliary block (malignant) glaucoma. Ophthalmology. 1995;102:1308–11.
10. Harbour JW, Rubsamen PE, Palmberg P. Pars plana vitrectomy in the management of phakic and pseudophakic malignant glaucoma. Arch Ophthalmol. 1996;114:1073–8.
11. Lois N, Wong D, Groenewald C. New surgical approach in the management of pseudophakic malignant glaucoma. Ophthalmology. 2001;108:780–3.
12. Fujii GY, De Juan EJ, Humayun MS, Pieramici DJ, Chang TS, Awh C, et al. A new 25-gauge instrument system for transconjunctival sutureless vitrectomy surgery. Ophthalmology. 2002;109:1807–13.
13. Fujii GY, De Juan EJ, Humayun MS, Chang TS, Pieramici DJ, Barnes A, et al. Initial experience using the transconjunctival sutureless vitrectomy system for vitreoretinal surgery. Ophthalmology. 2002;109:1814–20.
14. Eckardt C. Transconjunctival sutureless 23-gauge vitrectomy. Retina. 2005;25:208–11.
15. Wimpissinger B, Kellner L, Brannath W, Krepler K, Stolba U, Mihalics C, et al. 23-Gauge versus 20-gauge system for pars plana vitrectomy: a prospective randomised clinical trial. Br J Ophthalmol. 2008;92:1483–7.
16. Chylack LJ, Wolfe JK, Singer DM, Leske MC, Bullimore MA, Bailey IL, et al. The Lens Opacities Classification System III. The Longitudinal Study of Cataract Study Group. Arch Ophthalmol. 1993;111:831–6.
17. Park UC, Park KH, Kim DM, Yu HG. Ahmed glaucoma valve implantation for neovascular glaucoma after Vitrectomy for proliferative diabetic retinopathy. J Glaucoma. 2011;20:433–8.
18. Van Aken E, Lemij H, Vander Haeghen Y, de Waard P. Baerveldt glaucoma implants in the management of refractory glaucoma after vitreous surgery. Acta Ophthalmol. 2010;88:75–9.
19. Fine HF, Iranmanesh R, Iturralde D, Spaide RF. Outcomes of 77 consecutive cases of 23-gauge transconjunctival vitrectomy surgery for posterior segment disease. Ophthalmology. 2007;114:1197–2002.
20. Lakhanpal RR, Humayun MS, de Juan Jr E, Lim JI, Chong LP, Chang TS, et al. Outcomes of 140 consecutive cases of 25-gauge transconjunctival surgery for posterior segment disease. Ophthalmology. 2005;112:817–24.
21. Yanyali A, Celik E, Horozoglu F, Oner S, Nohutcu AF. 25-Gauge transconjunctival sutureless pars plana vitrectomy. Eur J Ophthalmol. 2006;16:141–7.
22. Byeon SH, Chu YK, Lee SC, Koh HJ, Kim SS, Kwon OW. Problems associated with the 25-gauge transconjunctival sutureless vitrectomy system during and after surgery. Ophthalmologica. 2006;220:259–65.
23. Chu TG, Green RL. Suprachoroidal hemorrhage. Surv Ophthalmol. 1999;43:471–86.
24. Healey PR, Herndon L, Smiddy W. Management of suprachoroidal hemorrhage. J Glaucoma. 2007;16:577–9.
25. Nagpal M, Wartikar S, Nagpal K. Comparison of clinical outcomes and wound dynamics of sclerotomy ports of 20, 25, and 23 gauge vitrectomy. Retina. 2009;29:225–31.
26. Woo SJ, Park KH, Hwang JM, Kim JH, Yu YS, Chung H. Risk factors associated with sclerotomy leakage and postoperative hypotony after 23-gauge transconjunctival sutureless vitrectomy. Retina. 2009;29:456–63.
27. Liu X, Li M, Cheng B, Mao Z, Zhong Y, Wang D. Phacoemulsification combined with posterior capsulorhexis and anterior vitrectomy in the management of malignant glaucoma in phakic eyes. Acta Ophthalmol. 2013;91:660–5.
28. Spierer O, Siminovsky Z, Loewenstein A, Barak A. Outcomes of 20-gauge transconjunctival sutureless vitrectomy. Retina. 2011;31:1765–71.

7

The serum angiotensin converting enzyme and lysozyme levels in patients with ocular involvement of autoimmune and infectious diseases

Ozlem Sahin[1*], Alireza Ziaei[2], Eda Karaismailoğlu[3] and Nusret Taheri[4]

Abstract

Background: Increased serum levels of angiotensin converting enzyme and lysozyme are considered as inflammatory markers for diagnosis of sarcoidosis which is an autoimmune inflammatory disease. The purpose of this study is to evaluate the significance of differences in serum angiotensin converting enzyme and lysozyme levels of patients with ocular involvement of other autoimmune inflammatory and infectious diseases.

Methods: This is a prospective study involving patients with ankylosing spondylitis, behcet's disease, presumed sarcoidosis, presumed latent tuberculosis, presumed latent syphilis, and control group. The serum levels of angiotensin converting enzyme and lysozyme were analyzed by enzyme-linked immunosorbent assay. Bonnferoni analysis was used to assess pairwise comparisons between the groups.

Results: There was a significant increase in serum angiotensin converting enzyme level in patients with presumed sarcoidosis compared to ankylosing spondylitis ($p = 0.0001$), behcet's disease ($p = 0.0001$), presumed latent tuberculosis ($p = 0.0001$), presumed latent syphilis ($p = 0.0001$), and control group ($p = 0.0001$). The increase in serum lysozyme level was significant for patients with presumed sarcoidosis with respect to ankylosing spondylitis ($p = 0.0001$), behcet's disease, ($p = 0.0001$) presumed latent tuberculosis ($p = 0.001$), presumed latent syphilis ($p = 0.033$), and control group ($p = 0.0001$).

Conclusion: Elevated serum angiotensin converting enzyme levels are significant for patients with presumed sarcoidosis compared to ocular involvement of other autoimmune diseases such as behcet's disease and ankylosing spondylitis, and ocular involvement of infectious diseases such as presumed latent tuberculosis and presumed latent syphilis. However, elevated serum lysozyme level might be also detected in ocular involvement of infectious diseases such as presumed latent tuberculosis and presumed latent syphilis.

Trial registration: Trial Registration number: NCT02627209. Date of registration: 12/09/2015.

Keywords: Angiotensin converting enzyme, Lysozyme, Ankylosing spondylitis, Behcet's disease, Sarcoidosis, Syphilis, Tuberculosis, Ocular inflammation

* Correspondence: ozlem1158@yahoo.com
[1]Department of Ophthalmology/Uveitis, Dunya Goz Hospital Ltd., Ankara, Turkey
Full list of author information is available at the end of the article

Background

The renin angiotensin system (RAS) is an important hormonal system which promotes inflammation through the axis of angiotensin converting enzyme (ACE)-angiotensin peptides-distinct receptor subtypes [1]. Hyperactivation of the RAS system has been disclosed to involve in inflammatory responses of the eye [2, 3]. Increased serum ACE activity has been reported especially in uveitis associated with sarcoidosis, and also infectious uveitis such as recurrent toxoplasmic and toxocaral iridocyclitis and choroioretinitis [4, 5]. Lysozyme is an enzyme that hydrolyses glycosidic bonds, and it is revealed to degrade the peptidoglycans in the bacterial cell wall [6]. Muramidase activity of lysozyme has been shown to limit the inflammation caused by rapidly degrading peptidoglycans at the site of infection [7]. Elevated levels of serum lysozyme have been reported in granulomatous uveitis especially sarcoidosis and tuberculosis [8]. The purpose of this study is to evaluate the significance of differences in serum ACE and lysozyme levels of patients with ocular involvement of autoimmune diseases such as HLAB27$^+$ ankylosing spondylitis (AS), HLAB51$^+$ behcet's disease (BD) and presumed sarcoidosis and ocular involvement of infectious diseases such as QuantiFERON(®)-TB Gold$^+$ presumed latent tuberculosis (TB) and presumed latent syphilis compared to control group by using pairwise comparisons between the groups.

Methods

Study patients

This is a prospective study involving 76 patients with AS, 72 patients with BD, 31 patients with presumed sarcoidosis, and 68 patients with presumed latent TB, 11 patients with presumed latent syphilis, and 22 control subjects having refractive errors only. Institutional review board/ethics committee approval was obtained from the Dunya Goz Hospital Institutional Board (DGH-070) Ankara, Turkey. This study adhered to the tenets of the Declaration of Helsinki. The written informed consent was obtained for all individuals who enrolled in this study. The patients had ocular manifestations including acute or chronic granulomatous or non-granulomatous iritis or iridocyclitis, intermediate, posterior or panuveitis, retinitis, retinal vasculitis, choroiditis and papillitis. The uveitis was not always granulomatous inside the the group of presumed ocular sarcoidosis. The international criteria for the diagnosis of presumed ocular sarcoidosis and international study criteria for BD were used [9, 10]. Inclusion criteria for all patients involve the presence of ocular signs associated with a positive test for HLAB27 for patients with AS, a positive test for HLAB51 for the patients with BD, a negative tuberculin skin test in BCG-vaccinated patients, positive findings on chest x-ray or chest CT or abnormal results on whole body Gallium 67 scintigraphy

for the patients with presumed sarcoidosis, a positive test for QuantiFERON(®)-TB Gold In-Tube (Cellestis limited, Melbourne, Australia) and a positive tuberculin skin test for the patients with presumed latent TB. Presumed latent syphilis was diagnosed on the basis of negative serum venereal disease research laboratory test (VDRL) and rapid plasma reagin test, (RPR) positive serum fluorescent treponemal antibody absorption (FTAABS) and microhemagglutination assay for Treponema pallidum, (MHA-TP), negative cerebrospinal fluid (CSF) FTAABS, and improvement in level of ocular inflammation after treatment with specific therapy for syphilis [11]. The difference in the levels of ACE in granulomatous and a non-granulomatous groups were not compared. The connection of increased serum lysozyme levels between systemic diseases such as sarcoidosis was not studied. The exclusion criteria for the patient and control groups were using ACE inhibitors, systemic steroids, immunosuppressive or immunomodulatory therapies.

Blood sampling

Blood samples were collected from the patients by using a standard aseptic technique. Native blood was incubated for 60 min at room temperature; serum fractions (separated by centrifugation at $1500\,g$ for 15 min) were stored at −20 °C.

Serum ACE activity measurement using spectrophotometric assay

Serum ACE activity was measured as described by Beneteau et al [12]. ACE activity was determined with an artificial substrate (FAPGG, (N-[3-(2-furyl) acryloyl]-L-phenylalanyl-glycylglycine; Sigma-Aldrich) in a reaction mixture containing 25 mM HEPES (N-2-hydroxyethylpiperazine-N-2-ethanesulfonic acid), 0.5 mM FAPGG, 300 mM NaCl, and the desired dilution of serum at pH 8.2. Measurements were performed in 96-well plates (Greiner-Bio One) at 37 °C. Changes in optical density (340 nm) were measured at 5-min intervals for at least 90 min with a plate reader (NovoStar plate reader; BMG Labtech). Optical density values were plotted as a function of reaction time and fitted by linear regression (GraphPad Prism 5.0). The fit and the data were accepted when r^2 was >0.90. ACE activity was calculated with the equation:

$$activity = (S/k)D$$

where S is the rate of observed decrease in optical density (1/min), k is the change in optical density upon the complete cleavage of 1 μmol of FAPGG, and D is the dilution of the serum. ACE activity is given in units where 1 U is equivalent to the cleavage of 1 μmol of FAPGG in 1 min. The reference range for serum ACE level was between 8 and 52 U/L for adults, and between 13 and 100 U/L for children less than 18 years of age.

Serum lysozyme activity measurement using radial immunodiffusion

Serum lysozyme activity was measured by using radial immunodiffusion as described by Mancini G. et al. [13]. Human 'NL' Nanorid plate, No GT073.3, (Binding Site Ltd., Birmingham, UK) and lysozyme - NL 2.1–21* GT073.3 NANORID™ kits (Binding Site Ltd., Birmingham, UK) were used. The precipitation ring diameters were measured using Digital Rid Plate Reader. (Binding Site Ltd., Birmingham, UK) The reference range for serum lysozyme was between 9.6 and 16.8 mg/L for all age groups.

Statistical analysis

Statistical analysis was performed by using SPSS for Windows 13.0.1 (SPSS Inc., Chicago, IL, USA) statistical software products. All results were expressed as mean ± SD. All statistical analyses were performed two-tailed and $p < 0.05$ was considered as significant. One-way ANOVA and Tukey's tests were used for age distribution, and Chi Square test is used for sex distribution. Multivariate analysis of covariance was used to determine the significance of differences in serum levels of ACE and lysozyme with age as the covariate. Bonnferoni analysis was used to assess pairwise comparisons between the groups.

Results

Demographics of the patient and control groups

The age range, mean, standard deviation (SD), and the lower and upper bounds of 95 % confidence interval (CI) values for mean values of age for patients with AS, BD, presumed sarcoidosis, presumed latent TB, presumed latent syphilis, and control group were shown in Table 1. The age range of total 280 subjects was between 9 and 86 with a mean (SD) of 42.892 (16.013). The mean

(SD) ages of patients with AS, BD, presumed sarcoidosis, presumed latent TB, presumed latent syphilis and control group were 41.868 (12.536), 38.277 (14.681), 41.000 (18.954), 52.735 (15.525), 44.272 (14.553), and 33.090 (15.377) years respectively (Table 1). The sex distribution and percentages within the groups were shown in Table 2. The total of 280 subjects 139 (49.6 %) were female and 141 (50.4 %) were male. The sex distribution and percentages of the patients with AS, BD, presumed sarcoidosis, presumed latent TB, presumed latent syphilis, and control group were 35 (46.10 %) female and 41 (53.9) male, 43 (59.7 %) female and 29 (40.3 %) male, 13 (41.9 %) female and 18 (58.1 %) male, 36 (52.9 %) female and 32 (47.1 %) male, 4 (36.4 %) female and 7 (63.6 %) male, and 8 (36.4 %) female and 14 (63.6 %) male respectively (Table 2).

Serum ACE and lysozyme activities of the patient and control groups

The mean (SD) values of serum ACE and lysozyme levels of the patients with AS, BD, presumed sarcoidosis, presumed latent TB, presumed latent syphilis and control group were shown in Table 3. The mean (SD) values of serum ACE for patients with AS, BD, presumed sarcoidosis, presumed latent TB, presumed latent syphilis and control group were 29.363 (2.012), 31.227 (15.225), 58.164 (35.110), 33.061 (15.065), 30.527 (16.016) and 20.704 (7.962) U/L respectively (Table 3). The estimated marginal means of serum ACE levels in groups were disclosed in Fig. 1. According to this graph, the lowest value for the estimated marginal mean of serum ACE level is 21.251 U/L for control group, and the highest value is 58.274 U/L for the patients with presumed sarcoidosis. The estimated marginal mean values of serum ACE level for the patients with AS, BD, presumed latent TB and presumed latent syphilis were 29.360, 31.392, 32.500 and 30.452 U/L respectively which were lower than the estimated marginal mean value of ACE for presumed sarcoidosis, but higher than the estimated

Table 1 The sample size, age range, mean value, standard deviation, the lower and upper bounds of 95 % confidence interval for mean age of the patients with ocular involvement of ankylosing spondylitis, behcet's disease, presumed sarcoidosis, presumed latent tuberculosis, presumed latent syphilis and control group

Groups	n	Min age	Max age	Mean age	SD	95 % CI for Mean Lower Bound	95 % CI for Mean Upper Bound
AS	76	15	74	41.868	12.536	37.003	44.733
BD	72	9	75	38.277	14.681	34.827	41.727
P. Sarcoidosis	31	10	72	41.000	18.954	34.047	47.952
TB	68	21	86	52.735	15.525	48.977	56.493
P. Syphilis	11	22	67	44.272	14.553	34.495	54.050
Control	22	12	68	33.090	15.377	26.272	39.908
Total	280	9	86	42.892	16.013	41.009	44.776

n Sample size, *Min* minimum, *Max* maximum, *SD* standard deviation, *CI* confidence interval, *AS* ankylosing spondylitis, *BD* behcet's disease, *TB* presumed latent tuberculosis, *P. Sarcoidosis* presumed sarcoidosis, *P. Syphilis* presumed latent syphilis

Table 2 The sex distribution and sample size of patients with ocular involvement of ankylosing spondylitis, behcet's disease, presumed sarcoidosis and presumed latent tuberculosis, presumed latent syphilis and control group

Groups	Female	Male	n
AS	35 (46.1 %)	41 (53.9 %)	76
BD	43 (59.7 %)	29 (40.3 %)	72
P. Sarcoidosis	13 (41.9 %)	18 (58.1 %)	31
TB	36 (52.9 %)	32 (47.1 %)	68
P. Syphilis	4 (36.4 %)	7 (63.6 %)	11
Control	8 (36.4 %)	14 (63.6 %)	22
Total	139 (49.6)	141 (50.4)	280

n sample size, *AS* ankylosing spondylitis, *BD* behcet's disease, *TB* presumed latent tuberculosis, *P. Sarcoidosis* presumed sarcoidosis, *P. Syphilis* presumed latent syphilis

marginal mean value of ACE for control group (Fig. 1). The mean (SD) values of serum lysozyme level for patients with AS, BD, presumed sarcoidosis, presumed latent TB, presumed latent syphilis and control group were 14.096 (4.586), 14.244 (5.358), 20.712 (6.780), 15.259 (8.516), 14.018 (6.679) and 12.927 (4.720) mg/L respectively (Table 3). The estimated marginal means of serum lysozyme levels in groups were disclosed in Fig. 2. According to this graph, the lowest value for the estimated marginal mean of serum lysozyme level was13.200 mg/L

Table 3 The sample size, mean value, standard deviation of serum angiotensin converting enzyme levels of the patients with ocular involvement of ankylosing spondylitis, behcet's disease, presumed sarcoidosis, presumed latent tuberculosis, presumed latent syphilis and control group

Groups	Mean value	SD	95 % CI Lower bound	95 % CI Upper bound
Serum ACE Level (U/L)				
AS	29.363	2.012	25.403	33.324
BD	31.486	2.091	27.369	35.603
P. Sarcoidosis	58.270	3.151	52.067	64.472
TB	32.504	2.254	28.066	36.942
P. Syphilis	30.449	5.285	20.044	40.854
Control	21.254	3.800	13.772	28.736
Serum Lysozyme Level (mg/L)				
AS	14.124	0.718	12.710	15.538
BD	14.371	0.747	12.901	15.841
P. Sarcoidosis	20.765	1.125	18.550	22.979
TB	14.987	0.805	13.402	16.571
P. Syphilis	13.980	1.887	10.265	17.695
Control	13.196	1.357	10.525	15.868

ACE angiotensin converting enzyme, *AS* ankylosing spondylitis, *BD* behcet's disease, *CI* confidence interval, *TB* presumed latent tuberculosis, *P. Sarcoidosis* presumed sarcoidosis, *P. Syphilis* presumed latent syphilis, *SD* standard deviation

for control group, and the highest value was 20.776 mg/L for patients with presumed sarcoidosis. The estimated means of serum lysozyme levels of patients with AS, BD, presumed latent TB and presumed latent syphilis were 14.122, 14.374, 14.998 and 13.989 mg/L respectively which were lower than the estimated marginal mean value of lysozyme for presumed sarcoidosis, and higher than the estimated marginal mean value of serum lysozyme for control group (Fig. 2).

Pairwise comparisons of the mean differences of serum ACE levels between groups

The mean (SD) differences of serum ACE levels between the patients with presumed sarcoidosis and AS, BD, presumed latent TB, presumed latent syphilis and control group were 28.907 (3.735), 26.784 (3.770), 25.776 (3.898), 27.821 (6.155), and 37.016 (4.918) U/L respectively. (Table 4) The increase in serum ACE level was significant for patients with presumed sarcoidosis compared to patients with AS ($p = 0.0001$), BD ($p = 0.0001$), presumed latent TB ($p = 0.0001$), presumed latent syphilis ($p = 0.0001$), and control group ($p = 0.0001$). The mean (SD) differences of serum ACE levels between control group and AS, BD, presumed latent TB, presumed latent syphilis were −8.110 (4.288), −10.232 (4.285), −11.250 (4.528), and −9.195 (6.520) respectively (Table 4). There were no significant differences of serum ACE levels between control group and AS ($p = 0.895$), control group and BD ($p = 0.264$), control group and TB, ($p = 0.204$) control group and presumed latent syphilis. ($p = 1.000$) (Table 4) Pairwise comparison of mean (SD) difference of serum ACE level between AS and BD was −2.123 (2.894), between AS and presumed latent TB was −3.141 (3.038), between AS and presumed latent syphilis was −1.086 (5.656), between BD and presumed latent TB was −1.018 (3.149), between BD and presumed latent syphilis was 1.037 (5.689), and between presumed latent TB and presumed latent syphilis was 2.055 (5.734) respectively (Table 4). No significant differences of serum ACE levels revealed between AS and BD ($p = 0.689$), between AS and presumed latent TB ($p = 1.000$), between AS and presumed latent syphilis ($p = 0.996$), between BD and presumed latent TB ($p = 1.000$), between BD and presumed latent syphilis ($p = 0.817$), and between presumed latent TB and presumed latent syphilis ($p = 0.504$), (Table 4).

Pairwise comparisons of the mean differences of serum lysozyme levels between groups

The mean (SD) differences of serum lysozyme levels between patients with presumed sarcoidosis and AS, BD, presumed latent TB, presumed latent syphilis and control group were 6.641 (1.334), 6.394 (1.346), 5.778 (1.392), 6.785 (2.198), and 7.568 (1.756) mg/L respectively (Table 5). The increase in serum lysozyme level was

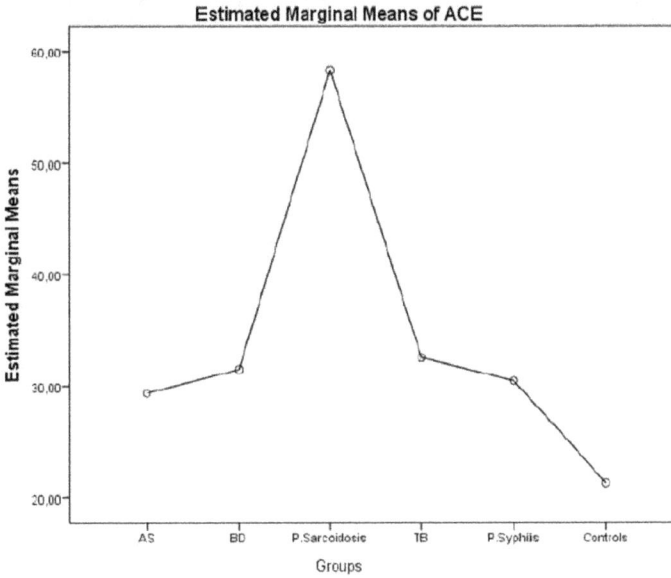

Fig. 1 The estimated marginal means of serum angiotensin converting enzyme levels of patients with ocular involvement of ankylosing spondylitis, behcet's disease, presumed sarcoidosis, presumed latent tuberculosis, presumed latent syphilis and control group

significant for patients with presumed sarcoidosis with respect to AS ($p = 0.0001$), BD ($p = 0.0001$), presumed latent TB ($p = 0.001$), presumed latent syphilis ($p = 0.033$), and control group ($p = 0.0001$) (Table 5) The mean (SD) differences of serum lysozyme levels between control group and AS, BD, presumed latent TB, presumed latent

syphilis were –0.928 (1.531), –1.175 (1.530), –1.790 (1.617), and –0.784 (2.328) respectively (Table 5). There were no significant differences of serum lysozyme levels between control group and AS ($p = 1.000$), control group and BD ($p = 1.000$) control group and presumed latent TB ($p = 1.000$), control group and presumed latent syphilis

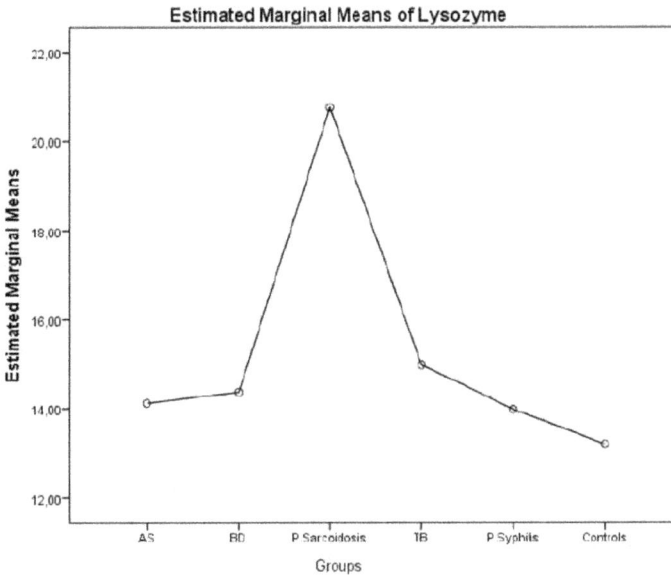

Fig. 2 The estimated marginal means of serum lysozyme levels of patients with ocular involvement of ankylosing spondylitis, behcet's disease, presumed sarcoidosis, presumed latent tuberculosis, presumed latent syphilis and control group

Table 4 Pairwise comparison of the mean difference values of serum angiotensin converting enzyme levels of the patients with ocular involvement of ankylosing spondylitis, behcet's disease, presumed sarcoidosis, presumed latent tuberculosis, presumed latent syphilis and control group

Pairwise Comparison	Mean Difference	Standard Deviation	Sig^b	95 % CI Lower Bound	95 % CI Upper Bound
AS - BD	−2.123	2.894	0.689	−10.691	6.446
AS - P. Sarcoidosis	−28.907	3.735	0.0001	−39.969	−17.845
AS - TB	−3.141	3.038	1.000	−12.137	5.856
AS - P. Syphilis	−1.086	5.656	0.996	−17.836	15.665
AS - Control	8.110	4.288	0.895	−4.590	20.809
BD - AS	2.123	2.894	0.689	−6.446	10.691
BD – P. Sarcoidosis	−26.784	3.770	0.0001	−37.948	−15.620
BD - TB	−1.018	3.149	1.000	−10.343	8.306
BD - P. Syphilis	1.037	5.689	0.817	−15.812	17.885
BD - Control	10.232	4.285	0.264	−2.458	22.922
P. Sarcoidosis - AS	28.907	3.735	0.0001	17.845	39.969
P. Sarcoidosis - BD	26.784	3.770	0.0001	15.620	37.948
P. Sarcoidosis - TB	25.766	3.898	0.0001	14.222	37.310
P. Sarcoidosis–P. Syphilis	27.821	6.155	0.0001	9.593	46.048
P. Sarcoidosis–Control	37.016	4.918	0.0001	22.453	51.580
TB - AS	3.141	3.038	1.000	−5.856	12.137
TB - BD	1.018	3.149	1.000	−8.306	10.343
TB - P. Sarcoidosis	−25.766	3.898	0.0001	−37.310	14.222
TB - P. Syphilis	2.055	5.734	0.504	−14.925	19.095
TB - Control	11.250	4.528	0.204	−2.159	24.660
P. Syphilis - AS	1.086	5.656	0.996	−6.124	5.837
P. Syphilis - BD	−1.037	5.689	0.817	−17.885	15.812
P. Syphilis–P. Sarcoidosis	−27.821	6.155	1.000	−19.035	14.925
P. Syphilis - Control	9.195	6.520	1.000	−10.113	28.504
Control - AS	−8.110	4.288	0.895	−20.809	4.590
Control - BD	−10.232	4.285	0.264	−22.922	2.458
Control –P. Sarcoidosis	−37.016	4.918	0.0001	−51.580	−22.453
Control - TB	−11.250	4.528	0.204	24.660	2.159
Control - P. Syphilis	−9.195	6.520	1.000	−28.504	10.113

The mean difference is significant at the 0.05 level

Sigb Adjustment for multiple comparisons Bonferroni, *DV* Dependent variable, *ACE* Angiotensin converting enzyme, *AS* ankylosing spondylitis, *BD* behcet's disease, *TB* presumed latent tuberculosis, *P. Sarcoidosis* presumed sarcoidosis, *P. Syphilis* presumed latent syphilis

($p = 1.000$) (Table 5). Pairwise comparison of mean (SD) difference of serum lysozyme level between AS and BD was −0.247 (1.033), between AS and presumed latent TB was −0.863 (1.085), between AS and presumed latent syphilis was 0.144 (2.020), between BD and presumed latent TB was −0.616 (1.124), between BD and presumed latent syphilis was 0.391 (2.031), and between presumed latent TB and presumed latent syphilis was 1.007 (2.047) (Table 5). There were no significant differences of serum lysozyme levels between AS and BD ($p = 1.000$), between AS and presumed latent TB ($p = 1.000$), between AS and presumed latent syphilis ($p = 1.000$), between BD and presumed latent TB ($p = 1.000$), between

BD and presumed latent syphilis ($p = 1.000$), and between presumed latent TB and presumed latent syphilis ($p = 1.000$) (Table 5).

Discussion

Previous studies have demonstrated the correlations of serum levels of inflammatory chemokines and cytokines with serum ACE and lysozyme activities in patients with ocular and pulmonary sarcoidosis [14, 15]. Chemokine (C-X-C motif) ligand 9 (CXCL9), also known as monokine induced by gamma interferon, (MIG) and C-X-C motif chemokine 10 (CXCL10) also known as interferon gamma-induced protein 10 (IP-10) have been reported

Table 5 Pairwise comparison of the mean difference values of serum lysozyme levels of the patients with ocular involvement of ankylosing spondylitis, behcet's disease, presumed sarcoidosis, presumed latent tuberculosis, presumed latent syphilis and control group

Pairwise Comparison	Mean Difference	Standard Deviation	Sig.b	95 % CI Lower Bound	95 % CI Upper Bound
AS - BD	−0.247	1.033	1.000	−3.306	2.812
AS - P. Sarcoidosis	−6.641	1.334	0.0001	−10.590	−2.691
AS - TB	−0.863	1.085	1.000	−4.075	2.349
AS - P. Syphilis	0.144	2.020	1.000	−5.837	6.124
AS - Control	0.928	1.531	1.000	−3.607	5.462
BD - AS	0.247	1.033	1.000	−2.812	3.306
BD − P. Sarcoidosis	−6.394	1.346	0.0001	−10.380	−2.408
BD - TB	−0.616	1.124	1.000	−3.945	2.713
BD - P. Syphilis	0.391	2.031	1.000	−5.625	6.407
BD - Control	1.175	1.530	1.000	−3.356	5.705
P. Sarcoidosis - AS	6.641	1.334	0.0001	2.691	10.590
P. Sarcoidosis - BD	6.394	1.346	0.0001	2.408	10.380
P. Sarcoidosis - TB	5.778	1.392	0.001	1.656	9.900
P. Sarcoidosis–P. Syphilis	6.785	2.198	0.033	0.277	13.293
P. Sarcoidosis − Control	7.568	1.756	0.0001	2.369	12.768
TB - AS	0.863	1.085	1.000	−2.349	4.075
TB - BD	0.616	1.124	1.000	−2.713	3.945
TB - P. Sarcoidosis	−5.778	1.392	0.001	−9.900	−1.656
TB - P. Syphilis	1.007	2.047	1.000	−5.056	7.069
TB - Control	1.790	1.617	1.000	−2.997	6.578
P. Syphilis - AS	−0.144	2.020	1.000	−6.124	5.837
P. Syphilis - BD	−0.391	2.031	1.000	−6.407	5.625
P. Syphilis − P. Sarcoidosis	−6.785	2.198	0.033	−13.293	−0.277
P. Syphilis - TB	−1.007	2.047	1.000	−7.069	5.056
P. Syphilis - Control	0.784	2.328	1.000	−6.110	7.678
Control - AS	−0.928	1.531	1.000	−5.462	3.607
Control - BD	−1.175	1.530	1.000	−5.705	3.356
Control − P. Sarcoidosis	−7.568	1.756	0.0001	−12.768	−2.369
Control - TB	−1.790	1.617	1.000	−6.578	2.997
Control - P. Syphilis	−0.784	2.328	1.000	−7.678	6.110

The mean difference is significant at the 0.05 level
Sigb Adjustment for multiple comparisons Bonferroni, *CI* Confidence Interval, *ACE* Angiotensin converting enzyme, *AS* ankylosing spondylitis, *BD* behcet's disease, *TB* presumed latent tuberculosis, *P. Sarcoidosis* presumed sarcoidosis, *P. Syphilis* presumed latent syphilis

to induce the recruitment of activated T helper (Th1) cells [16, 17]. Serum levels of CXCL9 and CXCL10 have been correlated with serum ACE levels in presumed ocular sarcoidosis [15]. Interleukin 12 (IL-12) p40, an essential component of IL-12 has been reported to induce differentiation of naïve Th cells into Th1 cells [15]. Serum concentrations of IL-12 p40 have been found significantly higher in pulmonary sarcoidosis than healthy subjects and have been correlated with serum levels of ACE and lysozyme [18]. This study compares for the first time the serum ACE and lysozyme levels of patients diagnosed with ocular involvement of autoimmune diseases such as AS, BD and presumed sarcoidosis and

ocular involvement of infectious diseases such as presumed latent TB and presumed latent syphilis. Intraocular inflammation compatible with sarcoidosis associated with elevated serum ACE levels is considered suggestive for diagnosis of presumptive sarcoidosis in patients without having a tissue biopsy [16, 17, 19–21]. The serum ACE level is disclosed higher in children than in adults [21]. The World Association of Sarcoidosis and Other Granulomatous disorders (WASOG) considered an increased ACE might help in diagnosis of sarcoidosis in children [22]. The age range in sarcoidosis group in our study is between 10 and 72 with a mean age of 41. The estimated mean level of serum ACE of our patients with presumed sarcoidosis is 58.274 IU/L which is above the normal adult range of 8–52 IU/L. Serum ACE level has been compared between patients having sarcoidosis and sarcoidosis-like lung diseases including TB, fibrosing alveolitis, histiocytosis X, and pneumoconiosis [23]. Rise of serum ACE activity has been found in 93 % of patients with active sarcoidosis, 41 % of patients with TB and 56 % of patients with nonspecific inflammatory lung diseases including fibrosing alveolitis, histiocytosis X, and pneumoconiosis [23]. Serum ACE level has not been studied before in the ocular involvement of presumed latent TB. Our study revealed the estimated marginal mean of serum ACE level in patients with presumed latent TB as 32.500 U/L. Pairwise comparison of serum ACE levels between patients with presumed latent TB and presumed sarcoidosis disclosed a statistically significant difference for patients with presumed sarcoidosis with respect to presumed latent TB ($p = 0.0001$). There was also no significant difference of elevated serum ACE levels between patients with presumed latent TB and control group ($p = 0.204$).

The serum activity of ACE has been compared for patients with BD, Vogt-Koyanagi-Harada's disease and sarcoidosis [24]. Significant elevation of serum ACE activity has been observed only for patients with sarcoidosis [24]. Our study revealed the estimated marginal mean of serum ACE level for patients with BD as 31.392 U/L. A significant elevation of serum ACE level in patients with presumed sarcoidosis with respect to BD has been disclosed in our study ($p = 0.0001$). Serum levels of ACE activity have been compared in patients with rheumatoid arthritis, osteoarthritis, ankylosing spondylitis, psoriatic arthritis and BD, and no statistically significant differences have been found from those of normal controls [25]. The serum ACE activity has not been investigated in HLAB27 positive AS related uveitis. Our study disclosed the estimated marginal mean of serum ACE level in patients with AS as 29.363 U/L. Our study revealed a statistically significant difference in serum ACE level for patients with presumed sarcoidosis compared to patients with AS ($p = 0.0001$). No significant difference of elevated serum ACE levels was found between AS and control group. ($p = 1.000$) Elevated serum lysozyme levels have been included in the criteria for diagnosis of ocular sarcoidosis [26]. The serum levels of ACE and lysozyme have been reported increased in 40 and 42 % of patients with biopsy-proven ocular sarcoidosis respectively [27]. The levels of at least one of the serum markers ACE and lysozyme were found elevated in 58 % of patients with biopsy-proven sarcoidosis [27]. The estimated marginal means of serum ACE and lysozyme levels for the patients with AS, BD, presumed sarcoidosis, presumed latent TB, presumed latent syphilis and control group disclosed on Graph 1 and Graph 2 in our study have similar curves with minimum

values for control group and maximum values for presumed sarcoidosis. The sensitivity of serum lysozyme for predicting sarcoidosis was reported as 79.1 % and the sensitivity of serum ACE for predicting sarcoidosis was reported as 59 % [28]. However, the specificity of serum lysozyme level has been reported to be less for sarcoidosis than serum ACE level, and it has been considered that the diagnostic value of serum lysozyme for sarcoidosis might be limited [28]. In another study considering the predictive value of serum ACE and lysozyme levels in diagnosis of ocular sarcoidosis, the sensitivity of increased serum ACE level was found as 84 %, specificity was 95 %, and predictivity was 47 %. However, the sensitivity of increased serum lysozyme levels was 60 %, specificity was 76 %, and spredictivity was 12 % [29]. Both studies showed that increased serum lysozyme levels might be less predictive for ocular sarcoidosis. Our study revealed the estimated marginal means of serum lysozyme for patients with AS, BD, presumed sarcoidosis, presumed latent TB, presumed latent syphilis and control group as 14.124, 14.371, 20.765,14.987, 13.980, and 13.196 mg/L respectively. Pairwise comparisons of the serum lysozyme levels between patients with presumed sarcoidosis and AS and BD revealed statistically significant differences for presumed sarcoidosis ($p = 0.0001$ and $p = 0.0001$ respectively). Pairwise comparison of the serum lysozyme levels between patients with presumed sarcoidosis and presumed latent TB revealed a statistically significant difference for sarcoidosis with the p value 0.001 which was greater than the p value of pairwise comparison of the serum ACE levels between patients with presumed sarcoidosis and presumed latent TB. Pairwise comparison of the serum lysozyme levels between the patients with presumed sarcoidosis and presumed latent syphilis revealed a statistically significant difference for presumed sarcoidosis with the p value 0.033 which was also greater than the p value of pairwise comparison of the serum ACE levels between patients with presumed sarcoidosis and presumed latent syphilis. Our study disclosed that increase in serum lysozyme levels is more significant than increase in serum ACE levels for patients with infectious uveitis such as presumed latent TB and presumed latent syphilis. This study also revealed that the increase in serum lysozyme levels is less specific than increase in serum ACE levels for presumed sarcoidosis, and elevated serum lysozyme levels might be much more commonly detected in infectious uveitis such as presumed latent TB and presumed latent syphilis than autoimmune uveitis such as AS and BD.

Conclusions

Elevated serum ACE levels are significant for patients with presumed sarcoidosis compared to ocular involvement of other autoimmune diseases such as BD and AS, and ocular involvement of infectious diseases such as presumed latent TB and presumed latent syphilis. However, elevated serum lysozyme levels might be also detected in ocular involvement of infectious diseases such as presumed latent TB and presumed latent syphilis.

Abbreviations
ACE: angiotensin converting enzyme; AS: ankylosing spondylitis; BD: behcet's disease; CI: confidence interval; CSF: cerebrospinal fluid; CXCL: chemokine; D: dilution of the serum. ACE activity is given in units where 1 U is equivalent to the cleavage of 1 μmol of FAPGG in 1 min; FAPGG: N-[3-(2-furyl) acryloyl]-L-phenylalanyl-glycylglycine; FTAABS: fluorescent treponemal antibody absorption; IP: interferon gamma-induced protein; k: change in optical density upon the complete cleavage of 1 μmol of FAPGG; MHA-TP: microhemagglutination assay for Treponema pallidum; RAS: renin angiotensin system; RPR: rapid plasma reagin; S: rate of observed decrease in optical density; SD: standard deviation; Th: T helper; VDRL: venereal disease research laboratory test; WASOG: World Association of Sarcoidosis and Other Granulomatous disorders.

Competing interests
The authors declare that they have no competing interests.

Authors' contributions
OS carried out the clinical examinations, diagnosis, treatment and follow-up the patients. AZ participated in design and coordination of the study. EK carried out the statistical analysis of the study. NT carried out the biochemical analysis of the sera of the patients and control groups. All authors have read and approved the final version of the manuscript.

Acknowledgements
Reha Alpar, M.D. Professor of Biostatistics, Hacettepe University Medical Faculty, for his contributions to the statistical evaluations of this study. There is no fund supporting this study.

Author details
[1]Department of Ophthalmology/Uveitis, Dunya Goz Hospital Ltd., Ankara, Turkey. [2]Department of Ophthalmology, Boston University School of Medicine, Boston, MA, USA. [3]Department of Biostatistics, Hacettepe University Medical Faculty, Ankara, Turkey. [4]Department of Biochemistry, Middle East Technical University, Health Sciences, Ankara, Turkey.

References
1. Chappell MC, Marshall AC, Alzayadneh EM, Shaltout HA, Diz DI. Update on the Angiotensin Converting Enzyme 2-Angiotensin (1–7)-Mas Receptor Axis: Fetal programming, sex differences, and intracellular pathways. Front Endocrinol (Lausanne). 2014;4:201.
2. Miyazaki A, Kitaichi N, Ohgami K, Iwata D, Jin XH, Iwabuchi K, et al. Anti-inflammatory effect of angiotensin type 1 receptor antagonist on endotoxin-induced uveitis in rats. Graefes Arch Clin Exp Ophthalmol. 2008;246:747–57.
3. Kurihara T, Ozawa Y, Ishida S, Okano H, Tsubota K. Renin-Angiotensin system hyperactivation can induce inflammation and retinal neural dysfunction. Int J Inflam. 2012. doi:10.1155/2012/581695.
4. Bonfiolli AA, Orefice F. Sarcoidosis. Semin Ophthalmol. 2005;20:177–82.
5. Mulak M, Misiuk-Hojlo M, Slowik M. The behavior of angiotensin converting enzyme in patients with uveitis. Klin Oczna. 1999;101:5–8.
6. Nash JA, Ballard TN, Weaver TE, Akinbi HT. The peptidoglycan degrading property of lysozyme is not required for bacteriocidal activity in vivo. J Immunol. 2006;177:519–26.
7. Majcherczyk PA, Langen H, Heumann M, Fountoulakis M, Glauser P, Moreillion P. Digestion of Streptococcus pneumonia cell walls with its major peptidoglycan hydrolase releases branched stem peptides carrying proinflammatory activity. J Biol Chem. 1999;274:12537–43.
8. Sen DK, Sarin GS. Immunoassay of serum muramidase (lysozyme) in ocular diseases. Indian J Ophthalmol. 1987;35:103–7.
9. Herbort CP, Rao NA, Mochizuki M, members of Scientific Committee of First International Workshop on ocular sarcoidosis. International criteria for the diagnosis of ocular sarcoidosis: results of the first international Workshop on ocular sarcoidosis (IWOS). Ocul Immunol Inflamm. 2009;17:160–9.
10. [No authors listed] Evaluation of the diagnostic ('classification') criteria in Behcet's disease-towards internationally agreed criteria. The International Study Group for Behcet's disease. Br J Rheumatol 1992;31:299–308.
11. Morshed MG. Current trend on syphilis diagnosis: issues and challenges. Adv Exp Med Biol. 2014;808:51–64.
12. Beneteau B, Baudin B, Morgant G, Giboudeau J, Baumann FC. Automated kinetic assay of angiotensin-converting enzyme in serum. Clin Chem. 1986;32:884–6.
13. Mancini G, Carbonara AO, Heremans JF. Immunochemical quantitation of antigens by single radial immunodiffusion. Immunochemistry. 1965;2:235–54.
14. Takeuchi M, Oh-I K, Suzuki J, Hattori D, Takeuchi A, Okunuki Y, et al. Elevated serum levels of CXCL9/monokine induced by interferon- Gamma and CXCL10/interferon gamma-inducible protein-10 in ocular sarcoidosis. Invest Ophthalmol Vis Sci. 2006;47:1063–8.
15. Trinchieri G. Interleukin-12: a cytokine produced by antigen-presenting cells with immunoregulatory functions in the generation of T-helper cells type 1 and cytotoxic lymphocytes. Blood. 1994;84:4008–27.
16. Murdoch C, Finn A. Chemokine receptors and their role in inflammation and infectious diseases. Blood. 2000;95:3032–43.
17. Gerard C, Rollins BJ. Chemokines and disease. Nat Immunol. 2001;2:108–15.
18. Ichimura S et al. Increased circulating interleukin-12 (IL-12) p40 in pulmonary sarcoidosis. Clin Exp Immunol. 2003;132:152–7.
19. Stavrou P, Linton S, Young DW, Murray PI. Clinical diagnosis of ocular sarcoidosis. Eye (Lond). 1997;11:365–70.
20. Weinreb RN, O'Donnell JJ, Sandman R, Char DH, Kimura SJ. Angiotensin-converting enzyme in sarcoid uveitis. Invest Ophthalmol Vis Sci. 1979;18:1285–7.
21. Power WJ, Neves RA, Rodriquez A, Pedrosa-Seres M, Foster CS. The value of combined serum angiotensin-converting enzyme and gallium scan in diagnosing ocular sarcoidosis. Ophthalmology. 1995;102:2007–11.
22. Deverriere G, Flamans-Klein A, Firmin D, Azouzi O, Courville P, Le Roux P. Early onset pediatric sarcoidosis, diagnostic problems. Arch Pediatr. 2012;19:707–10.
23. Hunninghake GW, Costabel U, Ando M, Baughman R, Cordier JF, du Bois R, et al. ATS/ERS/WASOG statement on sarcoidosis. Sarcoidosis Vasc Diffuse Lung Dis. 1999;16:149–73.
24. Adamovich VN, Borisov SE, Zubkov AA, Danilov SM, Sakharov II, Atochina EN. Serum angiotensin converting enzyme in the diagnosis of sarcoidosis and other lung diseases. Probl Tuberk. 1991;10:18–22.
25. Fukami R, Ohba S, Ishida K, Nakamura S, Konno M, Ohno S. Serum adenosine deaminase and angiotensin converting enzyme activity in patients with endogenous uveitis. Nihon Ganka Gakkai Zasshi. 1994;98:287–92.
26. Lowe JR, Dixon JS, Guthrie JA, McWhinney P. Serum and synovial fluid levels of angiotensin converting enzyme in polyarthritis. Ann Rheum Dis. 1986;45:921–4.
27. Tomita H, Sato S, Matsuda R, Suquira R, Kawaquichi H, Niimi T, et al. Serum lysozyme levels and clinical features of sarcoidosis. Lung. 1999;177:161–7.
28. Birnbaum AD, Oh FS, Chakrabarti A, Tessler HH, Goldstein DA. Clinical features and diagnostic evaluation of biopsy-proven ocular sarcoidosis. Arch Ophthalmol. 2011;129:409–13.
29. Baarsma GS, La Hey E, Glasius E, de Vries J, Kijlstra A. The predictive value of serum angiotensin converting enzyme and lysozyme levels in the diagnosis of ocular sarcoidosis. Am J Ophthalmol. 1987;104:211–7.

8

A retrospective analysis of eleven cases of invasive rhino-orbito-cerebral mucormycosis presented with orbital apex syndrome initially

Nan Jiang, Guiqiu Zhao[*], Shanshan Yang, Jing Lin, Liting Hu, Chengye Che, Qian Wang and Qiang Xu

Abstract

Background: Rhino-orbito-cerebral mucormycosis(ROCM) is an invasive fungal infection that usually occurs in immunocompromised patients and sometimes presents as orbital apex syndrome(OAS) initially. It is rapidly fatal without an early diagnosis and treatment. We report the cases of invasive ROCM presenting with OAS initially in order to raise the attention of clinicians.

Methods: We retrospectively investigated eleven cases of invasive ROCM presenting initially with OAS admitted between January 2006 and December 2013. We analyzed clinical features, results of laboratory and radiological examinations, nasal endoscopy, aggressive surgical excision and debridement, and medical management outcomes of each case.

Results: A total of eleven cases of invasive ROCM with OAS as an initial sign were presented. Mucormycosis was accompanied by type II diabetes mellitus in nine cases, renal transplant in one case, and injury caused by traffic accident in one case. Anterior rhinoscopy revealed palatine or nasal necrotic lesions in all patients, and transethmoidal optic nerve decompression was carried out in three patients at the same time. CT scan revealed rhino-orbital-cerebral involvement in every patient. All patients were given intravenous amphotericin B. Nine patients underwent surgical debridement of necrotic tissue. Three patients survived.

Conclusions: ROCM is a severe, emergent and fatal infection requiring multidisciplinary management. It may often present with OAS initially. For ophthalmologist, mucormycosis must be considered in immunocompromised patients presenting with OAS initially, and anterior rhinoscopy is imperative before hormonotherapy, even in the cases absent of ketoacidosis induced by diabetes mellitus.

Keywords: Rhino-orbito-cerebral mucormycosis, Orbital apex syndrome, Ocular manifestations, Diabetes mellitus, Immunocompromise

Background

Mucormycosis is a rare and severe opportunistic fungal infection resulted from a fungus of the order mucorales. At present, the incidence of fungal infections is increasing. Mucormycosis is the second most frequent fungal infection following aspergillus [1–3]. This fungal infection can rapidly progress in individuals who are immunologically or metabolically compromised through vascular thrombosis or central nervous system involvement [4]. The most common co-morbidities include diabetes mellitus, lymphoid malignancy, burn, severe trauma, renal failure and steroid therapy [5, 6].

The rhino-orbital-cerebral presentation is the most frequent. The diagnosis is often made late and relies on anatomopathological and mycological examinations, especially for some patients presenting with atypical symptoms initially for example swelling lid, nasal stuffiness, vision loss *et al*. Rhino-orbital-cerebral mucormycosis (ROCM) may be rapidly fatal if not recognized early and treated promptly.

* Correspondence: zhaoguiqiu_good@126.com
Department of Ophthalmology, the Affiliated Hospital of Qingdao University, Qingdao, Shandong Province, China

Early diagnosis and appropriate medical management are vital to save the life. In this paper, we retrospectively presented eleven cases of ROCM with ocular symptoms initially and discussed clinical features, results of laboratory investigations, radiological examinations and treatment outcomes of each case.

Methods

Eleven ROCM patients with orbital apex syndrome(OAS) initially presenting to our hospital between January 2006 and December 2013 were retrospectively investigated. These studies were conducted in full conformance with the principles of the Declaration of Helsinki in 1995 or with the laws of China, which ever afforded the greater protection to the study participant. Written informed consents were obtained from the Institutional Research Ethics Committee at the Affiliated Hospital of Qingdao University and eleven patients for publication of this research article and any accompanying images.

Evaluation at presentation included a detailed history, clinical signs, ENT, ophthalmic, and neurological examination to assess the extent of disease, nasal endoscopy with biopsy, and results of laboratory and radiological examinations.

The diagnosis of mucormycosis was made by histological examination of biopsy samples and finding filaments of the Mucorales order. CT and MRI scan revealed rhino-orbital-cerebral involvement in every patient. Treatment with systemic amphotericin B was started as soon as the diagnosis of mucormycosis was established. Treatment was also instituted to stabilize the underlying metabolic derangement and surgical debridement was indicated.

Results

Out of 11 cases of ROCM followed and treated in our hospital, three were female and eight were male. The mean age of the patients was 53.7 years (range: 45–60 years). Diabetes was the most frequent risk factor, presenting in nine patients. One patient presented with renal transplant, and one was injured by traffic accident .Of 11 cases of mucormycosis with rhino-orbito-cerebral involvement, all had OAS. Vision was altered in all patients including blindness in eight and only perception of light/hand moving in three cases.

The main clinical signs on physical examination were progressively decreased vision ($n = 11$), involvement of cranial nerves ($n = 11$), blepharoptosis ($n = 11$), exophthalmia ($n = 9$), periorbital edema ($n = 9$), and facial swelling ($n = 8$) (Fig. 1).

Table 1 shows main clinical features, locations of the involvements, imaging manifestation, and therapeutic data of the cases.

Table 2 shows clinical signs and symptoms of the cases of mucormycosis.

All the patients underwent CT/MRI scan of the paranasal sinuses, orbit and craniocerebrum. Pansinusitis was found in eight patients, and maxilloethmoidal sinusitis was found in three patients. The thickening sinus mucosa and extension of lesions to the orbits were observed in all patients. Four patients presented with thrombosis of cavernous sinuses. Extensionto frontal lobes, dilatation of the ventricular system and cortical grooves, and thrombophlebitis of the right lateral sinus were observed in one patient each. MRI performed in one patient revealed lesion predominantly located in sphenoid sinus, involving the left orbital apex (Fig. 2).

On anterior rhinoscopy all patients had black blood stained debris in the region of inferior and middle turbinate along with necrosis on endoscopy. Direct examination was performed after PAS staining. Tissue specimens for culture were obtained from all cases. The culture was made on Sabouraud chloramphenicol medium with and without cycloheximide. In ten cases, the diagnosis of mucormycosis was based on positive histopathological findings for mucormycosis (Fig. 3). In three cases, Mucor spp. was isolated from tissue cultures and it was pathologically verified in all patients of mucormycosis. The histological examination revealed large non-septate mycelial filaments, sometimes branched at a right angle with images of angioinvasion within necrotic and inflammatory material.

Duration of illness between the first clinical signs and diagnosis ranged from 10 days to 50 days. At the early stage, the nasal and sinus phase was neglected by all patients. Once diagnosis, all patients had received antifungal treatment with amphotericin B, at 0.3 mg/kg per day initially with close renal function monitoring, gradually up to maximum dose at 1 mg/kg per day for an average of 4–6 weeks. During the course, three patients presented with severe renal insufficiency induced by amphotericin B treatment leading to treatment interruption and switched to itraconazole. For the patients accompanied with diabetes mellitus or renal transplantation, insulin therapy with a strict surveillance of glycemia or the therapy with improvement of renal function was prescribed. Meanwhile, nine cases received surgical debridement of necrotic tissue associated to drug therapy.

Finally, one patient with trauma had been rapidly transferred to the ICU for severe skin and soft tissue infection, and died of septicemia and acute respiratory insufficiency. The patient with renal transplantation refused further treatment and died of renal failure. The outcome was favorable for three patients with diabetes mellitus, 12, 18, and 24 months later, respectively. Three patients had fulminating disease and early mortality due to intracranial and pulmonary infection. One died of ventricular arrhythmia disorder, one died of neurological distress, and one case was due to hemorrhagic shock.

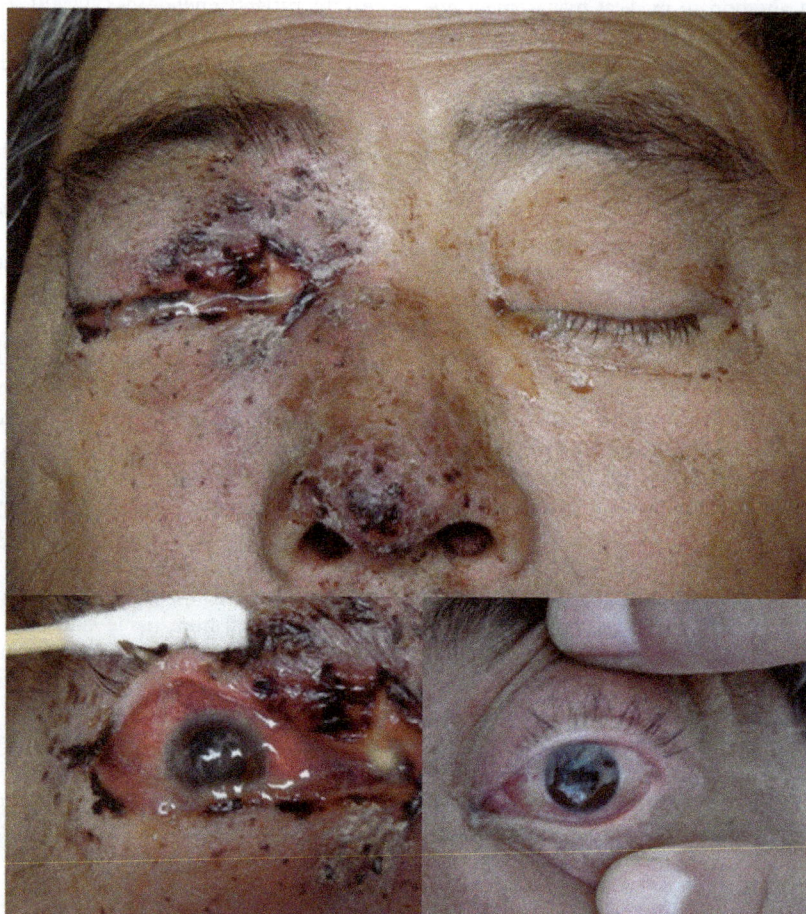

Fig. 1 Pre-operative aspect of patient exhibiting bilateral periorbital edema with facial swelling, exophthalmia, blepharoptosis,and Ocular purulent secretion

Discussion

Mucormycosis is a rare filamentous and fatal fungal infection mostly encountered among immuno-suppressed patients [7, 8]. The most common risk factors accompanied with mucormycosis are diabetes mellitus, especially ketoacidosis, immunosuppressive conditions like hematologic malignancies and organ transplantations [9–11]. Nine patients (81.8 %) had diabetes mellitus, in which neutrophils had an impaired ability of phagocytosis and chemotaxis [12]. Presence of diabetic ketoacidosis increases predisposition to mucormycosis. Acidosis disrupts iron binding of transferrin, resulting in increased proportion of unbound iron, which may promote growth of the fungus [13, 14]. Another accompanying disease is renal transplantation. The least frequently accompanying disease is haematological malignity.

Mucormycosis presents in various distinct forms depending on the immunological status of the host and the affected site. Among the various localizations, the rhino-orbital-cerebral presentation is the most frequent (40 %) [15, 16]. The fungus invades the wall of the blood vessels, causing mechanical and toxic damage to the intima leading to thrombosis, and later it invades the lymphatics and veins. These thromboses cause emboli and vascular obstruction responsible for tissue necrosis.

The infection progressively spreads from the nasal mucosa to the nose, facial sinuses, the palate, orbits and brain. It evolves in three stages: nasal and sinus involvement often pauci or asymptomatic unnoticed by the patient, orbital involvement motivating the patient for consultation, and finally cerebral involvement.

OAS is a rare syndrome with retro-orbital pain, complete ophthalmoplegia, and visual loss. In the etiology of OAS, inflammatory, infectious, neoplastic, iatrogenic/traumatic and vascular pathologies should

Table 1 main clinical features, locations of the involvements, imaging manifestation, and therapeutic data of the cases

	N
Cases	11
Mean age (range)	53.7 (45–60)
Gender(F/M)	3/8
Accompanying disease	
Diabetes mellitus	9
Renal transplant	1
Trauma	1
Locations of the involvements	
Rhinocerebral	11
Sino-orbital	0
Rhino-orbital-cerebral	11
Clinical involvement	
Orbital apex syndrome	11
Imaging manifestation(CT/MRI)	
Thickening in sinus Mucosa	11
Inflammation in the periorbital muscles	11
Involvement of the cavernous sinus	4
Occlusion of the internal carotid artery	2
Sings of cerebral infarct	2
Rhinoscopy	11
Therapy	
Surgical debridement	8
Amphotericin B.	11
Outcomes	
Survive with sequeale	3
Death	8

Table 2 Clinical features and radiological features of the cases of mucormycosis

Signs/symptoms	n	%
Fever	9	81.8
Headache	7	63.6
Consciousness	6	54.5
Cranial nerve palsy	11	100
Decreased vision	11	100
Exophthalmia	9	81.8
Diplopia	9	81.8
Blepharoptosis	11	100
Periorbital edema	9	81.8
Facial swelling and pain	8	72.7
Ocular purulent secretion	7	63.6
Nasal blockage/crusting	6	54.5
Blood stained discharge	5	45.5

be considered [17]. Fungal infections can cause extensive tissue damage potentially leading to permanent vision loss and death if not treated [18]. Species of Fusarium, Aspergillus, Candida, dematiaceous fungi, Mucorales and Scedosporium predominate. Diagnosis is aided by recognition of typical clinical features and by direct microscopic detection of fungi in scrapes, biopsy specimens, and other samples. Culture confirms the diagnosis. Histopathological, immunohistochemical, or DNA-based tests may also be needed [19]. For example, ROCM, also known as mucormycosis, is commonly caused by the non-septate filamentous fungus, Rhizopus oryzae [20]. Patients with ROCM present acutely and progress rapidly. Another fungal orbital infection important to understand is sino-orbital aspergillosis. Sino-orbital Aspergillus infection can occur acutely or chronically and can affect both the immunocompetent and immunocompromised [21, 22]. Invasive Aspergillus infection in the

immunocompetent host usually presents in a more indolent but progressive course. CT imaging can show heterogenous soft tissue enhancement with focal bony destruction with intraluminal calcification being indicative of an Aspergillus infection [23, 24].

For mucormycosis with a late diagnosis, the evolution is marked by extension to the orbits. The orbital involvement is related to the vascular tropism of the fungus inducing arteriole thrombosis affecting the orbit wall, oculomotor and optical nerves responsible for blindness with or without thrombosis of the ophthalmic artery. It is unilateral and marked by orbital pain, diplopia, ophthalmoplegia, periorbital edema, chemosis, exophthalmia or even blindness. OAS may be firstly diagnosed. Eye fundus is a key examination for the diagnosis of ROCM. It may reveal a venous congestion or thrombosis of the artery or of the central vein of retina, optic atrophy or panophthalmia [16, 25–27]. In the OAS, the prognosis is good if treated early. There is mucosal invasion and hence radical debridement and antifungal therapy is imperative. If the inflammation can't be controlled, intracranial involvement occurs from invasion by way of superior orbital fissure, ophthalmic vessels, cribriform plate and not uncommonly, through carotid artery.

In the patients involved in our study, the clinical signs and symptoms of mucormycosis may vary with the involved organ widely. Mostly, the clinical presentation is atypical. Nasal discharge or nasal blockage may occur in a small proportion of the patients. Sometimes even eschar, typical presentation of rinocerebral mucormycosis may not appear. The patients reported here most frequently presented with ptosis, exophthalmia and examination of the revealed sinuses

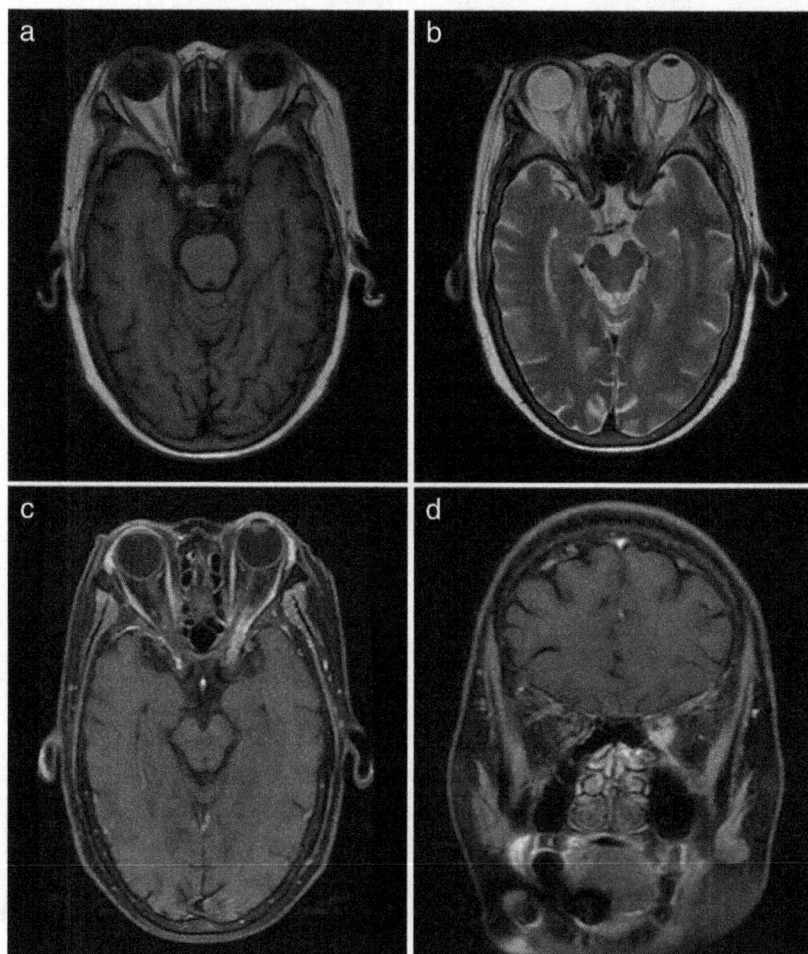

Fig. 2 MRI presentations of mucormycosis presented with orbital apex syndrome. **a**: Axial T1WI MR shows a isointensity lesion in the left orbital apex;**b**: Axial T2WI MR shows a hypointensity lesion in the left orbital apex and high signal in the sphenoid sinus; **c**: Axial contrast-enhanced T1WI MR shows a enhancing lesion in the left orbital apex; **d**: Coronal contrast-enhanced T1WI MR shows a enhancing lesion in the left orbital apex

eschar in most of cases. In such patients, MRI has the advantage of detecting early vascular and intracranial invasion.

Successful treatment of mucormycosis is based on three principles. First, early diagnosis is greatly imperative and can enormously reduce the patient's mortality. Second, necrotic tissues should be aggressively debrided or infected tissues should be resected. Last, medical treatment with antimycotic agents should be carried out [7]. Surgical therapy alone has a great influence on treatment outcome in cases of mucormycosis. In fact, Tedder *et al.* reported that the mortality rate was 11 % in patients who underwent surgery but 60 % in patients without surgical therapy [28]. Systemic antifungal therapy includes the use of high dose amphotericin B and is associated with an overall survival rate of 72 %. It is usually given in dextrose 5 % in water intravenously at a dose of 1.0–1.5 mg/kg daily since its usage is associated with renal toxicity and it requires careful monitoring of serum urea nitrogen, blood urea nitrogen, potassium, creatinine as well as creatinine clearance as an essential part of the therapy. Recently, studies have shown that liposomal amphotericin B and fluconazole, caspofungin can be combined with each other. Hyperbaric oxygen therapy is believed to improve neutrophilic killing by higher oxygen delivery, low dose of heparin, anti inflammatory medicine can be used with good success [29–31].

Prognosis is dependent on multiple factors and early initiation of treatment is an important element. A multidisciplinary approach consisting of dental specialists, ENT surgeons, ophthalmologists and neurologist is critical in

References

1. Denning DW, Stevens DA. Antifungal and surgical treatment of invasive aspergillosis: review of 2,121 published cases. Rev Infect Dis. 1990;12(6): 1147–201.
2. Hagensee ME, Bauwens JE, Kjos B, Bowden RA. Brain abscess following marrow transplantation: experience at the Fred Hutchinson Cancer Research Center, 1984–1992. Clin Infect Dis. 1994;19(3):402–8.
3. Pfaffenbach B, Donhuijsen K, Pahnke J, Bug R, Adamek RJ, Wegener M, et al. Systemic fungal infections in hematologic neoplasms. An autopsy study of 1,053 patients] Med Klin (Munich). 1994;89(6):299–304.
4. Gelston CD, Durairaj VD, Simoes EA. Rhino-orbital mucormycosis causing cavernous sinus and internal carotid thrombosis treated with posaconazole. Arch Ophthalmol. 2007;125(6):848–9.
5. Pagano L, Ricci P, Tonso A, Nosari A, Cudillo L, Montillo M, et al. Mucormycosis in patients with haematological malignancies: a retrospective clinical study of 37 cases. GIMEMA Infection Program (Gruppo Italiano Malattie Ematologiche Maligne dell'Adulto). Br J Haematol. 1997;99(2):331–6.
6. Walsh TJ, Groll AH. Emerging fungal pathogens: evolving challenges to immunocompromised patients for the twenty-first century. Transpl Infect Dis. 1999;1(4):247–61.
7. Eucker J, Sezer O, Graf B, Possinger K. Mucormycoses. Mycoses. 2001; 44(7–8):253–60.
8. Van den Saffele JK, Boelaert JR. Zygomycosis in HIV-positive patients: a review of the literature. Mycoses. 1996;39(3–4):77–84.
9. Almyroudis NG, Sutton DA, Linden P, Rinaldi MG, Fung J, Kusne S. Zygomycosis in solid organ transplant recipients in a tertiary transplant center and review of the literature. Am J Transplant. 2006;6(10):2365–74.
10. Kauffman CA, Malani AN. Zygomycosis: an emerging fungal infection with new options for management. Curr Infect Dis Rep. 2007;9(6):435–40.
11. Roden MM, Zaoutis TE, Buchanan WL, Knudsen TA, Sarkisova TA, Schaufele RL, et al. Epidemiology and outcome of zygomycosis: a review of 929 reported cases. Clin Infect Dis. 2005;41(5):634–53.
12. Reinhardt DJ, Kaplan W, Ajello L. Experimental cerebral zygomycosis in alloxan-diabetic rabbits I. Relationship of temperature tolerance of selected zygomycetes to pathogenicity. Infect Immun. 1970;2(4):404–13.
13. Sheldon WH, Bauer H. The development of the acute inflammatory response to experimental cutaneous mucormycosis in normal and diabetic rabbits. J Exp Med. 1959;110:845–52.
14. Waldorf AR, Ruderman N, Diamond RD. Specific susceptibility to mucormycosis in murine diabetes and bronchoalveolar macrophage defense against Rhizopus. J Clin Invest. 1984;74(1):150–60.
15. Hosseini SM, Borghei P. Rhinocerebral mucormycosis: pathways of spread. Eur Arch Otorhinolaryngol. 2005;262(11):932–8.
16. Prabhu RM, Patel R. Mucormycosis and entomophthoramycosis: a review of the clinical manifestations, diagnosis and treatment. Clin Microbiol Infect. 2004;10 Suppl 1:31–47.
17. Yeh S, Foroozan R. Orbital apex syndrome. Curr Opin Ophthalmol. 2004; 15(6):490–8.
18. Klotz SA, Penn CC, Negvesky GJ, Butrus SI. Fungal and parasitic infections of the eye. Clin Microbiol Rev. 2000;13:662–85.
19. Thomas PA. Current Perspectives on Ophthalmic Mycoses. Clin Microbiol Rev. 2003;16(4):730–97.
20. Ribes JA, Vanover-Sams CL, Baker DJ. Zygomycetes in human disease. Clin Microbiol Rev. 2000;13:236–301.
21. Levin LA, Avery R, Shore JW, Woog JJ, Baker AS. The Spectrum of orbital aspergillosis: A clinicopathological review. Surv Ophthalmol. 1996;41:142–54.
22. Kagen SL. Aspergillus: An inhalable contaminant of marihuana. N Engl J Med. 1981;304:483–4.
23. Stammberger H. Formation of roentgen dense structures in aspergillus mycoses of the paranasal sinuses. HNO. 1985;33:62–4.
24. Krennmair G, Lenglinger F, Muller-Schelken H. Computed tomography (CT) in the diagnosis of sinus aspergillosis. J Craniomaxillofac Surg. 1994;22:120–5.
25. Talmi YP, Goldschmied-Reouven A, Bakon M, Barshack I, Wolf M, Horowitz Z, et al. Rhino-orbital and rhino-orbito-cerebral mucormycosis. Otolaryngol Head Neck Surg. 2002;127(1):22–31.
26. Toumi A, Larbi Ammari F, Loussaief C, Hadhri R, Ben Brahim H, Harrathi K, et al. Rhino-orbito-cerebral mucormycosis: five cases. Med Mal Infect. 2012; 42(12):591–8.

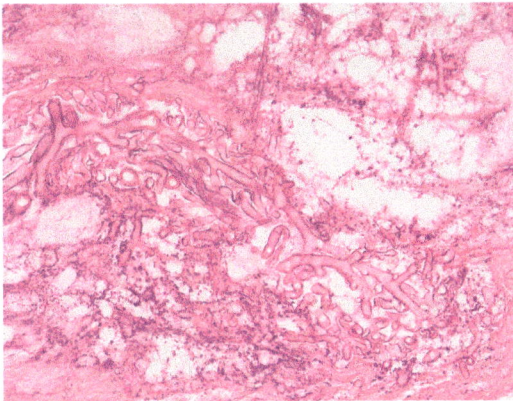

Fig. 3 Nasal biopsy showing mycelial filaments of variable thickness and necrosis (PAS;×200)

successful management of a patient with mucormycosis. Hence the general approach is to treat early, aggressively and with all modalities available.

Conclusions

Mucormycosis is a severe, emergent and fatal infection requiring multidisciplinary management. It is a disease with various presentations, and sometimes its manifestations are atypical. For ophthalmologist, it should be kept in mind when dealing with the case of OAS, even exophthalmia, progressive periorbital or facial edema or necrosis, with or without involvement of cranial nerves in the patients accompanied with immunodeficiency disorders. The diagnosis relies on histological and mycological examination data. Early diagnosis and urgent antifungal treatment associated to surgery are of extreme importance for successful eradication of infection and for patient survival.

Abbreviations
OAS: Orbital apex syndrome; ROCM: Rhino-orbital-cerebral mucormycosis.

Competing interests
All authors declare that they have no competing interests.

Authors' contributions
NJ, GZ conceived of the work that led to the assembly and review of the acquired data, and the interpretation and submission of the results. SY, JL, LH drafted and revised the manuscript and CC, QW, QX provided a critical review of the content. All authors approved the manuscript for submission.

Acknowledgements
The authors wish to acknowledge Dr. Jianbao Ju for his guidance of diagnosis and treatment of our patients. This work was supported by grants from National Natural Science Foundation of China (81170825, 81470609), Specialized Research Fund for the Doctoral Program of Higher Education (20123706110003) and grants from the Youth Natural Science Foundation of Shandong Province (ZR2013HQ007) and the Key Project of Natural Science Foundation of Shandong Province(ZR2012FZ001).

27. Turunc T, Demiroglu YZ, Aliskan H, Colakoglu S, Arslan H. Eleven cases of
     mucormycosis with atypical clinical manifestations in diabetic patients.
     Diabetes Res Clin Pract. 2008;82(2):203–8.
28. Tedder M, Spratt JA, Anstadt MP, Hegde SS, Tedder SD, Lowe JE. Pulmonary
     mucormycosis: results of medical and surgical therapy. Ann Thorac Surg.
     1994;57(4):1044–50.
29. Cagatay AA, Oncu SS, Calangu SS, Yildirmak TT, Ozsut HH, Eraksoy HH.
     Rhinocerebral mucormycosis treated with 32 gram liposomal amphotericin
     B and incomplete surgery: a case report. BMC Infect Dis. 2001;1:22.
30. Couch L, Theilen F, Mader JT. Rhinocerebral mucormycosis with cerebral
     extension successfully treated with adjunctive hyperbaric oxygen therapy.
     Arch Otolaryngol Head Neck Surg. 1988;114(7):791–4.
31. Kocak R, Tetiker T, Kocak M, Baslamisli F, Zorludemir S, Gonlusen G.
     Fluconazole in the treatment of three cases of mucormycosis. Eur J Clin
     Microbiol Infect Dis. 1995;14(6):559–61.

9

Spontaneous resolution of foveal detachment in traction maculopathy in high myopia unrelated to posterior vitreous detachment

Tso-Ting Lai[1], Tzyy-Chang Ho[1] and Chung-May Yang[1,2]*

Abstract

Background: Foveal detachment associated with foveoschisis usually takes a progressive course, and is associated with a poor visual outcome. The purpose of this study was to report the spontaneous resolution of foveal detachment in patients with myopic traction maculopathy without posterior vitreous detachment.

Methods: A retrospective study involving eight cases of high myopia with foveoschisis and foveal detachment in which the subfoveal fluid had spontaneously resolved. The clinical characteristics and optical coherence tomography (OCT) findings were described.

Results: All cases involved predominant schisis in the outer retina, with six showing internal limiting membrane detachment. The average central foveal thickness was 445.1 μm, and the average foveal detachment height was 271.5 μm. None of the cases involved traction of the vitreomacular interface or posterior vitreous detachment (PVD), either before or after the resolution of foveal detachment. In seven cases, the mean best-corrected visual acuity improved after foveal reattachment.

Conclusions: Spontaneous reattachment not associated with PVD can occur in cases of high myopic traction maculopathy, especially in those without obvious vitreomacular traction.

Keywords: Foveal detachment, High myopia, Foveoschisis, Optical coherence tomography, Posterior vitreous detachment

Background

Myopic foveoschisis is a complication of high myopia that can affect visual function. Studies have suggested that this condition usually takes a progressive course, with only a minority of cases remaining stable during follow-up [1–3]. Foveal detachment occurs in 34.5–72.0 % of patients with this condition, either at the time of diagnosis or during follow-up [1–3]; this is usually associated with a poor visual outcome [1]. However, a recent study involving 207 patients showed a much more stable clinical course, with the myopic foveoschisis progressing in only

11.6 % of cases during a follow-up period of more than 2 years [4]. Moreover, several investigations have suggested that surgical interventions, such as gas tamponade or vitrectomy, improve anatomical and functional outcomes in patients with this condition [1, 2, 5–7]. Nonetheless, complications such as macular hole formation have been reported [1, 5, 6], and functional outcomes may not parallel structural improvements [8, 9].

With regard to pathogenesis, foveoschisis is related to strong pre-retinal traction combined with axial length elongation [1, 3, 10–12]. In a previous report involving spontaneous resolution of macular detachment, a complete posterior vitreous detachment (PVD) occurred *before* the reattachment of the macula; for this reason, the investigators suggested that the PVD contributed to the reattachment [8]. Similarly, another recent study

* Correspondence: chungmay@ntu.edu.tw
[1]Department of Ophthalmology, National Taiwan University Hospital, No. 7, Chun-Shan S. Rd., Taipei City 100, Taiwan
[2]College of Medicine, National Taiwan University, No.1 Jen-Ai Rd. Sec. 1, Taipei City 100, Taiwan

suggested that rupture of the internal limiting membrane (ILM) reduces traction and leads to resolution of schisis and foveal detachment [4]. In this study, which involved eight patients, we report the spontaneous resolution of foveal detachment in myopic tractional maculopathy that is unassociated with PVD or ILM rupture. In addition, we present the clinical course, as well as the findings from optical coherence tomography (OCT). Finally, various factors that may be associated with this spontaneous improvement are discussed.

Methods

We retrospectively reviewed the cases of eight consecutive patients with myopic foveoschisis in whom a foveal detachment had spontaneously resolved; all patients had been diagnosed between January 2009 and December 2014. OCT images were traced backward to the patients' original visits. All patients had been followed up by the Department of Ophthalmology at the National Taiwan University Hospital, and written informed consent had been obtained from all patients. Approval for this study was obtained from the National Taiwan University Hospital Research Ethics Committee, and it adhered to the tenets of the Declaration of Helsinki.

High myopia was defined as myopia of ≥ 6 diopters, and/or axial length ≥ 26 mm; spontaneous resolution of foveal detachment was defined as reattachment of the fovea without any surgical intervention (gas injection or vitrectomy). Clinical data were collected by retrospective chart review in all cases; these data included patient age, gender, auto-refraction, best-corrected visual acuity (BCVA), axial length (measured using the LENSTAR LS 900; Haag-Streit USA Inc., Mason, OH, USA), and findings from both slit-lamp and dilated fundus examinations. Findings from serial OCT images (spectral domain OCT,

Cirrus™; HD-OCT, Carl Zeiss Meditec, Inc., Dublin, CA, USA; or RTVue™ RT100 version 3.5; Optovue Inc., Fremont, CA, USA) were recorded during the follow-up period. These included inner plexiform layer (IPL) retinoschisis [3], outer retinal retinoschisis, lamellar hole, ILM detachment, inner segment/outer segment (IS/OS) junction defect, and vitreoretinal interface traction. We carefully reviewed all the OCT images, which were obtained from a 5-line raster scan of the fovea, as well as from a macular cube scan of the entire macular area. Retinoschisis on the OCT images was classified according to the extent of outer schisis, as described by Shimada [4]: no macular retinoschisis (S0), extra-foveal retinoschisis (S1), fovea-only retinoschisis (S2), foveal and partial macular area retinoschisis (S3), entire macular area retinoschisis (S4). The height of the foveal detachment was defined as the largest distance, measured manually, from the surface of the retinal pigment epithelium (RPE) to the photoreceptor cell ellipsoid zone. The longest of these measurements in the series of OCT images was chosen as the foveal detachment height for each particular patient. The central foveal thickness (CFT) was measured at the same site, and was defined as the distance between the RPE and the inner retinal surface. Again, the longest of these measurements in the series of OCT images was chosen as the central foveal thickness [7]. The presence of PVD was determined by OCT examination, funduscopic findings, or clinical records of previous ocular surgery. In patients who had developed foveal detachment during follow-up after an initial presentation of only foveoschisis (patient Nos. 1–4 in Table 1), the duration of foveal detachment was defined as the interval between the first date on which OCT had shown foveal detachment and the first date on which it had shown complete resolution of foveal detachment.

Table 1 Clinical features of patients with myopic foveoschisis combined with a foveal detachment that spontaneously resolved

Patient no.	Age (years)	Gender	RE (Diopter)	Axial length (mm)	Chorioretinal atrophy	Clinical course	Serial BCVA[a] (logMAR)	Duration of FD (months)
1	61–65	Woman	IOL	28.78	D + P	FS → FS + FD → FS	0.8 / 0.8 / 0.8	31
2	51–55	Woman	−18.37	30.47	D	FS → FS + FD → FS	0.7 / 1.0 / 0.8	27
3	41–45	Woman	−17.0	31.05	D + P	FS → FS + FD → FS	0.5 / 1.3 / 1.0	24
4	41–45	Man	−13.25	29.85	D	FS → FS + FD → FS	0.1 / 0.3 / 0.05	6
5	66–70	Man	−6.37	28.32	D	FS + FD → no FS/FD[b]	NA / 2.0 / 1.5	NA
6	41–45	Woman	−13.0	28.36	D	FS + FD → FS	NA / 0.4 / 0.1	NA
7	51–55	Woman	−11.75	NA	D	FS + FD → FS	NA / 2.0 / 1.0	NA
8	66–70	Woman	IOL	30.36	D	FS + FD → FS	NA / 0.5 / 0.3	NA
Mean ± SD	54.6 ± 10.0		−13.3 ± 3.9	29.6 ± 1.0				22.0 ± 9.6

BCVA best-corrected visual acuity, D diffuse atrophy, FD foveal detachment, FS foveoschisis, IOL intraocular lens, NA not available, P patchy atrophy, RE refractive error, RPE retina pigment epithelium, SD standard deviation
[a]The serial BCVA was recorded in the following order: with FS but before FD–during FS and FD–after FD had resolved
[b]In patient No. 5, the FS and FD both resolved completely during follow-up

Statistical analysis

The change in BCVA (measured in logarithm of the minimum angle of resolution [logMAR]) after resolution of the foveal detachment was analyzed using the student's t-test for paired samples; p-values < 0.05 were considered statistically significant.

Results

The clinical characteristics of the patients are listed in Table 1. The mean age was 54.6 ± 10.0 years (range = 44–68 years). The average spherical equivalent measured was −13.3 ± 3.9 diopters (range = −18.37–6.37) and the average axial length measured was 29.6 ± 1.0 mm (range = 28.32–31.05). The refractive error before cataract surgery was not available for patient Nos. 1 and 8. Diffuse chorioretinal atrophy was noted in all cases, while patchy atrophy over the macular area was noted in patient Nos. 1 and 3. Four patients had an initial presentation of foveoschisis and foveal detachment; the other four developed foveal detachment during the follow-up period. The mean duration of foveal detachment in the latter four cases was 22.0 ± 9.6 months (range = 6–31 months). In seven of the eight patients, BCVA improved after the subretinal fluid had resolved, and mean BCVA was significantly better after foveal detachment had resolved compared with when the fovea was detached ($p < 0.05$).

The OCT findings are summarized in Table 2, and Fig. 1 shows a typical example of such findings. All patients had S4 retinoschisis, except for patient No. 5, who had foveal and partial macular area retinoschisis, which was therefore classified as S3. None of the patients had visible vitreoretinal interface traction (epiretinal membrane or vitreomacular traction). In all patients, except for

No. 4, the IS/OS junction was disrupted after the retina had reattached. Patient 6 presented with retinoschisis, foveal detachment, and an inner lamellar hole at the initial visit. In addition, the lamellar hole continued to increase in size for as long as the schisis persisted, despite the resolution of subretinal fluid. An *outer* lamellar hole was noted at initial presentation in patient No. 8, who also had foveal detachment and schisis. All cases of retinoschisis mainly involved the outer retina; ILM detachment was noted in six cases. After the foveal detachment had resolved, the schisis remained the same in four cases, became less prominent in three cases, and completely resolved in one case. The average height of foveal detachment was 271.5 ± 68.2 μm (range = 191–396 μm). The mean CFT was 445.1 ± 79.6 μm (range = 330–550 μm). Two representative cases are presented here:

Report of cases
Patient No. 5

A 68-year-old man without any specific underlying disease was referred to our clinic and received scleral buckling to treat retinal detachment in the right eye. During the preoperative evaluation, poor vision in the left eye was noted, with BCVA being 2.0 logMAR. Fundoscopy revealed a typical myopic fundus with diffuse atrophy. OCT showed foveal detachment with foveoschisis in the left eye (Fig. 2). The schisis mainly occurred in the outer retina, without notable ILM detachment or lamellar hole formation. Furthermore, there was no macular hole or visible premacular traction. The axial lengths were 27.40 mm and 28.32 mm in the right and left eyes, respectively. The subretinal fluid, as well as the schisis in the left eye, gradually decreased during follow-up, and the

Table 2 Optical coherence tomography findings from patients with myopic foveoschisis and foveal detachment that spontaneously resolved

Patient no.	Classification[a]	ERM/VMT	ILM detachment	Retinoschisis	LH	Persisted schisis	IS/OS junction disruption	FD (μm)	CFT (μm)
1	S4	Removed[b]	+	Outer	-	+	+	272	493
2	S4	-	+	Inner & outer[c]	-	+	+	230	482
3	S4	-	+	Outer	-	Partial[d]	+	230	341
4	S4	-	+	Outer	-	+	-	191	499
5	S3	-	-	Outer	-	-	+	371	499
6	S4	-	+	Inner & outer[c]	+[e]	+	+	242	367
7	S4	-	-	Outer	-	Partial[d]	+	240	330
8	S4	-	+	Outer	+[f]	Partial[d]	+	396	550

CFT central foveal thickness, ERM epiretinal membrane, FD the height of foveal detachment, ILM internal limiting membrane, IS/OS inner segment/outer segment, LH lamellar hole, VMT vitreomacular traction

+ = present; − = absent

[a]The classification of retinoschisis was based on the extent of outer retinoschisis described by Shimada [4], where schisis involving the fovea and partial macula was classified as S3, and schisis involving the entire macula area was classified as S4

[b]In patient No. 1, the ERM was removed via vitrectomy without ILM peeling one month before the development of foveal detachment

[c]In patient Nos. 2 and 6, the retinoschisis involved both the inner (inner plexiform layer) and outer retina

[d]In patient Nos. 3, 7, and 8, the retinoschisis had decreased, with some residual schisis in the outer retina

[e]In patient No. 6, an inner lamellar hole was noted at initial presentation, with enlargement during follow-up

[f]In patient No. 8, an outer lamellar hole was noted at initial presentation

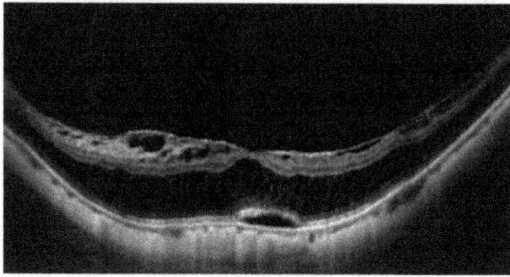

Fig. 1 Optical coherence tomography (OCT) image from patient No. 2. Representative OCT image from patient No. 2 showing typical findings: ILM detachment, retinoschisis, disruption of the IS/OS junction, and foveal detachment. The schisis was more prominent in the outer retina, and no vitreoretinal interface traction or outer laminar break was seen

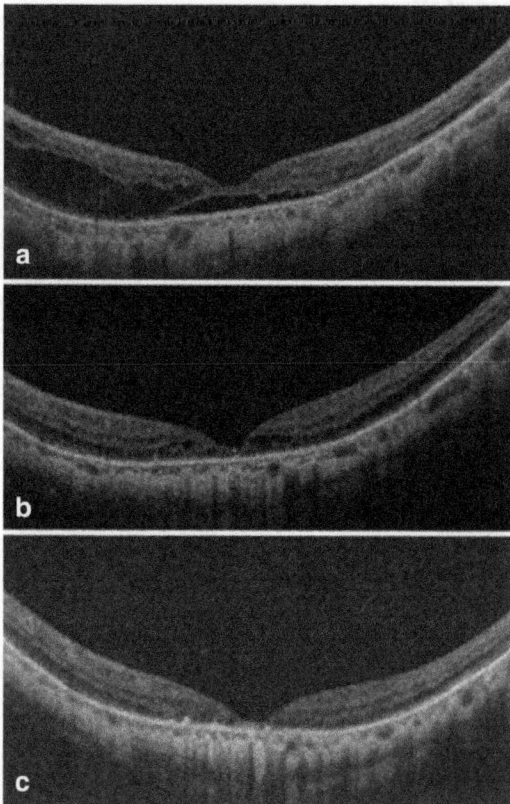

Fig. 2 Serial optical coherence tomography (OCT) images from patient No. 5. Serial OCT images from a 68-year-old man (patient No. 5) demonstrate spontaneous resolution of foveoschisis and foveal detachment. **a** At presentation, OCT showed foveoschisis of the outer retina combined with foveal detachment. **b** One year later, the subretinal fluid had resolved spontaneously, and the severity of schisis had decreased. **c** Four months after the detachment had resolved, OCT revealed complete resolution of foveoschisis, as well as some tissue loss in the outer retina and disruption of the IS/OS junction

retina had reattached one year later. Specifically, the schisis had resolved completely four months after the reattachment of the fovea—OCT revealed an attached retina with a disruption of the IS/OS junction. The patient's BCVA in the left eye was 1.5 logMAR at the last visit, 23 months after the initial presentation.

Patient No. 6

A 44-year-old woman with high myopia presented with a history of vitrectomy to treat retinal detachment in the right eye. She complained of decreased vision in the left eye, which had persisted for one month prior to her initial visit to our hospital. Fundoscopy revealed a tessellated fundus with diffuse atrophy in the left eye; OCT showed foveoschisis with foveal detachment, as well as an inner lamellar hole (Fig. 3). Moreover, ILM detachment was also noted on the OCT image. The patient's BCVA was 0.4 logMAR, and her axial length was 28.36 mm in the left eye. Six months later, the retina had reattached without treatment, and the patient's BCVA had improved to 0.1 logMAR. Although foveoschisis persisted, and the lamellar hole continued to enlarge during the subsequent two years, no macular hole formed. The final BCVA in the left eye was 0.4 logMAR, with cataract progression.

Discussion

The evolution of foveoschisis in high myopia can be diverse. For instance, it is generally believed that the condition takes a progressive course in most cases; however, in a recent study involving the most patients with myopic retinoschisis reported in any investigation to date, the disease had progressed in only 24 (11.6 %) of 207 eyes during follow-up [4], with retinal detachment developing in 7 of those 24. The same researchers reported that the schisis had spontaneously improved in 8 of the 207 eyes, and it had completely resolved in 6 of those. In this study, we analyzed eight cases of foveoschisis in which foveal detachment spontaneously resolved during follow-up without obvious changes in the vitreoretinal relationship. These clinical courses imply that myopic foveoschisis, and the foveal detachment associated with it, has a more complex etiology.

The pathogenesis of foveoschisis is related to strong traction on the retina, which is in turn caused by rigidity of the ILM, posterior vitreous, epiretinal membrane, and retinal vessels [3, 10]. Increases in the axial length, which are associated with pathological myopia, also play a role in generating tractional force from the tissues listed above. Previous studies have associated various factors with the development of foveal detachment and foveoschisis: axial length > 31 mm, macular chorioretinal atrophy, and vitreoretinal interface factors [12], as well as ILM detachment, and IPL retinoschisis [3]. However, the average

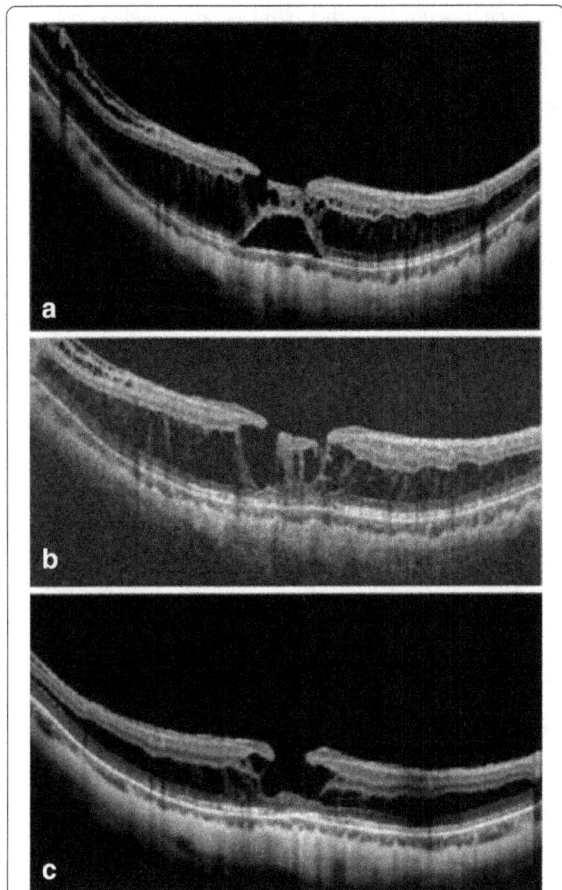

Fig. 3 Serial optical coherence tomography (OCT) images from patient No. 6. The serial OCT images from a 44-year-old woman with high myopia (patient No. 6) show spontaneously resolved foveal detachment and enlarged inner lamellar hole. **a** The OCT at initial presentation showed retinoschisis, mainly over the outer retina, and ILM detachment. An inner lamellar hole was also present. No vitromacular interface traction was noted. **b** The retina had reattached 6 months later, without operation, with disruption to the IS/OS junction visible on the same image. The schisis, ILM detachment, and inner lamellar hole persisted. **c** After 44 months, the macula remained attached, while the inner lamellar hole had enlarged without the formation of a macular hole. The retinoschisis over the outer retina was still visible, as was the disruption to the IS/OS junction

axial length measured in our study was 29.6 mm, and only one patient had an axial length over 31 mm. In addition, none of our patients had any traction in the vitromacular interface that was visible by either fundoscopy or OCT. The relatively short axial length, as well as the absence of visible vitromacular interface factors, indicates less severe traction on the retina, which may contribute to the spontaneous resolution of foveal detachment in our study.

Using OCT, Fujimoto et al. showed a higher incidence of ILM detachment and IPL retinoschisis in foveoschisis patients with foveal detachment than in those without detachment [3]. These findings may suggest that a stronger inward traction is generated at the vitreous membrane, as well as at the rigid ILM, and that this is transmitted to the outer retina through the columnar structure in the layers of the retinoschisis. Likewise, Shimada et al. reported two cases of ILM disruption prior to spontaneous resolution of retinoschisis, and assumed that the disruption of the already detached ILM releases the severe traction [4]. In our study, the retinoschises were mainly confined to the outer retina, and ILM detachment was noted in six eyes (75 %). No disruption of any detached ILM was noted in our study, at least in the scanning area. The lack of IPL retinoschisis in six of our eight cases may indicate a less severe traction, and this may serve as a predictive factor for spontaneous resolution of the subretinal fluid.

The lower foveal detachment height and shorter CFT provide further evidence for less severe traction in our patients than in those from a previous study who had foveoschisis and foveal detachment that showed a progressive course and required surgery [7]. In our previous study on the treatment of foveoschisis, the average heights of foveal detachment (576.9 ± 378.6 μm) and CFT (762.8 ± 314.7 μm) were significantly greater than in this study ($p < 0.05$). Thus, we would suggest a quantitative measurement of these two parameters before considering surgical treatment.

A previous study from Shimada et al. found that the formation of an outer lamellar hole predisposes a patient to foveal detachment in myopic retinoschisis [13]. In none of our patients did any lamellar hole occur during the follow-up period, except for patient No. 8, who had an outer lamellar hole at the initial presentation. Foveal detachment developed *during* the follow-up period in four cases in our study, and the OCT images from these cases showed no evidence of outer lamellar hole formation before the retinal detachment. However, it is uncertain whether this really indicates a favorable disease process; it may simply have been due to inadequate scanning, because only a small cubic region of the macular area was examined. One eye in our series had an inner lamellar hole, which enlarged after the subretinal fluid resolved. The enlarged opening of the hole in this eye may have released some of the traction; in fact, loss of the columnar structure of the retina, caused by the hole itself, may actually have decreased transmission of the inward traction. Both factors may have played a role in the resolution of the foveal detachment.

In one previous report in which macular detachment spontaneously resolved, complete PVD occurred before the reattachment of macula; the investigators therefore postulated PVD as a contributing factor to the reattachment [8]. Indeed, PVD occurred in four of the eight eyes with decreased or resolved retinoschisis that were reported by Shimada et al. [4], and in three of the four eyes reported by Hirota et al. in which traction maculopathy had resolved [9]. Nonetheless, no such association was observed in our study. One of our patients had received pars plana vitrectomy (PPV) long before the macular detachment, and PVD was induced during that operation; in none of the others was PVD found, whether by OCT or fundoscopy. This was true both before and after the foveal detachment had resolved. Although there was no obvious evidence of vitreomacular membrane or PVD in our cases, even after all the OCT images had been carefully reviewed, it remains possible that posterior hyaloid detachment was not detected by OCT before the resolution of foveal detachment [12]. Nonetheless, as our cases were different from those of previous reports, we believe a different mechanism may have been involved in the formation of foveal detachment, and factors other than PVD may have been responsible for the resolution of macular detachment in the eyes without detectable vitreomacular interface tractions.

In previous studies, PPV with or without ILM peeling has been used to treat foveal detachment and foveoschisis [1, 2, 5, 6]; the procedure is generally associated with a positive visual outcome. A less invasive procedure using the gas tamponade has also been proposed to treat myopic foveoschisis with foveal detachment, and also results in favorable outcomes [7]. However, macular hole formation is not an uncommon complication after vitrectomy to treat myopic foveoschisis [1, 5, 6], especially in those with IS/OS junction defect [6]. In our study, although seven of the eight patients had IS/OS junction defect, none developed macular hole after their foveal detachment had resolved spontaneously.

Subretinal fluid was the main cause of visual impairment among our patients; visual acuity improved significantly after the retina reattached, even in those with longstanding subretinal fluid and IS/OS junction defect. Nonetheless, the final visual acuity was poor in most cases, because of the duration for which the subretinal fluid and the disruption to the IS/OS junction had persisted.

The present study was limited by its small number of patients. Furthermore, as it was retrospective in nature, it lacked a well-designed control group. Nonetheless, the investigation constituted a longitudinal follow-up, over a relatively long period, of patients with foveoschisis and foveal detachment. Furthermore, our report presents the common OCT findings in such cases. We found that foveal detachment can spontaneously resolve through previously unreported mechanisms; this should be taken into consideration before surgery is planned, especially in eyes with a relatively short axial length, a predominant outer segment retinoschisis, or no obvious vitreomacular

interface traction. Further studies are needed, using a greater number of cases and well controlled approaches, to determine the exact predictive factors for this different clinical course.

Conclusions

Spontaneous reattachment of foveal detachment and resolution of foveoschisis can occur in cases with high myopic traction maculopathy without evidence of PVD, especially in those without obvious vitreomacular tractions. This possibility should be taken into consideration before surgery is planned in such cases.

Abbreviations
BCVA: best-corrected visual acuity; CFT: central foveal thickness; ILM: internal limiting membrane; IPL: inner plexiform layer; IS/OS: inner segment/outer segment; OCT: optical coherence tomography; PPV: pars plana vitrectomy; PVD: posterior vitreous detachment.

Competing interests
None of the authors have any competing interests, financial or otherwise.

Authors' contributions
TL, TH, and CY were involved in management, analysis, interpretation, and preparation of the data, as well as interpretation and preparation of the manuscript. All authors read and approved the final manuscript.

Acknowledgements
The authors received no grant support in reporting these clinical observations.

References
1. Gaucher D, Haouchine B, Tadayoni R, Massin P, Erginay A, Benhamou N, et al. Long-term follow-up of high myopic foveoschisis: natural course and surgical outcome. Am J Ophthalmol. 2007;143(3):455–62.
2. Fang X, Weng Y, Xu S, Chen Z, Liu J, Chen B, et al. Optical coherence tomographic characteristics and surgical outcome of eyes with myopic foveoschisis. Eye. 2009;23(6):1336–42.
3. Fujimoto M, Hangai M, Suda K, Yoshimura N. Features associated with foveal retinal detachment in myopic macular retinoschisis. Am J Ophthalmol. 2010;150(6):863–70.
4. Shimada N, Tanaka Y, Tokoro T, Ohno-Matsui K. Natural course of myopic traction maculopathy and factors associated with progression or resolution. Am J Ophthalmol. 2013;156(5):948–57e1.
5. Kobayashi H, Kishi S. Vitreous surgery for highly myopic eyes with foveal detachment and retinoschisis. Ophthalmology. 2003;110(9):1702–7.
6. Gao X, Ikuno Y, Fujimoto S, Nishida K. Risk factors for development of full-thickness macular holes after pars plana vitrectomy for myopic foveoschisis. Am J Ophthalmol. 2013;155(6):1021–7e1.
7. Wu TY, Yang CH, Yang CM. Gas tamponade for myopic foveoschisis with foveal detachment. Graefe's archive for clinical and experimental ophthalmology. Graefes Arch Clin Exp Ophthalmol. 2013;251(5):1319–24.
8. Polito A, Lanzetta P, Del Borrello M, Bandello F. Spontaneous resolution of a shallow detachment of the macula in a highly myopic eye. Am J Ophthalmol. 2003;135(4):546–7.
9. Hirota K, Hirakata A, Inoue M. Dehiscence of detached internal limiting membrane in eyes with myopic traction maculopathy with spontaneous resolution. BMC Ophthalmol. 2014;14(1):39.
10. Kuhn F. Internal limiting membrane removal for macular detachment in highly myopic eyes. Am J Ophthalmol. 2003;135(4):547–9.
11. Sayanagi K, Morimoto Y, Ikuno Y, Tano Y. Spectral-domain optical coherence tomographic findings in myopic foveoschisis. Retina. 2010;30(4):623–8.

12.   Wu PC, Chen YJ, Chen YH, Chen CH, Shin SJ, Tsai CL, et al. Factors
       associated with foveoschisis and foveal detachment without macular hole
       in high myopia. Eye. 2009;23(2):356–61.
13.   Shimada N, Ohno-Matsui K, Yoshida T, Sugamoto Y, Tokoro T, Mochizuki M.
       Progression from macular retinoschisis to retinal detachment in highly
       myopic eyes is associated with outer lamellar hole formation. Br J
       Ophthalmol. 2008;92(6):762–4.

10

Effects of intraocular lenses with different diopters on chromatic aberrations in human eye models

Hui Song, Xiaoyong Yuan and Xin Tang[*]

Abstract

Background: In this study, the effects of intraocular lenses (IOLs) with different diopters (D) on chromatic aberration were investigated in human eye models, and the influences of the central thickness of IOLs on chromatic aberration were compared.

Methods: A Liou-Brennan-based IOL eye model was constructed using ZEMAX optical design software. Spherical IOLs with different diopters (AR40e, AMO Company, USA) were implanted; modulation transfer function (MTF) values at 3 mm of pupil diameter and from 0 to out-of-focus blur were collected and graphed.

Results: MTF values, measured at 555 nm of monochromatic light under each spatial frequency, were significantly higher than the values measured at 470 to 650 nm of polychromatic light. The influences of chromatic aberration on MTF values decreased with the increase in IOL diopter when the spatial frequency was ≤12 c/d, while increased effects were observed when the spatial frequency was ≥15 c/d. The MTF values of each IOL eye model were significantly lower than the MTF values of the Liou-Brennan eye models when measured at 555 nm of monochromatic light and at 470 to 650 nm of polychromatic light. The MTF values were also found to be increased with the increase in IOL diopter.

Conclusion: With higher diopters of IOLs, the central thickness increased accordingly, which could have created increased chromatic aberration and decreased the retinal image quality. To improve the postoperative visual quality, IOLs with lower chromatic aberration should be selected for patients with short axial lengths.

Keywords: Intraocular lens, Computer simulation, Diopter, Chromatic aberration, Modulation transfer function

Background

In polychromatic light, the retinal image quality is affected by interactions between monochromatic and chromatic aberrations. Some study had shown that ocular longitudinal chromatic aberration (LCA) was low intersubject variability and the LCA was independence of the presence of high order aberration [1]. Chromatic aberration has attracted increasing attention in intraocular lenses (IOLs) implantation for cataract surgeries. Recent studies have demonstrated that correcting monochromatic aberrations and chromatic aberrations at the same time could improve visual acuity and contrast

sensitivity [2–4]. Applegate et al. [5] also demonstrated that correction of spherical aberrations could increase the contrast sensitivity of the retina by 12-fold, and correcting chromatic aberration could increase contrast sensitivity by 5-fold, while correcting both spherical and chromatic aberrations simultaneously could strikingly increase contrast sensitivity by 25-fold.

In Weeber's study, subjects were implanted with an IOL correcting both LCA and spherical aberration (SA) in one eye and an IOL correcting only SA in the fellow eye. Although this study included a small number of subjects, it showed a tendency for better visual performance in the eyes where both aberrations were corrected [6]. Considering that the LCA causes a substantial defocus over the visible range of about 2 diopters (D), the additional correction of this aberration should

* Correspondence: tangprofessor@aliyun.com
Tianjin Eye Hospital, Tianjin Key Laboratory of Ophthalmology and Vision Science, Clinical College of Ophthalmology, Tianjin Medical University, No. 4 Gansu Rd, Heping District, Tianjin 300020, China

further improve visual quality even considering the protective mechanisms [7]. Perez-Merino et al. have reported the chromatic difference of focus in two groups of pseudophakic eyes implanted with IOLs of different materials, and found statistical difference, consistent with Abbe number of IOL materials in the 532–787 nm range [8].

Chromatic aberration is not only associated with Abbe number, which is widely known by researchers, but some other factors, including IOL shapes (thickness and radii of curvature) and the value of the refractive index material, could also affect chromatic aberrations [9]. Investigating the effects of IOLs with different diopters on chromatic aberrations in human eyes could help to further improve patients' visual quality as well as the design of IOLs [10].

In the present study, Liou-Brennan-based IOL eye models [11] were constructed using ZEMAX optical design software (ZEMAX Development Corporation, Bellevue, WA, USA), and IOLs were implanted to investigate the effects of IOLs with different diopters on the modulation transfer function (MTF) values in monochromatic and polychromatic light.

Methods

Construction parameters of the Liou-Brennan eye model
The Liou-Brennan eye model was used as the control (Table 1, Fig. 1), while for the treatment, another eye model, namely an IOL eye model that was constructed according to the process of constructing the control eye model, except for the gradient of the refractive index lens, was replaced by certain IOLs. All the study was approved by the Research Ethics Committee at the Tianjin Eye Hospital.

Optical parameters of IOLs
To simulate and investigate the retinal image quality of human eye models after implantation of IOLs with different diopters (–10 D, 0 D, 10 D, 20 D, and 30 D), traditional spherical IOLs AR40e, (Abbott Medical Optics, Santa Ana, CA, US) were used in the present study. The optical parameters of these IOLs are listed in Table 2.

Construction of the eye models
The construction of a physical model of the human eyes is based on the anatomical features of humans and on experimental results [12]. The Liou-Brennan eye model has been regarded as the most comprehensive and accurate human model that best fulfills the physiological status of human eyes [13]. The parameters of the Liou-Brennan eye model were entered into the ZEMAX optical design software to construct models of natural and aphakic eyes. Then, IOLs with different diopters were implanted to replace the natural lenses (the posterior surface of the IOL coincided with the posterior surface of the natural lens) to construct the IOL eye model. The vitreous chamber depth was optimized until the out-of-focus blur was 0 (indicating that parallel rays could focus on the retina). The transmission of light through the optical systems was simulated according to the ray-tracing theory (Fig. 2). The axial lengths of the IOLs with different diopters are listed in Table 2.

Modulation transfer function (MTF) is the difference between monochromatic and polychromatic MTF in the same space frequencies. With an IOL diopter increase, the optical zone increases in thickness, resulting in the optical path leading to increased color. A% represents the magnitude of this change. The MTF values at 3 mm of pupil diameter for each of the IOLs were collected with monochromatic (555 nm) and polychromatic (470–650 nm) light under different spatial frequencies and were graphed. Yellow-green light with a wavelength of 555 nm was chosen as the monochromatic light in the present study, while for polychromatic light, we chose light with wavelengths ranging from 470 to 650 nm (including monochromatic light with wavelengths of 470, 510, 555, 610, and 650 nm and with weights of 0.091, 0.503, 1, 0.503, and 0.107, respectively). All of the MTF values were collected using the ZEMAX Optical Design Program.

Comparison of the MTF curves
Origin software, version 7.0, was used for the data processing and graphing. The trends and difference were compared among the MTF curves that were constructed with the data collected under same conditions. Student's t test was used to compare the differences between the 2

Table 1 Construction parameters of the Liou-Brennan eye model

Surface	Radius of curvature (mm)	Asphericity	Thickness (mm)	Refractive index (555 nm)
1	7.77	−0.18	0.50	1.376
2	6.40	−0.60	3.16	1.336
3(pupil)	12.40	−0.94	1.59	Grad A[a]
4	Infinity	—	2.43	Grad P[a]
5	−8.10	+0.96	16.27	1.336

[a]:Grad A and P represent different formulas for calculating gradient refractive index formula

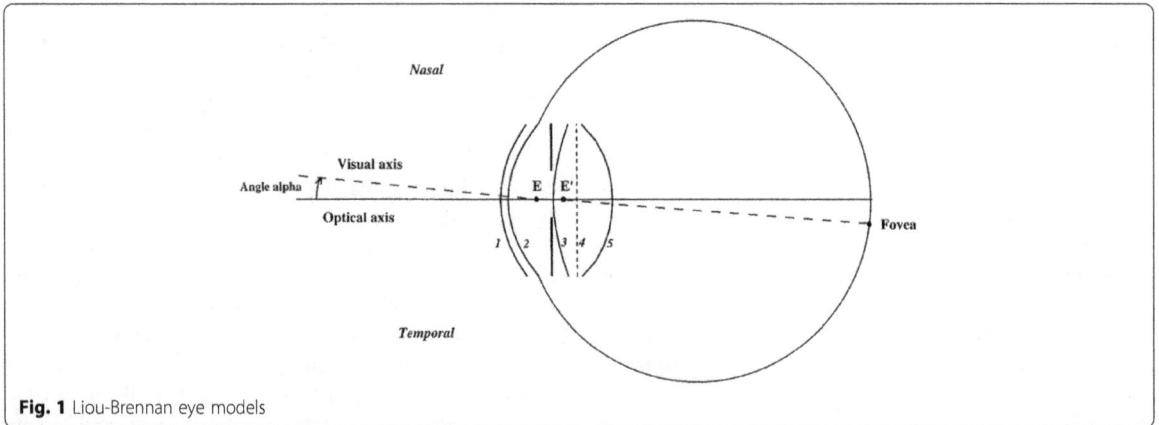

Fig. 1 Liou-Brennan eye models

groups. One-way ANOVA test was used to make comparisons between multiple groups (>3 groups), and the Dunnett test was further used to compare different IOLs groups with the Liou group. Statistical significance was set at $p < 0.05$.

Results

Comparisons of the MTF values of the IOL eye model under monochromatic and polychromatic light

MTF values at 3 mm of pupil diameter, measured at 555 nm of monochromatic light under each spatial frequency (ranging from 0 to 60 c/d), were significantly higher than the values at 470–650 nm of polychromatic light (Fig. 3a–f). In addition, the differences between the MTF values that were measured under monochromatic (555 nm) and polychromatic (470–650 nm) light increased with the IOL diopter (i.e., the central thickness of the IOLs increased with the diopters, and the axial length decreased accordingly) (Fig. 3a–e). We also found that the A-value increased with the spatial frequencies (SFs), indicating the increased influence of chromatic aberration on MTF values (Table 3). In contrast, the A-value decreased (indicating that the influence of chromatic aberration on MTF values decreased) with the increase of IOL diopters when the MTF values were measured at 3 mm of pupil diameter with spatial frequencies ≤12 c/d. However, the A-value was found to be increased with the IOL diopters when the spatial frequencies were ≥15 c/d (Table 3).

Comparisons of the MTF values between the IOL and Liou-Brennan eye models under monochromatic and polychromatic light

The MTF values of most of the IOL eye models were significantly lower than those of the Liou-Brennan eye models when measured under monochromatic light (555 nm), with pupil diameter of 3 mm and spatial frequencies between 0 and 60 c/d, and F values from 10, 20, 30, 40, 50, and 60 c/d were 3.96, 14.35, 29.07, 37.36, 51.34, 69.39 with $p < 0.05$ respectively. However, the MTF value of the IOL eye model with 30 D was slightly higher than the MTF value of the Liou-Brennan eye model when measured with the spatial frequencies ≥50 c/d. The MTF values of the IOL eye models increased with the IOL diopter (Fig. 4a). When measured under polychromatic light (470–650 nm), the MTF values of the IOL eye models were significantly lower than those of the Liou-Brennan eye models, with pupil diameter of 3 mm and spatial frequencies between 0 and 60 c/d with F values 3.38, 8.91, 17.15, 28.69, 47.45, and 64.65 ($p < 0.05$), but the differences between the IOL and Liou-Brennan eye models were substantially less than those under monochromatic light (555 nm). We also

Table 2 Optical parameters and axial lengths of IOLs with different diopters

Diopters (D)	Refractive index	Curvature radius of the anterior surface (mm)	Central thickness (mm)	Curvature radius of the posterior surface (mm)	Axial length (mm)
+30.00	1.470	6.1951	1.224	−15.7226	22.6597
+20.00	1.470	11.6078	0.977	−15.7226	24.9205
+10.00	1.470	26.7716	0.760	−26.7716	27.7042
0.00	1.470	38.1000	0.533	38.0492	31.3168
−10.00	1.470	50.8000	0.397	10.5918	36.4486

IOL intraocular lens

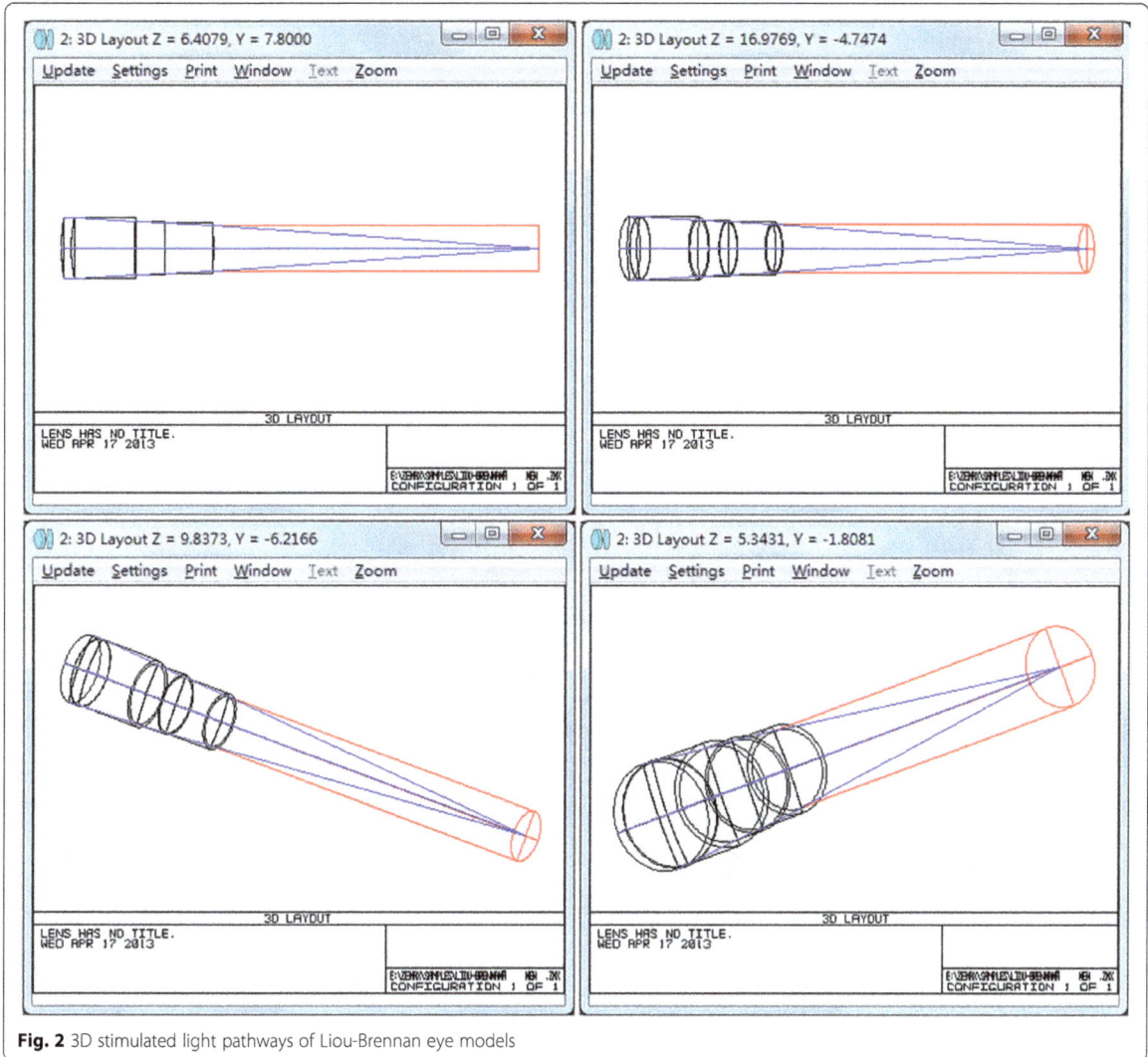

Fig. 2 3D stimulated light pathways of Liou-Brennan eye models

observed that the MTF values increased with IOL diopters, as measured under monochromatic light (Fig. 4b).

Discussion
Parameters of IOL eye model
The pupil plays an important role in optical imaging [14]. Studies [3, 4, 15, 16] have demonstrated that correcting spherical and chromatic aberrations simultaneously could increase visual acuity and contrast sensitivity under white light as well as provide better visual quality with a broader range of pupil diameters. Decreased visual quality was closely associated with increased spherical aberration of IOLs after the implantation of traditional spherical IOLs [17]; however, a diameter of the pupil of 3 mm is very close to the pupil diameter in diffraction-limited systems (pupil diameter less than 2.5 mm), indicating that the influence from chromatic aberration is even greater than other factors, compared with eyes with their own optical aberrations. Campbell and Gubisch reported that whereas for 4 mm pupils the effect of spherical and chromatic aberration was approximately equal, monochromatic aberrations had a larger effect for large pupils [18]. In the present study, the differences between the MTF values for pupils with diameters less than 3 mm that were measured under monochromatic and polychromatic light were found to increase with diopters, which could have been caused mainly by chromatic aberration. The IOL material and its unique dependency between refractive index and wavelength are of critical importance for the optical performance of IOLs in polychromatic light [19]. As chromatic aberration is associated with the material of

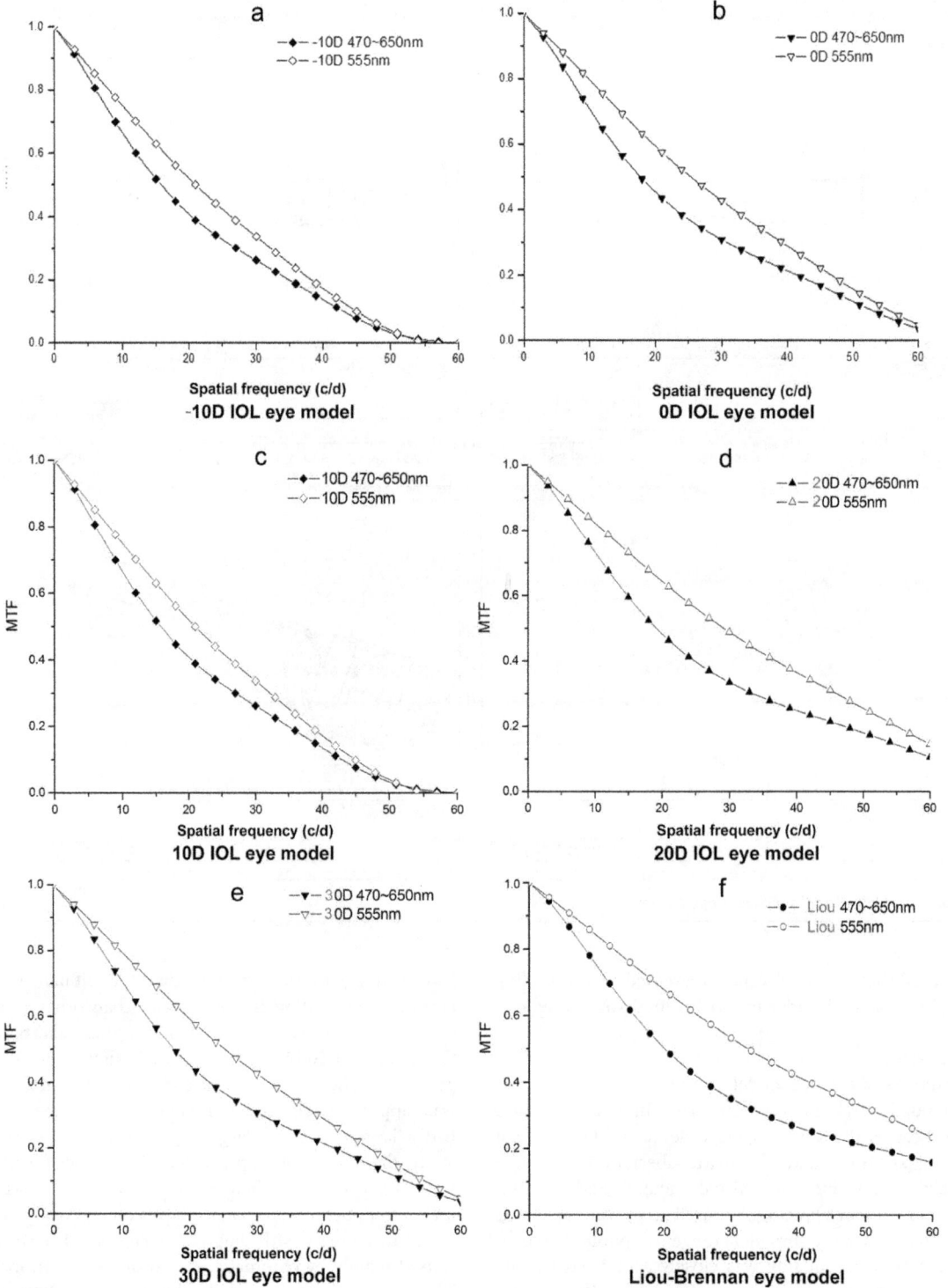

Fig. 3 Modulation transfer function (MTF) curves of the IOLs from −10 diopters (D) to 30 D and Liou-Brennan eye models under monochromatic and polychromatic light. **a**. -10 D IOL eye model, **b**. 0 D IOL eye model, **c**. 10 D IOL eye model, **d**. 20 D IOL eye model, **e**. 30 D IOL eye model, **f**. Liou-Brennan eye model

Table 3 A-value of the IOL eye models with different diopters at 3 mm of the pupil diameter

SF (c/d)	30D	20D	10D	0D	−10D
3	1.241	1.285	1.353	1.449	1.595
6	4.495	4.595	4.752	4.991	5.344
9	8.951	9.077	9.270	9.556	9.923
12	13.909	14.019	14.128	14.271	14.341
15	19.031	18.892	18.768	18.548	17.954
24	31.353	30.192	28.620	26.333	22.675
33	37.830	35.336	32.098	27.644	21.559
42	40.159	36.569	31.629	25.449	21.245
51	40.562	35.455	28.944	24.503	11.747
60	39.331	32.501	27.721	23.957	——

IOL intraocular lens, *SF* spatial frequencies, *MTF* modulation transfer function, *D* diopter, A value = $\Delta MTF/MTF_1$; $\Delta MTF = MTF_1-MTF_2$; MTF_1 represents the MTF values measured under 555 nm of monochromatic light, MTF_2 represents the MTF values measured under 470–650 nm of polychromatic light

thus could provide very limited value for clinical investigations. Lower spatial frequencies could affect outline identification more than higher spatial frequencies, and most of the information that is received by the eyes is from low spatial frequencies [23]. Because excellent retinal image contrast is also required under low spatial frequencies, in addition to higher cut-off spatial frequencies [24], 0–60 c/d of the spatial frequencies were chosen for the investigation in the present study.

The retina is most sensitive to yellow light with a wavelength of 555 nm under photopic conditions [25]; while for polychromatic light, we chose light with wavelengths ranging from 470 to 650 nm (including monochromatic light with wavelengths of 470, 510, 555, 610, and 650 nm and with weight of 0.091, 0.503, 1, 0.503, and 0.107, respectively). The MTF values were measured under monochromatic and polychromatic light and were compared to investigate the effects of chromatic aberration on retinal image qualities.

the IOL, in the present study, only AR40e IOLs were chosen because they were the same type and were designed with the same materials.

Retinal image quality in the human eyes is dependent on the features of neural pathways. Studies have demonstrated that the cut-off spatial frequency is approximately 60 c/d under photopic conditions [20]; however, when the spatial frequency was increased to 32 c/d, some healthy adults could not detect the gratings, suggesting that they had very low contrast sensitivity [21]. Qu et al. also demonstrated that MTF could be used to reflect the contrast sensitivity of the optical system of the eyes [22]. The MTF values of the eyes of healthy adults are very low at a spatial frequency of 32 c/d and

Visual qualities of the IOL eye models

In the present study, we investigated the effects of IOLs on the chromatic aberrations of human eyes with different refraction states. The findings demonstrated that the MTF values were significantly lower when measured under polychromatic light than when measured under monochromatic light for each of the IOLs, without influences from other factors, suggesting that chromatic aberrations could reduce retinal image quality. Polychromatic MTF contains information on both monochromatic and chromatic aberrations [26]. While the monochromatic MTF of the eye clearly exceeds the polychromatic MTF and there is evidence that, in the absence of both chromatic and monochromatic aberrations, visual performance exceeds that

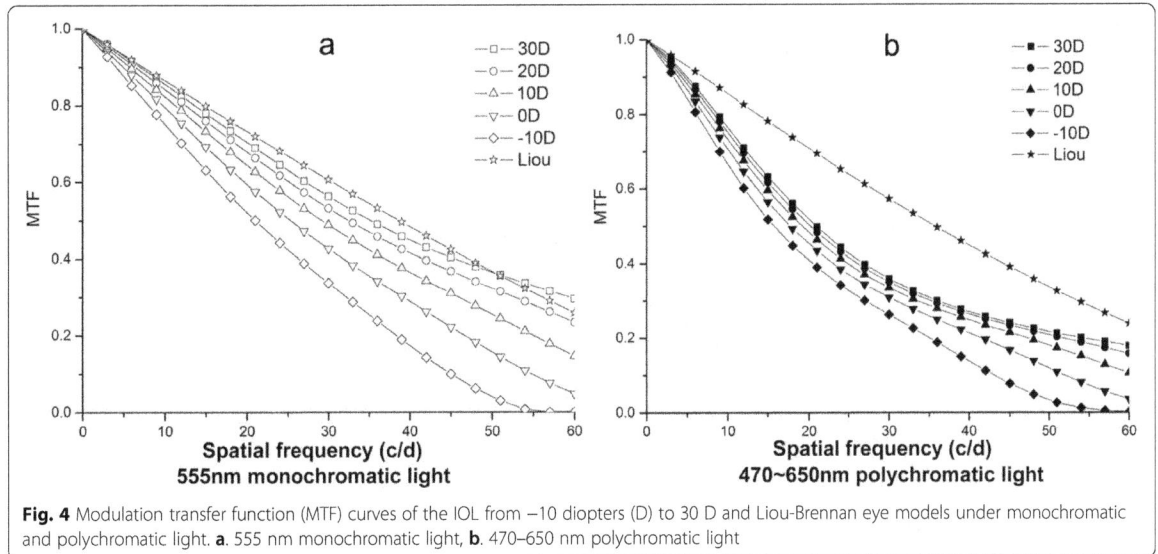

Fig. 4 Modulation transfer function (MTF) curves of the IOL from −10 diopters (D) to 30 D and Liou-Brennan eye models under monochromatic and polychromatic light. **a**. 555 nm monochromatic light, **b**. 470–650 nm polychromatic light

with noncorrected chromatic aberrations [8, 27, 28]. In addition, we also found that the difference between the MTF values that were measured under monochromatic and polychromatic light increased with the diopters of the IOLs (indicating that the central thickness of the IOLs increased), suggesting the increased influences of chromatic aberrations on retinal image quality. The findings of the present study also suggested that shorter axial length required IOLs with higher diopters, which could result in higher chromatic aberrations. Therefore, for patients with short axial length who require IOLs with high diopters, IOLs with low chromatic aberration should be selected to improve the postoperative visual quality.

However, with the increase in IOL diopters, the influence of chromatic aberrations on the MTF values decreased when the spatial frequencies were ≤12 c/d for pupils with diameters of 3 mm, which could also reflect the effects of chromatic aberrations on the retinal image quality decreasing at medium or low spatial frequency when IOL with higher central thickness was used. Generally, most of the information that is received by the eyes is from low spatial frequencies, and lower spatial frequencies could affect outline identification more than higher spatial frequencies [23]. In another study performed by Nio et al., the findings showed that the contrast sensitivity of normal human eyes peaked at medium and low spatial frequencies (4–8 c/d) [21]. Therefore, for elderly patients undergoing cataract extraction and IOL implantation, IOLs with higher diopters could reduce the effects of chromatic aberrations on retinal image quality while identifying the outlines of objects, whereas IOLs with lower diopters could increase the effects.

The findings of the present study demonstrated that the MTF values of all of the IOL eye models were lower than those of the Liou-Brennan eye models, under either monochromatic or polychromatic light, suggesting that the implantation of IOLs could reduce the retinal image quality of human eyes [8, 29], although the difference was not that significant for the "common" implanted IOL-powers (from 15 D to 25 D). The differences between the MTF values in the IOL eye models and the Liou-Brennan eye models were not as high under polychromatic light than under monochromatic light (555 nm), suggesting that the introduction of chromatic aberrations could further decrease retinal image quality. Interestingly, we found that the MTF values increased with the IOL diopters, either under 555 nm of monochromatic light or under polychromatic light, which could have been caused by the interactions of monochromatic aberrations and chromatic aberrations in the eye models. In addition, the axial length of the eye model could change after the implantation of IOLs, as well as optimization of optical aberrations and out-of-

focus images, which could in turn affect the MTF values. Moreover, with the increase in diopters of the IOLs, the central thickness also increased. Because the thicknesses of IOLs with higher diopters are closer those in the Liou-Brennan eye models (4.02 mm) with the increased IOL diopters, the MTF values of the IOL eye models could also approach the MTF values of the Liou-Brennan eye models. However, no studies have investigated the detailed mechanisms, and further studies are warranted to validate the above-mentioned theories.

Conclusion

The present study showed that IOLs with different diopters affected chromatic aberrations of the eye when the diameter of the pupil was 3 mm. The chromatic aberrations increased when IOLs with higher diopters (which also indicates higher central thickness) were implanted, thus reducing retinal image quality. The implantation of IOLs with relative high diopters for patients with less axial depth created relatively high chromatic aberrations, which could influence the visual quality of the patients. Interestingly, the increase in IOL diopters was mirrored by the decrease in the influence of the chromatic aberrations on visual quality at medium or low spatial frequencies. However, contradictory results were found at high spatial frequencies. The visual quality of the IOL eye model further decreased due to the effects of chromatic aberrations. The findings of the present study provided evidence for the designing of IOLs in the near future.

Abbreviations

IOLs: intraocular lenses; D: diopter; MTF: modulation transfer function; SF: spatial frequencies; LCA: longitudinal chromatic aberration; SA: spherical aberration.

Competing interests

The authors declare that they have no competing or financial interests.

Authors' contributions

HS has been involved in designing the study and acquisition of the most data, and drafting the manuscript of this study. XY made contributions in adjusting the experimental designs, analyzing the results and revising the manuscript. XT supervised the study designs, analysed and interpreted the results, and did extensive contribution to the manuscript draft. All authors read and approved the final manuscript.

Acknowledgments

This study was supported by the Key Projects of the Bureau of Health, Tianjin (2012KR17, 10KG108).

References

1. Vinas M, Dorronsoro C, Cortes D, Pascual D, Marcos S. Longitudinal chromatic aberration of the human eye in the visible and near infrared from wavefront sensing, double-pass and psychophysics. Biomed Opt Express. 2015;6(3):948–62.
2. Artal P, Manzanera S, Piers P, Weeber H. Visual effect of the combined correction of spherical and longitudinal chromatic aberrations. Opt Express. 2010;18:1637–48.

3. Weeber HA, Piers PA. Theoretical performance of intraocular lenses correcting both spherical and chromatic aberration. J Refract Surg. 2012;28:48–52.
4. Sabesan R, Zheleznyak L, Yoon G. Binocular visual performance and summation after correcting higher order aberrations. Biomed Opt Express. 2012;3:3176-89.
5. Applegate RA, Thibos LN, Hilmantel G. Optics of aberroscopy and super vision. J Cataract Refract Surg. 2001;27:1093–107.
6. Weeber HA, Pohl R, Mester U, Piers PA. Visual performance of pseudophakic eyes corrected for spherical and chromatic aberrations with an achromatic intraocular lens. Invest Ophthalmol Vis Sci. 2013;54:808.
7. Schwarz C, Canovas C, Manzanera S, Weeber H, Prieto PM, Piers P, et al. Binocular visual acuity for the correction of spherical aberration in polychromatic and monochromatic light. J Vis. 2014;14:1–11.
8. Perez-Merino P, Dorronsoro C, Llorente L, Duran S, Jimenez-Alfaro I, Marcos S. In vivo chromatic aberration in eyes implanted with intraocular lenses. Invest Ophthalmol Vis Sci. 2013;54:2654–61.
9. Siedlecki D, Ginis HS. On the longitudinal chromatic aberration of the intraocular lenses. Optom and Vis Sci. 2007;84:984–9.
10. López-Gil N, Bradley A. The potential for and challenges of spherical and chromatic aberration correction with new IOL designs. Br J Ophthalmol. 2013;97(6):677–8.
11. Liou HL, Brennan NA. Anatomically accurate, finite model eye for optical modeling. J Opt Soc Am A Opt Image Sci Vis. 1997;14:1684–95.
12. Piers PA, Weeber HA, Artal P, Norrby S. Theoretical comparison of aberration-correcting customized and aspheric intraocular lenses. J Refract Surg. 2007;23:374–84.
13. Liang J, Williams DR. Aberration and retinal image quality of the normal human eye. J Opt Soc Am A Opt Image Sci Vis. 1997;14:2873–83.
14. Thibos LN, Bradley A, Still DL, Zhang X, Howarth PA. Theory and measurement of ocular chromatic aberration. Vision Res. 1990;30:33–49.
15. Awwad ST, El-Kateb M, McCulley JP. Comparative higher-order aberration measurement of the LADARWave and Visx WaveScan aberration at varying pupil sizes and after pharmacologic dilation and cycloplegia. J Cataract Refract Surg. 2006;32:203–14.
16. Ravikumar S, Bradley A, Thibos LN. Chromatic aberration and polychromatic image quality with diffractive multifocal intraocular lenses. J Cataract Refract Surg. 2014;40(7):1192–204.
17. Guirao A, Redondo M, Arta LP. Optical aberrations of the human cornea as a function of age. J Opt Soc Am A Opt Image Sci Vis. 2000;17:1697–702.
18. Campbell FW, Gubisch RW. The effect of chromatic aberration on visual acuity. J Physiol. 1967;192:345–58.
19. Siedlecki D, Jozwik A, Zajac M, Hill-Bator A, Turno-Krecicka A. In vivo longitudinal chromatic aberration of pseudophakic eyes. Optom Vis Sci. 2014;91:240–6.
20. Sekiguchi N, Williams DR, Brainard DH. Efficiency in detection of isoluminant and isochromatic interference fringes. J Opt Soc Am A Opt Image Sci Vis. 1993;10:2118–33.
21. Nio YK, Jansonius NM, Fidler V, Geraghty E, Norrby S, Kooijman AC. Age-related changes of defocus-specific contrast sensitivity in healthy subjects. Opthal Physiol Opt. 2000;20:323–34.
22. Qu J, Lv F, Mao X. Evaluation of visual correction. Chin J Ophthalmol. 2003;6:325–7.
23. Wang Y, Zhao K. Wavefront Aberration and Clinical Vision Correction. Beijing: People's Medical Publishing House; 2011.
24. Kornowski JA, Petersik JT. Effect on face recognition of spatial-frequency information contained in inspection and test stimuli. J Gen Psychol. 2003;130:229–44.
25. Zhao H, Mainster MA. The effect of chromatic dispersion on pseudophakic optical performance. Br J Ophthalmol. 2007;91:1225–9.
26. Williams CS, Becklund OA. Introduction to the optical transfer function. Bellingham: SPIE Press; 1989.
27. McLellan JS, Marcos S, Prieto PM, Burns SA. Imperfect optics may be the eye's defense against chromatic blur. Nature. 2002;417:174–6.
28. Ravikumar S, Thibos LN, Bradley A. Calculation of retinal image quality for polychromatic light. J Opt Soc Am A Opt Image Sci Vis. 2008;25:2395–407.
29. Franchini A. Compromise between spherical and chromatic aberration and depth of focus in aspheric intraocular lenses. J Cataract Refract Surg. 2007;33:497–509.

11

Use of flucinolone acetonide for patients with diabetic macular oedema: patient selection criteria and early outcomes in real world setting

Ibrahim Elaraoud[1]*, Walter Andreatta[1], Andrej Kidess[2], Ajay Bhatnagar[1], Marie Tsaloumas[2], Fahad Quhill[3] and Yit Yang[1,4]

Abstract

Introduction: Fluocinolone acetonide slow release implant (Iluvien®) was approved in December 2013 in UK for treatment of eyes which are pseudophakic with DMO that is unresponsive to other available therapies. This approval was based on evidence from FAME trials which were conducted at a time when ranibizumab was not available. There is a paucity of data on implementation of guidance on selecting patients for this treatment modality and also on the real world outcome of fluocinolone therapy especially in those patients that have been unresponsive to ranibizumab therapy.

Method: Retrospective study of consecutive patients treated with fluocinolone between January and August 2014 at three sites were included to evaluate selection criteria used, baseline characteristics and clinical outcomes at 3-month time point.

Results: Twenty two pseudophakic eyes of 22 consecutive patients were included. Majority of patients had prior therapy with multiple intravitreal anti-VEGF injections. Four eyes had controlled glaucoma. At baseline mean VA and CRT were 50.7 letters and 631 μm respectively. After 3 months, 18 patients had improved CRT of which 15 of them also had improved VA. No adverse effects were noted. One additional patient required IOP lowering medication. Despite being unresponsive to multiple prior therapies including laser and anti-VEGF injections, switching to fluocinolone achieved treatment benefit.

Conclusion: The patient level selection criteria proposed by NICE guidance on fluocinolone appeared to be implemented. This data from this study provides new evidence on early outcomes following fluocinolone therapy in eyes with DMO which had not responded to laser and other intravitreal agents.

Keywords: Fluocinolone Acetonide, Iluvien, Diabetic macular oedema, Patient selection, early clinical outcome, visual acuity, central retinal thickness

Background

Diabetic Macular Oedema (DMO) is one of the leading causes of blindness in the working-age population [1, 2] In the UK, 17.7 % of severe sight impairment certifications in adults aged 16–64 has been attributed to diabetes [3]. Several landmark clinical trials have established the firm position of intravitreal anti-VEGF agents as the first line therapy of choice for DMO [4–6]. Intravitreal corticosteroids have also been shown to be effective in achieving visual gain and reduction of oedema in DMO and with reduced frequency of injections needed [7–9], but with associated risks of causing steroid induced cataract or ocular hypertension and glaucoma. Current guidelines therefore, recommend their use only in those eyes which have either chronic oedema not responsive to laser or those eyes with oedema that have not responded to repeated injections of anti-VEGF agents [10, 11].

* Correspondence: i_melaroud@hotmail.com
[1]Wolverhampton Eye Infirmary, New Cross Hospital, Wednesfield Road, Wolverhampton WV10 0QP, UK
Full list of author information is available at the end of the article

There are currently three corticosteroid agents that have been used for DMO; triamcinolone [7], fluocinolone implant releasing 0.2 µg/day of fluocinolone acetonide (ILUVIEN®, Alimera Sciences Limited, Aldershot, UK) [8] and dexamethasone implant containing 700 µg of dexamethasone (Ozurdex®, Allergan, Inc., Irvine, CA, USA) [9]. The United Kingdom was one of the first countries to approve the use fluocinolone implant for treatment of DMO but current National Institute for Care and Health Excellence (NICE) guidance recommends its use only in pseudophakic eyes with DMO that has been unresponsive to other available therapy [10]. Due to this unique selection criteria and early exposure to this technology, the setting in our National Health Service in the United Kingdom is therefore ideal for reporting the implementation of this guidance, in particular, the early experiences in patient selection behaviour by clinicians and also early clinical outcomes in the real world. Such data may be useful for developing future strategies for reducing the frequency of side effects, design of follow-up regimen that can further justify the use of such a unique treatment with its prolonged duration of action.

This retrospective study reports the initial real world experience of implementation of TA301 in the clinical setting, in particular, the patient level criteria used for selection of patients for intravitreal fluocinolone implant, the initial treatment response and the short term safety profile.

Methods

Consecutive patients treated at each of three hospital departments using fluocinolone implant for DMO according to NICE guidance (TA301) between January 2014 and August 2014 were identified at each site using their respective patient database systems for tracking patients on intravitreal therapies. The study involved collection of data retrospectively from case notes and OCT scans performed as part of patients' standard care pathways at each institution, approval by Ethics Committee was not required according to the institutional review policies at each site. Case notes review was performed and data were collected at baseline, which was at the time of fluocinolone implant and at the visit nearest to the 3 month time-point of follow-up. At the baseline time-point, data were collected on demographics, visual acuity (treated and fellow eyes), OCT parameters, IOP, IOP lowering medication use, presence of co-existing ocular pathology and prior laser for DMO and DR or intravitreal therapy and duration of DMO. At the 3 month time-point, data were collected on visual acuity (treated eyes), IOP, IOP lowering medication use and OCT parameters. Snellen visual acuity was converted using a standard estimation method so that all acuity data was presented in terms of

number of ETDRS letters. The type of conversion method we used would convert 6/60 to 35 letters and 6/6 to 85 letters as obtained when an ETDRS acuity is used at 2 meters for acuity scoring. [12, 13]. Descriptive statistics were used to present the data to demonstrate the spectrum of baseline characteristics with particular emphasis on the types of prior therapies which had been attempted on these eyes prior to using fluocinolone. Short term follow-up data was analysed to show the initial efficacy and occurrences of any serious adverse events.

Results

A total of 22 patients (14 M:8 F) aged between 42 and 85 years (mean 67.2 years) were included. Nineteen patients had Type-2 and 3 patients had Type-1 diabetes mellitus; mean duration of diabetes was 17.9 years (range: 3–60). All patients had unilateral fluocinolone implants ie; 11 right and 11 left eyes treated.

Visual acuity conversion for Snellen fraction to ETDRS was required for five patients. In all other patients, acuity scores were captured directly using ETDRS chart. Treated eyes had mean baseline visual acuity of 50.7 letters and mean CRT of 631 µm. Twenty two eyes had foveal eversion and 13 eyes had pre-existing vitreo-retinal interface abnormalities. Majority of eyes had prior laser of either macular or pan retinal photocoagulation. All 22 eyes had prior intravitreal therapy. Thirteen eyes had prior ranibizumab or bevacizumab, 3 eyes had both ranibizumab and bevacizumab and 6 eyes had prior intravitreal triamcinolone for DMO. Mean duration of DMO was 26.2 months (range: 9-47). All patients had a minimum of 8 weeks wash out period after using Anti-VEGF before having the fluocinolone implant.

Fellow eyes had visual acuities ranging from NPL to 85 letters. In 11 patients, the fellow eye had visual acuities equal to or worse than treated eyes. Baseline characteristics of 22 treated eyes are shown in Table 1. From these characteristics, it is evident that the eyes that were selected had moderately low visual acuities, severe macular thickening, presence of other co-existing pathologies such as epiretinal membranes and controlled glaucoma.

At the 3 month time-point, mean change in BCVA for all patients was +6.4 ETDRS letters (SD: ±7.2; range: -11 to +25). A gain of >0 letters was seen in 21 eyes (95.4 %); 0-4 letters in 4 eyes (18.1 %), 5-9 letters in 7 eyes (31.8 %) and ≥10 letters in 6 eyes (27.2 %), CRT after three months reduced by 148.9 µm (SD: ±240.6; range: -714 to +385 µm). A total of 18 out of 22 eyes (81.8 %) showed some reduction in CRT at 3-months. In the 4 eyes without CRT improvement, the mean increase in CRT was 134.75 µm (SD: ±169.8; range: +26 to +385 µm).

Table 1 Baseline parameters of Fluocinolone Acetonide implant treated eyes

Parameter	Value
Visual Acuity (ETDRS letters)	Range (2–85), Mean (50.7)
Central Retinal Thickness (Micrometers)	Range (373–1052) .Mean (631)
Duration of DMO(Months)	Range (9-47). Mean (26.2)
Foveal eversion	21
Pseudophakia	22
Eyes with one co-existing pathology	ERM(n = 11)
	VMT(n = 2)
	Glaucoma/Ocular hypertension (n = 4)
	NVD n = 1
	NVE n = 1
Eyes with >1 co-existing pathologies	3
Eyes on IOP lowering drugs	4
Eyes with prior macular laser only	15
Eyes with prior vitrectomy for DMO/ERM	1
Eyes with prior intravitreal therapy	Ranibizumab only– n = 11
	Bevacizumab only n = 2
	Rani and Beva n = 3
	Triamcinolone n = 6
Eyes with prior PRP	9

Overall, 15 patients (68.2 %) showed some improvement in both visual acuity and CRT, 3 patients (13.6 %) showed some visual gain without any reduction in CRT, another 3 patients (13.6 %) achieved a reduction in CRT without any corresponding visual gain and 1 patient (4.5 %) did not show any improvement in visual acuity or CRT.

Of the 5 eyes which had undergone prior vitrectomy, visual acuity was improved by +7.2 letters (range: 0 to +14) and CRT reduced by 176.8 (range:-714 to +385). Four of 5 eyes showed both a reduction in CRT with improved visual acuity but one patient had reduced CRT (-345) with no gain in visual acuity.

One patient worsened by 11 letters and had increase in CRT of 385 µm; this particular patient had received prior treatment with macular laser and four ranibizumab and one triamcinolone intravitreal injections.

Mean baseline IOP was 16.9 mmHg (SD: ±3.1; range 10–22 mmHg), with the mean change of 0.3 mmHg (SD: ±3.1; range: -7 to +5 mmHg) at month 3. No cases with substantial elevation in IOP were documented in the short follow up period. Of 22 eyes, four eyes, were receiving IOP-lowering drops (timolol and/or latanoprost) prior to fluocinolone implant. Following implant an additional one eye needed IOP lowering medication.

Discussion

Our study set out to evaluate two important aspects in the use of fluocinolone acetonide in the real world clinical setting for treatment of DMO; firstly, the characteristics of patients selected for treatment by clinicians and secondly, the early treatment response seen in their patients.

In terms of selection, we found that fluocinolone implant was used infrequently in patients with DMO. In all three sites, there were only 22 procedures performed in three sites in the 8-month period following approval of fluocinolone by NICE. Given the large number of patients needing repeated injections of ranibizumab for DMO at these sites [14], this infrequent use of fluocinolone suggests that clinicians had a high threshold for using fluocinolone for DMO. The majority of patients did have severe oedema with mean CRT of over 600 µm. The majority of eyes had prior macular laser and all eyes had prior intravitreal therapy. This finding supports the fact that clinicians are following the NICE guidance criterion of unresponsiveness to other available therapy [10]. Six eyes had prior intravitreal triamcinolone but no anti-VEGF. This reflects the general acceptability of switching between corticosteroid agents especially if prior triamcinolone did not cause uncontrolled glaucoma [15]. This may be an observation of a growing trend to use a shorter acting intravitreal corticosteroid such as triamcinolone as a steroid challenge in these patients, a trend which has been adopted by the American Food and Drug Administration (FDA) when fluocinolone was approved to be used in DMO [11]. Another criterion stipulated by NICE guidance is that the treated eyes had to be pseudophakic. In this survey, all treated eyes were already pseudophakic indicating that clinicians are following NICE guidance recommendation carefully. We were also interested to evaluate whether clinicians were reluctant to use fluocinolone in better seeing eyes. With 11 out of 22 eyes being the better seeing eye, it does not appear to be the case that there was any reluctance in the selection behaviour of clinicians to avoid fluocinolone in better seeing eyes. However the majority of eyes had foveal eversion on OCT. This may be a future additional criterion of severity of oedema that could be used to select the most justifiable cases for fluocinolone therapy. All patients in this study had chronic DMO of more than 2 years, Authors could not identify any particular pattern between chronicity of DMO and early response/failure of this cohort of patients although admittedly is a short follow up period.

In terms of early outcome, we found promising results with 18 out of 22 eyes reported to have visual gain and 18 out of 22 eyes with at least a reduction in CRT at month 3 time-point. Figure 1 shows a dramatic reduction of CRT from 960 µm to 246 µm 3 months post

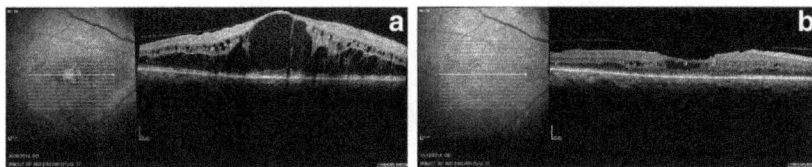

Fig. 1 a Spectral Domain OCT at baseline showing extensive intraretinal fluid with foveal eversion. **b** Spectral Domain OCT at three months showing significant resolution of intraretinal fluid and the re-formation of the foveal dip

fluocinolone. Given the majority of patients had prior injections of ranibizumab or bevacizumab in this study, this highlights the additional value that can be gained by switching from anti-VEGF to intravitreal fluocinolone in unresponsive cases. This also serves as new evidence for switching from ranibizumab to fluocinolone as some patients in the FAME trial had rescue bevacizumab but not ranibizumab and there have been no published series to our knowledge of visual outcome when switching from ranibizumab to fluocinolone. In one case report of a single patient, with longstanding DMO which was unresponsive to ranibizumab, Bertelmann and Shulze reported reduction in oedema and gain in visual acuity following a switch from ranibizumab to fluocinolone implant [16]. The three month follow-up period is admittedly too short for evaluating the risk of IOP rise. In this study, only one patient required commencement of IOP lowering medication at month 3 time-point. Based on available FAME data on IOP response, it is likely that more patients will subsequently develop elevated IOP.

There were limitations in the design of this real world study. The selection of patients for therapy is a complex process involving careful explanation and the confidence expressed by the treating clinician at counselling and a final decision made with the patient preference. It was possible that many other patients who were eligible for therapy but declined due to the risk factors involved. We could not capture those patients who declined treatment with our retrospective design and this study may represent the highest threshold for using fluocinolone at this early stage of implementing NICE guidance. We also captured basic baseline data on patient selection. We were unable in the scope of this study to capture the timescale and progression of DMO in these patients. We recognise that other factors, including the recent worsening of oedema or visual acuity and the frequency of previous visits do have an impact on tendency to use fluocinolone and these factors were not be captured uniformly in this retrospective design.

The strength of this study was the accuracy of the representation of those patients who were treated with fluocinolone. The sites selected were medium sized district general hospital settings as well as large teaching hospital centres which enables translation of our results to the majority of hospital eye departments. The inclusion of all consecutively treated patients in an 8-month period ensured a representative cohort of patients for reporting of a potentially wide spectrum of selection criteria used or variable response to treatment.

Conclusion

Numerous review articles have been published mentioning fluocinolone therapy for DMO but there is a paucity of published data on use of fluocinolone 0.2 µg/day or iluvien® outside the experience of the FAME trial [8, 17]. We are also unaware of any previously published case series describing the experience of switching from ranibizumab to fluocinolone. This study can hope to serve this small gap in our evidence base and also be of value for designing selection and follow-up protocols for treatment of patients with the fluocinolone implant.

Abbreviations
DMO: Diabetic macular oedema; VA: Visual acuity; CRT: Central retinal thinkness; Anti-VEGF: Anti-(vascular endothelial growth factor); NICE: National Institute for Health and Care Excellence; IOP: Intra ocular pressure; OCT: Ocular coherence tomography; EDTRS: Early treatment diabetic retinopathy study.

Competing interests
There was no financial support received related to this article.
IE, WA, AK, AB and MT have no conflicting interests.
Both FQ and YY serve as consultants and speakers for Alimera Science, Allergan, Bayer, Heidelberg and Novartis.

Authors' contributions
IE, WA, AK,AB,MT,FQ and YY all participated in the design of the study, IE, WA AK collected data, MT and FQ helped with statistical analysis and writing the methods and part of the discussion. IE and YY wrote and drafted the manuscript. All authors read and approved the final manuscript.

Acknowledgments
None to acknowledge.

Author details
¹Wolverhampton Eye Infirmary, New Cross Hospital, Wednesfield Road, Wolverhampton WV10 0QP, UK. ²Queen Elizabeth University Hospital Birmingham, Birmingham B15 2TH, UK. ³Royal Hallamshire Hospital, Glossop Road, Sheffield S10 2JF, UK. ⁴School of Life and Health Sciences, Aston University, Birmingham B4 7ET, UK.

References

1. Yau JW, Rogers SL, Kawasaki R, Lamoureux EL, Kowalski JW, Bek T, et al. Global prevalence and major risk factors of diabetic retinopathy. Diabetes Care. 2012;35:556–64.
2. Boyer DS, Hopkins JJ, Sorof J, Ehrlich JS. Anti-vascular endothelial growth factor therapy for diabetic macular edema. Ther Adv Endocrinol Metab. 2013;4:151–69.
3. Brand CS. Management of retinal vascular diseases: a patient-centric approach. Eye (Lond). 2012;26 Suppl 2:S1–16.
4. Brown DM, Nguyen QD, Marcus DM, Boyer DS, Patel S, Feiner L, et al. Long-term outcomes of ranibizumab therapy for diabetic macular edema: the 36-month results from two phase III trials: RISE and RIDE. Ophthalmology. 2013;120:2013–22.
5. Elman MJ, Ayala A, Bressler NM, Browning D, Flaxel CJ, Glassman AR, et al. Intravitreal ranibizumab for diabetic macular edema with prompt versus deferred laser treatment: 5-year randomized trial results. Ophthalmology. 2015;122(2):375–81. doi:10.1016/j.ophtha.2014.08.047. Epub 2014 Oct 28.
6. Diabetic Retinopathy Clinical Research Network, Wells JA, Glassman AR, Ayala AR, Jampol LM, Aiello LP, et al. Comparative effectiveness randomized clinical trial of aflibercept, bevacizumab, or ranibizumab for diabetic macular edema. N Engl J Med. 2015;372:1193–203. doi:10.1056/NEJMoa1414264.
7. Diabetic Retinopathy Clinical Research Network, Chew E, Strauber S, Beck R, Aiello LP, Antoszyk A, et al. Randomized trial of peribulbar triamcinolone acetonide with and without focal photocoagulation for mild diabetic macular edema: a pilot study. Ophthalmology. 2007;114(6):1190–6.
8. Campochiaro PA, Brown DM, Pearson A, Chen S, Boyer D, Ruiz-Moreno J, et al. Sustained delivery fluocinolone acetonide vitreous inserts provide benefit for at least 3 years in patients with diabetic macular edema. Ophthalmology. 2012;119:2125–32.
9. Ozurdex MEAD Study Group, Boyer D, Yoon Y, Belfort R, Bandello F, Maturi R, et al. Long-term benefit of sustained-delivery fluocinolone acetonide vitreous inserts for diabetic macular edema. Three-year, randomized, sham-controlled trial of dexamethasone intravitreal implant in patients with diabetic macular edema. Ophthalmology. 2011;118:626–35.
10. Fluocinolone acetonide intravitreal implant for treating chronic diabetic macular oedema after an inadequate response to prior therapy (rapid review of technology appraisal guidance 271). Accessed on 19 April 2015 <https://www.nice.org.uk/guidance/ta301>.
11. FDA approval of Flucinolone Acetonide in treatment of diabetic macular oedema. Accessed on 19 April 2015 http://www.accessdata.fda.gov/scripts/cder/drugsatfda/index.cfm?fuseaction=Search.DrugDetails>.
12. Gregori NZ, Feuer W, Rosenfeld PJ. Novel method for analyzing snellen visual acuity measurements. Retina. 2010;30(7):1046–50. doi:10.1097/IAE.0b013e3181d87e04. Jul-Aug.
13. Snellen - logMAR Visual Acuity Calculator. Last accessed 19 April 2015 <http://www.myvisiontest.com/logmar.php>.
14. Personal communications with F Quhill(Sheffield), A Bhatnagar (Wolverhampton and M Tsaloumas (Birmingham) 2015.
15. Levin DS, Han DP, Dev S, Wirostko WJ, Mieler WF, Connor TB, et al. Subtenon's depot corticosteroid injections in patients with a history of corticosteroid-induced intraocular pressure elevation. Am J Ophthalmol. 2002;133(2):196–202.
16. Thomas Bertelmann. Stephan Schulze long-term follow-up of patient with diabetic macular edema receiving fluocinolone acetonide intravitreal implant. Ophthalmol Ther. DOI 10.1007/s40123-015-0028-0.
17. Campochiaro PA1, Brown DM, Pearson A, Ciulla T, Boyer D, Holz FG, et al. Subtenon's depot corticosteroid injections in patients with a history of corticosteroid-induced intraocular pressure elevation. Ophthalmology. 2011;118(4):626–635.e2. doi:10.1016/j.ophtha.2010.12.028.

12

Partial thickness corneal tissue as a patch graft material for prevention of glaucoma drainage device exposure

Oriel Spierer[1][*][†], Michael Waisbourd[2][†], Yitzhak Golan[1], Hadas Newman[1] and Rony Rachmiel[1]

Abstract

Background: To protect from erosion of the tube in glaucoma drainage device (GDD), the tube is covered by a biologic tissue which is roofed by the conjunctiva. Sclera, pericardium, dura mater and cornea are available as a patch graft. Drawbacks of some of these materials may include high cost and poor appearance. The purpose of this study is to report the long-term outcomes of partial thickness corneal grafts to cover the tube and prevent its exposure, in GDD surgeries.

Methods: This was a retrospective review of all patients who underwent Ahmed glaucoma valve implantation and had a minimum follow-up of 12 months. The tube was covered by a 300-micron partial thickness corneal graft taken either from a previous Descemet stripping endothelial keratoplasty procedure or cut from a whole corneal graft button unsuitable for keratoplasty.

Results: Forty-four patients (45 eyes, mean follow-up of 27.6 ± 11.4 months) were enrolled. The partial thickness corneal grafts maintained clarity throughout follow-up with satisfactory cosmetic results. Mild conjunctival retraction occurred in 4 eyes (8.9 %) between 1 and 12 months after the surgery. Corneal graft melting occurred in 3 (6.7 %) eyes. Tube exposure and additional surgery to re-patch or suture the conjunctiva over the tube was needed in 1 (2.2 %) eye. None of the patients had graft infection or immunologic rejection.

Conclusions: Partial thickness corneal grafts have favorable long-term outcome as a patch for GDD tubes with low rates of tube exposure and other complications.

Keywords: Corneal patch graft, Glaucoma drainage device, DSEK, Conjunctival erosion, Tube exposure

Background

Glaucoma drainage device (GDD) surgeries are traditionally performed after failed trabeculectomy or in cases where trabeculectomy is at high risk for failure, such as in the management of complex glaucomas [1]. The more commonly used GDDs in current practice are the Ahmed, Baerveldt and Molteno implants [1]. A GDD is composed of a plate and a tube running along the sclera into the anterior chamber. To protect it from erosion, the tube is covered by a biologic tissue which is roofed by the conjunctiva. A GDD is, however, a foreign device that is implanted onto and into the eye and therefore bears surgical complications associated with foreign objects, among them conjunctival erosion that results in plate or tube exposure, diplopia and inflammation [2]. Covering the tube with a patch graft is intended to prevent the conjunctival erosion and the consequent tube exposure that put the eye under the risk of late endophthalmitis [3]. Sclera, pericardium, dura mater and cornea are available as a patch graft [4], but there are few reports that compare them [5, 6]. The use of a patch graft has some drawbacks, such as cost [7] and the fact that it is a foreign body with the potential to erode the overlying conjunctiva [7]. Specifically, the disadvantage of the scleral patch graft is its thickness [5], which may be a cosmetic issue. On the other hand, a pericardium patch might be too thin and a dura matter patch is expensive [5]. These shortcomings have

* Correspondence: oriels1@yahoo.com
[†]Equal contributors
[1]Department of Ophthalmology, Tel Aviv Sourasky Medical Center, Sackler Faculty of Medicine, Tel Aviv University, 6 Weizmann Street, Tel Aviv 64239, Israel
Full list of author information is available at the end of the article

led some investigators to seek other solutions which do not use patch grafts in GDD surgeries, but rather use a scleral tunnel for the tube [7, 8]. Using partial thickness corneal patch graft may resolve some of the above concerns. The purpose of this study was to report the long-term outcomes and complications of employing a partial thickness corneal graft to cover an Ahmed glaucoma valve implant.

Methods

Data collection

Demographic and perioperative data were collected through a retrospective record review of all patients who underwent GDD surgery with partial thickness corneal graft covering between 2007 and 2011 at the Tel Aviv Sourasky Medical Center. Inclusion criteria were age above 18 years at the time of surgery and a minimum follow-up of 12 months. Patients were excluded if they had undergone a previous GDD surgery or if they had a past or current ocular surface disease that could affect the healing of the covering conjunctiva. Patients who had concomitant surgeries, such as pars plana vitrectomy or cataract surgery, were also excluded.

Corneas were obtained from the Tel Aviv Sourasky Medical Center Lions Eye Bank after being approved for transplantation. Corneas were stored in Eusol-C Corneal Storage Media (AL.CHI.MI.A.SRL, Padova, Italy). Tissue evaluation included serology for hepatitis B and C, as well as for HIV. All surgeries were performed by one surgeon (RR) who was also responsible for the clinic visits that included intraocular pressure (IOP) measurements with Goldmann applanation tonometry (AT 900, Haag-Streit AG, Koeniz, Switzerland) before and periodically after surgery. The study followed the tenets of the Declaration of Helsinki and was approved by the ethics committee of the Tel-Aviv Sourasky Medical Center.

Surgical technique

All GDDs were implanted through a fornix-based incision using the FP7 Ahmed glaucoma valve (New World Medical, Inc., Rancho Cucamonga, CA), with the plate secured 8–12 mm from the corneoscleral limbus. Thirty-three eyes (73.3 %) underwent superotemporal GDD implantation, 11 eyes (24.4 %) underwent inferotemporal implantation, and 1 eye (2.2 %) underwent inferonasal implantation.

After priming, the tube was inserted through a scleral track posterior to the limbus by a 23-gauge needle, and introduced by an inserter into the anterior chamber. Viscoelastic was injected into the anterior chamber to maintain its proper depth. The partial thickness corneal graft, which was used to cover the tube, was sutured to the sclera with four 10-0 nylon sutures. The conjunctiva was closed meticulously with 8-0 vicryl and 10-0 nylon

sutures, taking care to ensure that it fully covered the corneal graft.

A partial thickness corneal graft was taken either from a previous Descemet stripping endothelial keratoplasty (DSEK) procedure or cut from a whole corneal graft button. Corneal grafts prepared for a DSEK procedure were cut by an automated microkeratome system (Moria ALTK System, Antony, France) with a 300 micron head passed to create a lamellar dissection. This formed an anterior cap mainly composed of stroma and a posterior endothelial lamellar donor graft. The posterior corneal lamella was used for the DSEK procedure, while the anterior corneal lamella was either discarded or used to cover the tube in the GDD surgery of a different patient. In other cases, a partial thickness corneal graft was prepared from a full-thickness corneal graft that was unsuitable for keratoplasty (i.e., donor age >80 years, low graft clarity, endothelial cell count <2000 cells/mm^2 and expired tissue [7–60 days from harvesting]).

Statistical analysis

All the data were recorded on Microsoft Excel™ spreadsheets. A paired-samples t-test was used to compare mean pre- and postoperative IOPs. Bonferroni correction for multiple comparisons and a mixed model for repeated measures were also used. Analyses were two-tailed, and significance was set at the 5 % level. Statistical analysis was performed with SPSS™ software V.21 (SPSS, Inc., Chicago, IL).

Results

Forty-four patients (45 eyes), comprised of 25 males and 19 females with a mean postoperative follow-up of 27.6 ± 11.4 months (range 12–60 months) fulfilled the inclusion criteria and were included in the analysis. Their demographic characteristics and clinical data are summarized in Table 1. The glaucoma subtypes of the study population are summarized in Table 2. The postoperative IOP levels at the different follow-ups were consistently lower ($P < 0.001$) than the preoperative IOP values (Table 1). These differences remained significant after Bonferroni correction for multiple comparisons and application of a mixed model for repeated measures. The mean IOP reduction (i.e., the last recorded preoperative IOP compared to the last recorded postoperative IOP) was 50 %. The mean number of topical anti-glaucoma medications decreased from 3.0 ± 0.9 (range 1–4) to 1.3 ± 1.2 (range 0–4) on the last postoperative follow-up.

Thirty-three (73.3 %) partial thickness corneal grafts were retrieved from previous DSEK procedures and 12 grafts (26.7 %) were prepared during the GDD surgery from full corneal grafts that were unsuitable to serve as an optical corneal graft. The mean corneal patch diameter was 8.3 ± 0.2 mm (range 8.0–.0 mm). The conjunctiva that

Table 1 Demographic and clinical data of 44 patients (45 eyes) who underwent glaucoma drainage device surgery

Male/female (%)		56.8/43.2
Age (years)		71.0 ± 10.8 (range 34–92)
Preop.duration of glaucoma (months)		116.2 ± 105.8 (range 1–396)
Trabeculectomies before surgery (n)		0.9 ± 0.9 (range 0–4)
Right/left eye (%)		55.6/44.4
Mean intraocular pressure (mmHg)		
	Preoperative	30.1 ± 8.1
	Postop. day 1	10.9 ± 5.4*
	Postop. week 1	10.5 ± 5.2*
	Postop. month 1	12.7 ± 5.8*
	Postop. month 3	14.1 ± 6.4*
	Postop. month 6	13.3 ± 5.3*
	Postop. year 1	13.8 ± 4.9*
	Postop. year 2	12.8 ± 3.6*
	Postop. final visit	14.5 ± 4.9*

Postop postoperative
*$P < 0.001$ (compared to preoperative)

covered the corneal patch graft had a button hole during surgery in 1 case (2.2 %). The conjunctival edges were approximated by 8-0 vicryl sutures. There were no other intra-operative complications.

None of the patients had graft infection or immunologic rejection and the partial thickness corneal grafts maintained clarity throughout follow-up. There were no GDD-related complications, such as diplopia, inflammatory reaction in the conjunctiva or plate exposure. Four eyes (8.9 %) had conjunctival retraction between 1 and 12 months after the surgery. As the conjunctival retraction was minimal, Seidel test was negative, and the tube was well-covered by the patch graft, these patients were observed without treatment. Conjunctival erosion with tube exposure occurred in 1 case (2.2 %) with superotemporal

Table 2 Subtype of glaucoma in 44 patients (45 eyes) who underwent glaucoma drainage device surgery

Subtype	n (%)
Pseudoexfoliation glaucoma	11 (25.5)
Open angle glaucoma	9 (20.5)
Neovascular glaucoma	9 (20.5)
Post penetrating keratoplasty glaucoma	6 (13.6)
Uveitic glaucoma	4 (9.1)
Chronic angle closure glaucoma	2 (4.5)
Malignant glaucoma	1 (2.3)
Angle recession	1 (2.3)
Normal tension glaucoma	1 (2.3)

GDDs. In this patient the corneal patch graft was also melting 1 month after surgery (Table 3). The patient underwent re-patching with another corneal graft and conjunctival closure. Three eyes (6.7 %) had corneal graft melting (Table 3): in one of them it occurred with conjunctival erosion and tube exposure as was described. In the other 2 patients graft melting occurred 12 and 33 months postoperatively. As the overlying conjunctiva was intact they were observed expectantly without the need for surgical intervention.

Discussion

Partial thickness corneal patch grafts covering GDD tubes have favorable long-term outcomes. According to our results, these grafts are associated with a 6.7 % rate of corneal graft melting and a 2.2 % rate of tube exposure. Only one case necessitated additional surgery to cover the exposed tube. A GDD transports aqueous humor from the eye through a tube to an episcleral plate located in one of the quadrants of the globe. The aqueous diffuses through the capsular wall and is absorbed by periocular lymphatics and capillaries [3, 9]. Post-surgical complications unique to GDDs include tube-endothelial contact which may cause significant corneal endothelial damage, fibrous encapsulation leading to filtration failure, continuing low-grade inflammation, and tube or plate migration or extrusion [2].

Conjunctival retraction leading to patch graft exposure is usually considered a minor complication, as long as the tube is well covered by the patch graft [10]. This condition, which does not require surgical intervention, was previously found in 33.5 % of eyes undergoing GDD implantation [10], compared with 8.9 % in the current study. Nevertheless, if the conjunctival retraction is significant and the tube is exposed, this may place the eye at risk for infection, especially if Seidel test is positive. Repairing the exposure in these cases may be challenging, especially if the conjunctiva is scarred.

Direct contact between the conjunctiva and the tube will cause the tube to erode the overlying conjunctiva over time and become exposed [7], putting the eye at risk of infection and endophthalmitis [3]. The most vulnerable site for tube erosion is at its entrance through the sclera, and the role of the patch graft is to prevent tube erosion [3]. Although this approach has been shown to decrease exposure rates, it does not always prevent this complication [7]. The reported rates for tube exposure or device extrusion range between 3 and 30.5 % [7, 10–13], putting our 2.2 % rate at the bottom of the scale. In the event of tube or plate exposure, the condition of the conjunctiva and patch graft needs to be assessed. The majority of those cases are effectively managed by conjunctival suturing with patch grafting, while poor conjunctiva quality may necessitate the use

Table 3 Description of 3 patients with partial thickness corneal patch graft melting

Characteristics	Patient 1	Patient 2	Patient 3
Gender	Male	Female	Male
Age (years)	74	66	79
Eye	Left	Right	Left
Type of glaucoma	Pseudo-exfoliation	Uveitic glaucoma	Pseudo-exfoliation
IOP before surgery (mmHg)	25	25	24
Trabeculectomies before surgery (n)	4	1	1
Location of Ahmed valve	Inferotemporal	Inferotemporal	Superotemporal
Medications before/after the surgery (n)	4/4	3/2	4/0
Corneal patch graft diameter (mm)	8.5	8.25	8.5
Complications during surgery	None	None	None
Post-surgery melting (months)	33	12	1
Follow-up duration (months)	42	36	32

IOP, intraocular pressure

of a conjunctival auto-graft, amniotic membrane or buccal graft [14, 15]. Re-patching with a different material should be considered in the event that the patch graft has melted [16]. However, removal of the plate or tube may nevertheless be necessary [13] as had been the case in one of our subjects. Causes for tube exposure have not been clearly elucidated in the literature [17], and the reported risk factors are inconsistent. Potential risk might be related to conjunctival status (as affected by aging, inflammation, and device mobility) [18], the number of previous ocular surgeries [18], the number of preoperative hypotensive medications [10], and a previous trabeculectomy [17]. Inferior quadrant implantation bears a higher risk of conjunctival erosion over the plate, possibly because of exposure or a shallower space within the inferior fornix and less conjunctiva and Tenon's capsule for implant coverage [10, 19, 20]. Another report suggested that tube exposure does not differ between Ahmed, Baerveldt, and Molteno implants [21]. However, since that report included 38 studies with many surgeons using different surgical techniques and different patch grafts, it is difficult to arrive at any firm conclusion from those data. The low rate of complications relevant to the conjunctiva and the partial thickness corneal graft in the current study makes it impossible for us to draw conclusions about the risk factors for graft patch melting and tube exposure. Two out of the 3 cases with melting had the implant placed inferiorly. Also, an immune-mediated process with resultant rapid melting may have contributed to the corneal melting in one of our patients who had underlying uveitis.

Considerations in the choice of patch graft material include biocompatibility, availability, immunologic safety, ease of use, cost and cosmetic appearance [22]. The use of allograft materials, among which the most common are sclera, pericardium, dura mater and cornea, has some disadvantages. Insofar as they are foreign bodies, they have a

prima facie potential to erode the overlying conjunctiva [7]. Secondly, they involve considerable cost [7]. The main disadvantage of preserved sclera is its thickness [5], which may be an issue of cosmetic appearance. Sterility and variable quality are other concerns [5]. When an autologous scleral patch graft is used, large areas of sclera may be thinned for harvesting the graft, thus carrying the risk of perforation as well [22]. As for a pericardium graft, it may be a priori too thin and also prone to more melting with longer follow-up [5]. Both pericardium and dura matter are expensive [5]. The use of gamma-irradiated cornea (VisionGraft) for the coverage of a glaucoma tube shunt was recently described as allowing for both decreased risk of disease transmission and improved availability [22]. However, prions are still a risk in these corneas and the high cost is a major obstacle. These drawbacks have led some investigators to seek other solutions, such as placing the tube in a scleral tunnel [8] with or without Tenon advancement and a conjunctival–Tenon flap [7]. These descriptions, however, are all derived from anecdotal reports and the conventional surgical method continues to be the use of a patch graft in GDD surgeries.

The biologic material used as a patch graft in GDD surgeries has at least some role in preventing tube erosion [6], but discussions of these issues are sparse. One report [5] stated that no material was more prone to erosion or melting than another when comparing donor sclera, dura mater and pericardium. Those authors, however, reported a high incidence of donor patch graft thinning (22–26 %) for all 3 of those materials. A corneal patch graft may have some advantages over other covering materials. Its tissue strength and rigidity make it particularly suitable for tectonic support of the ocular wall, and it may be less prone to melting compared to other patch grafts [4, 22, 23]. Moreover, its translucency gives the patient's eye a better cosmetic appearance [23], which is most relevant in cases where the GDD is placed in the inferior quadrants [22]. Migration, retraction and twisting are possible complications of the tube [24, 25], and they may be difficult to diagnose under an opaque patch graft, such as sclera or pericardium. The translucency of the cornea allows direct visualization of the underlying tube and greater facility in the diagnosis of possible complications [4]. It also facilitates laser suture lysis of the tying suture with non-valved tubes. We believe that the use of a partial thickness corneal graft offers satisfactory tectonic support and has some additional benefits over full thickness corneal grafts. The thin patch we use occupies little of the narrow space of the conjunctiva-sclera, thus minimizing the likelihood of the patch graft to erode the overlying conjunctiva. Indeed, none of our patients had that complication. The thin patch may also reduce the postoperative risk of dellen formation. Finally, the partial thickness corneal graft can be taken from a previous DSEK procedure or from a corneal graft that is unsuitable for optic corneal transplantation. This increases the availability of banked tissue without additional costs.

While a patch graft must be completely covered by the conjunctiva during the surgery, conjunctival laceration or button-hole formation may occur [10]. Simple suturing of the conjunctiva must then be carried out to ensure that the patch graft, tube and plate are entirely covered. This intra-operative complication occurred in one of our cases and was successfully dealt by prompt re-approximation of the conjunctival edges.

Limitations of this study include its retrospective nature, the relative small sample size and the lack of a control group with which to compare our results. Prospective randomized studies comparing partial thickness cornea to other patch graft materials are needed in order to determine which patch is less prone to conjunctival erosion and subsequent tube exposure. Cost considerations, the ideal thickness of the patch graft and its cosmetic appearance should also be taken into consideration. Since our analysis included only patients with follow-up of ≥12 months, complications occurring in patients with shorter follow-up were not reported, and this could have been a confounding factor. Although the mean postoperative follow-up time was more than 2 years, it was only 12 months in four patients. It is not clear whether a longer follow-up would reveal more cases of conjunctival dehiscence or corneal graft melting, but we consider it most probable that more of them would emerge over time. Some authors argued that these complications usually occur within the first 15-month postoperative period [5], while others held that these complications may occur even after 5 years [21]. Graft melting occurred 33 months after surgery in one of our patients, which suggests that patients who underwent GDD surgery should be examined regularly for years after surgery. The strict exclusion criteria that eliminated any cases of previous GDD surgery and patients with past and current ocular surface disease represent a strength of our study by allowing the evaluation of the partial thickness cornea as a patch graft without confounding factors that may influence conjunctival healing or erosion. Another strength is that all surgeries were done by one surgeon using the same technique, unlike most studies that evaluated the results and complications of GDDs placed by different surgeons using different techniques. Indeed, variations in techniques might affect tube exposure [6], making it difficult to draw any conclusions about the effectiveness of a specific patch graft in preventing the silicone tube exposure. We used a corneal patch that had an 8–9 mm diameter. The optimal size of a patch graft that will cover the tube completely from limbus to the plate has not yet been established, and this issue warrants further study.

Conclusions

A partial thickness corneal graft is a useful patch graft material for covering a GDD. It is associated with low rates of conjunctival retraction, graft melting, tube exposure and need for additional surgery.

Abbreviations
DSEK: descemet stripping endothelial keratoplasty; GDD: glaucoma drainage device; IOP: intraocular pressure.

Competing interests
The authors declare that they have no competing interests.

Authors' contributions
OS and MW contributed to the study design, were involved in data collection, conducted the data analysis, and drafted the manuscript. YG and HN contributed to the study design and were involved in data collection and interpretation of data. RR contributed to the study design and was involved in data management and interpretation of data. OS, MW, YG, HN and RR revised the manuscript critically for important intellectual content. All authors read and approved the final manuscript

Acknowledgments
There were no funding sources for the preparation of this manuscript.

Author details
[1]Department of Ophthalmology, Tel Aviv Sourasky Medical Center, Sackler Faculty of Medicine, Tel Aviv University, 6 Weizmann Street, Tel Aviv 64239, Israel. [2]Wills Eye Hospital, Philadelphia, PA, USA.

References
1. Minckler DS, Francis BA, Hodapp EA, Jampel HD, Lin SC, Samples JR, et al. Aqueous shunts in glaucoma: a report by the American Academy of Ophthalmology. Ophthalmology. 2008;115:1089–98.
2. Lim KS, Allan BD, Lloyd AW, Muir A, Khaw PT. Glaucoma drainage devices; past, present, and future. Br J Ophthalmol. 1998;82:1083–9.
3. Gedde SJ, Scott IU, Tabandeh H, Luu KK, Budenz DL, Greenfield DS, et al. Late endophthalmitis associated with glaucoma drainage implants. Ophthalmology. 2001;108:1323–7.
4. Singh M, Chew PT, Tan D. Corneal patch graft repair of exposed glaucoma drainage implants. Cornea. 2008;27:1171–3.

5. Smith MF, Doyle JW, Ticrney Jr JW. A comparison of glaucoma drainage implant tube coverage. J Glaucoma. 2002;11:143–7.
6. Lankaranian D, Reis R, Henderer JD, Choe S, Moster MR. Comparison of single thickness and double thickness processed pericardium patch graft in glaucoma drainage device surgery: a single surgeon comparison of outcome. J Glaucoma. 2008;17:48–51.
7. Tamcelik N, Ozkok A, Sarıcı AM, Atalay E, Yetik H, Gungor K. Tenon advancement and duplication technique to prevent postoperative Ahmed valve tube exposure in patients with refractory glaucoma. Jpn J Ophthalmol. 2013;57:359–64.
8. Kugu S, Erdogan G, Sevim MS, Ozerturk Y. Efficacy of long scleral tunnel technique in preventing Ahmed glaucoma valve tube exposure through conjunctiva. Semin Ophthalmol. 2015;30:1–5.
9. Gedde SJ, Parrish RK, Budenz DL, Heuer DK. Update on aqueous shunts. Exp Eye Res. 2011;93:284–90.
10. Geffen N, Buys YM, Smith M, Anraku A, Alasbali T, Rachmiel R, et al. Conjunctival complications related to Ahmed glaucoma valve insertion. J Glaucoma. 2014;23:109–14.
11. Huang MC, Netland PA, Coleman AL, Siegner SW, Moster MR, Hill RA. Intermediate-term clinical experience with the Ahmed Glaucoma Valve implant. Am J Ophthalmol. 1999;127:27–33.
12. Wilson MR, Mendis U, Paliwal A, Haynatzka V. Long-term follow-up of primary glaucoma surgery with Ahmed glaucoma valve implant versus trabeculectomy. Am J Ophthalmol. 2003;136:464–70.
13. Smith M, Buys YM, Trope GE. Replacement of Ahmed aqueous drainage devices in eyes with device-related complications. J Glaucoma. 2009;18:484–7.
14. Ainsworth G, Rotchford A, Dua HS, King AJ. A novel use of amniotic membrane in the management of tube exposure following glaucoma tube shunt surgery. Br J Ophthalmol. 2006;90:417–9.
15. Rootman DB, Trope GE, Rootman DS. Glaucoma aqueous drainage device erosion repair with buccal mucous membrane grafts. J Glaucoma. 2009;18:618–22.
16. Huddleston SM, Feldman RM, Budenz DL, Bell NP, Lee DA, Chuang AZ, et al. Aqueous shunt exposure: a retrospective review of repair outcome. J Glaucoma. 2013;22:433–8.
17. Koval MS, El Sayyad FF, Bell NP, Chuang AZ, Lee DA, Hypes SM, et al. Risk factors for tube shunt exposure: a matched case–control study. J Ophthalmol. 2013;2013:196215.
18. Byun YS, Lee NY, Park CK. Risk factors of implant exposure outside the conjunctiva after Ahmed glaucoma valve implantation. Jpn J Ophthalmol. 2009;53:114–9.
19. Pakravan M, Yazdani S, Shahabi C, Yaseri M. Superior versus inferior Ahmed glaucoma valve implantation. Ophthalmology. 2009;116:208–13.
20. Rachmiel R, Trope GE, Buys YM, Flanagan JG, Chipman ML. Intermediate-term outcome and success of superior versus inferior Ahmed Glaucoma Valve implantation. J Glaucoma. 2008;17:584–90.
21. Stewart WC, Kristoffersen CJ, Demos CM, Fsadni MG, Stewart JA. Incidence of conjunctival exposure following drainage device implantation in patients with glaucoma. Eur J Ophthalmol. 2010;20:124–30.
22. Lawrence SD, Netland PA. Gamma-irradiated cornea allograft for glaucoma surgery. J Glaucoma. 2013;22:355–7.
23. Spierer O, Rachmiel R, Lazar M, Alba M, Varssano D. Double use of corneal graft for Descemet stripping automated endothelial keratoplasty and coverage of glaucoma drainage device tube. J Glaucoma. 2012;21:490–2.
24. Anand A, Sheha H, Teng CC, Liebmann JM, Ritch R, Tello C. Use of amniotic membrane graft in glaucoma shunt surgery. Ophthalmic Surg Lasers Imaging. 2011;42:184–9.
25. Gupta VS, Sethi HS, Gupta M, Mehta A, Singh S, Yadav P, et al. Posterior migration of Ahmed glaucoma valve tube in a patient with Reiger anomaly: a case report. BMC Ophthalmol. 2010;10:23.

13

Diabetic macular morphology changes may occur in the early stage of diabetes

Yanwei Chen, Jianfang Li, Yan Yan[*] and Xi Shen[*]

Abstract

Background: The purpose of this study was to observe whether invisible morphological changes are presented in the two types of diabetes mellitus patients without diabetic retinopathy.

Methods: Twenty-six type 1 diabetes mellitus (T1DM) patients and 34 type 2 diabetes mellitus (T2DM) patients without diabetic retinopathy (DR) were recruited for this study. They underwent complete examinations that included stereoscopic color fundus photography and optical coherence tomography (OCT). The OCT patterns were used to measure the macular retinal thickness (RT), the ganglion cell and inner plexiform layer (GC-IPL) complex thickness, the inner nuclear layer (INL) thickness, the outer nuclear layer (ONL) thickness and the subfoveal choroidal thickness (SFCT) using the enhanced depth imaging (EDI) patterns and the retinal fiber layer (RNFL) thickness around the optic disc. All results were compared to those of age- and sex-matched control groups.

Results: In the patients with T1DM, the mean RT and GC-IPL complex thicknesses were significantly thinner than those of the control group ($p < 0.05$). The RNFL was found to be thinner at the 9 o'clock position around the optic disc in the patients compared with the control group. The SFCTs were similar in the controls and subjects. The INL and ONL were decreased in parts of the pericentral and peripheral areas in the T1DM patients ($p < 0.05$) and increased in the T2DM patients ($p < 0.05$).

Conclusions: This study demonstrated that in short-duration T1DM patients, the layers of the retina are affected and that the neural tissue has begun to be lost. As diabetes develops, neurodegeneration may cause vascular permeability, which causes thickening of the retinal layers.

Keywords: Diabetes retinopathy, Optical coherence tomography, Retinal morphology

Background

The global incidence of diabetes mellitus (DM) is increasing, and the number of patients is expected to reach 3.66 billion by 2030 [1]. Diabetic retinopathy (DR) is one of the most common and severe complications of DM and is also the leading cause of blindness. In America, 40 % of type 2 diabetes mellitus (T2DM) patients and 86 % of type 1 diabetes mellitus (T1DM) patients suffer from DR [2, 3]. In China, the incidence of DR is 27.9 % in urban areas and 43 % in rural areas [4, 5]. Thus, the early detection of DR is important for the preservation of useful acuity in later life.

The present examinations of DR included direct ophthalmoscopy, fundus photography, optical coherence

tomography (OCT) and fluorescence angiography. OCT is a noninvasive technique that was developed to be rapid in terms of its hardware and software attributes, and OCT exhibits high levels of accuracy and definition in the detection of early and small changes in retinal morphology. The newly updated Carl Zeiss OCT software version 6.0 integrates FastTrac retinal tracking, FoveaFinder, ganglion cell analysis, ONH and RNFL OU analyses, enhanced depth imaging (EDI) and other powerful functions that enable the acquisition of reliable data for clinical research.

In addition to the retinal layers, the choroid has also attracted much interest due to its vascular structure and supply of oxygen and nutrients to the outer retina. The EDI pattern is also useful for clearly displaying choroid thickness and structural abnormalities [6]. Increases and decreases in macular and choroid thicknesses have been observed in patients with and without diabetic retinopathy

* Correspondence: hz2004yan@163.com; carl_shen2005@126.com
The Department of Ophthalmology, RuiJin Hospital Affiliated Shanghai Jiao Tong University School of Medicine, Shanghai, China

in previous studies, and different mechanisms have been found to be responsible for these changes [7–11]. Our study aimed to fully utilize OCT to identify the types of morphological changes in DM patients without retinopathy.

Methods

Participants

This was a cross-sectional, case–control study. The design of this study followed of the principles of the Declaration of Helsinki and was approved by the Institutional Review Board of the RuiJin Hospital. Written informed consent was obtained from all participants or their parents (children who were under 16 years old). The patients were recruited from the outpatient clinic of the department of Endocrinology Medicine of the RuiJin Hospital affiliated with the Shanghai Jiao Tong University School of Medicine (Shanghai, China) between October 2013 and November 2014. The patients were diagnosed with type 1 or type 2 diabetes mellitus by an endocrine specialist and were treated with insulin or other medicines. The normal control subjects were selected from the medical examination center of the same hospital. They were age- and sex-matched to the patients; were free of all diagnoses of ocular disease, diabetes, or other systemic disease; and underwent a complete ophthalmologic examination that included a visual acuity assessment, slit-lamp examination with a handheld lens (Super Field; Volk Optical, Inc., Mentor, OH), intraocular pressure (IOP) assessment with a noncontact tonometer, and refraction, color fundus photograph (TRC-50IX; Topcon Corp.), and Cirrus high-definition optical coherence tomography (HD-OCT, Carl Zeiss Meditec, Dublin, California). The inclusion criteria were as follows: 1) a diagnosis of T1DM or T2DM with no clinical retinopathy as observed through dilated pupils by an experienced doctor using a stereoscopic slit lamp with a handheld lens; 2) a best-corrected visual acuity ≥20/25; and 3) refractive errors below -6 or above +3 diopter equivalent spheres. The exclusion criteria were significant media opacity, glaucoma, uveitis, ocular trauma or surgery history, and other serious systemic diseases. Additionally, age, sex, duration of diabetes (in years) were recorded, and fasting glucose and HbA1c levels were collected from the patients' recent blood reports (Tables 1 and 2).

OCT measurements

A Cirrus HD-OCT 4000 (software Version 6.0) was used to obtain the macular images. The patients placed their chins in a chinrest with their foreheads contacting a headrest and fixated on a green target. The macular cube 512×128 scan protocol was used to acquire all 128 OCT B-scans that covered an area of 6×6 mm and were 2 mm in length centered on the fovea. A mean retinal thickness (RT) map of nine zones from the internal limiting membrane to the retinal pigment epithelium was automatically measured. We defined the foveal area (A1) as a central circle with a diameter of 1 mm, the pericentral area (A2-A5) as a donut-shaped ring centered on the fovea with an inner diameter of 1 mm and an outer diameter of 3 mm, and the peripheral area (A6-A9) as a ring with an inner diameter of 3 mm and an outer diameter of 6 mm (Fig. 1a).

The ganglion cell analysis algorithm was used to measure the GC-IPL thickness within a 14.13 mm^2 elliptical annulus centered on the fovea based on the 3-dimensional data generated from the macular cube 512×128 scan protocol. The outer boundary of the retinal nerve fiber layer (RNFL) and the outer boundary of the inner plexiform layer were automatically segmented by the algorithm. The GC-IPL thicknesses of the superotemporal, superior, superonasal, inferotemporal, inferior and inferonasal sectors were automatically measured (Fig. 1b).

A one-line raster scan of the EDI pattern was performed to obtain high-quality images of the retina and macular choroid. The scan line was as close as possible to the fovea in the horizontal (0°) and vertical (90°) directions. Only images with signal strengths exceeding 6 were selected for the study. The thicknesses of the inner nuclear layer (INL) and the outer nuclear layer (ONL) were measured manually every 0.5 mm from the center to the periphery in the nasal and temporal directions. Each measurement was performed three times, and the mean values were determined. The choroid thickness was defined as the vertical distance from the hyper-reflective line of Bruch's membrane to the hyper-reflective line of the inner surface of the sclera. The subfoveal choroidal thickness (SFCT) was measured in the horizontally and vertically scanned images to obtain a mean value (Fig. 2).

Table 1 Characteristics of the subjects

Parameters	T1DM	Control	p value	T2DM	Control	p value
Female/Male	17/9	14/11	0.572	18/16	23/13	0.467
BCVA	0.00(log MAR)	0.00(log MAR)	0.922	0.05(log MAR)	0.05(log MAR)	0.669
IOP, mmHg	17.53±4.27	16.27±3.03	0.357	14.54±2.22	16.07±3.41	0.834
Age, years	21.8±5.3	23.1±4.8	0.397	59.7±13.9	57.0±7.5	0.183

All values are presented as the mean ± SD, and differences were considered statistically meaningful when $p < 0.05$

Table 2 Differences between T1DM and T2DM patients

Parameters	T1DM	T2DM	p value
Fasting blood glucose, mg/dL	6.22±1.30	6.37±1.37	0.248
HbA1c, %	7.84±2.39	6.56±0.65	0.072
DM duration, years	2.1±3.0	10.17±6.84	0.000*

All values are presented as the mean ± SD
*Statistically meaningful

The optic disc cube scan protocol was used to obtain the RNFL measurements from the T1DM patients. There were 200 A-scans, and from each of 200 B-scans, the software automatically determined the center of a disc with a radius of 1.73 mm. The RNFL thicknesses of 12 sectors of the optic disc that were defined like the hours on a clock were measured and calculated using this software. The data were recorded in the superior-to-temporal, inferior-to-nasal, and clockwise directions (Fig. 1c).

Statistical analysis

Statistical analyses were performed using SPSS software version 20.0 for IOS (IBM Corporation, Chicago, IL, USA). All data are expressed as the mean ± standard deviation (SD). A chi square test was used to assess the difference in the female/male ratio between the patients and controls. Analysis of variance (ANOVA) was used to assess the differences in mean age, BCVA, IOP, fasting glucose level, HbA1c and DM duration between the patients and controls. The mean RT, GC-IPL complex, INL, ONL and RNFL thicknesses in the diabetic patients and controls were compared using independent t tests. The results were considered statistically significant when $p < 0.05$.

Results

In total, 26 T1DM patients and 34 T2DM patients were analyzed in this study. Age- and sex-matched controls were 25 and 36 respectively (Table 1). Both eyes of all participants were scanned, and the left eyes were selected

for analysis. The mean RTs of all nine of the zones of the T1DM subjects were thinner than those of the control group, and the differences in zones A2 to A9 were statistically meaningful ($p < 0.05$); however, no significant changes were found in the T2DM patients (Table 3). All six sectors of the GCIPL complex in the T1DM patients were thinner than those in the control group, but these values were similar in the T2DM patients and controls (Table 4). The INL and ONL of the T1DM patients were both thinner at some of the tested points in the periphery and pericentral areas ($p < 0.05$) and slightly thicker in the fovea; the latter difference was not statistically meaningful (Figs. 3 and 4). In contrast, the opposite pattern of results was observed in the T2DM patients who displayed thicker layers (Figs. 5 and 6).

The SFCTs were 294.44 ± 60.96 μm in the T1DM patients and 303.16 ± 60.23 μm in the T1DM control group ($p = 0.64$). In the T2DM patients and their control group, these values were 284 ± 84.89 μm and 254 ± 67.36 μm, respectively ($p = 0.32$).

The RNFL thicknesses of the optic discs of the T1DM patients were significantly decreased at the 9 o'clock position ($p = 0.005$).

Discussion

Previous studies have reported changes in the macular retinal thickness and the thicknesses of different layers in patients with and without diabetic retinopathy [7–11]. The early diagnosis and early detection of functional changes related to DR that occur prior to retinal morphology changes are important for preventing DR. Some researchers have found that retinal neurodegeneration may occur in DR before any microcirculatory abnormalities can be detected [12, 13]. Neural apoptosis and the loss of ganglion cell bodies and glial reactivity are now considered to be the main factors in DR [14, 15].

In this study, we observed significant decreases in the RTs of the A2 to A9 zones and the thickness of all

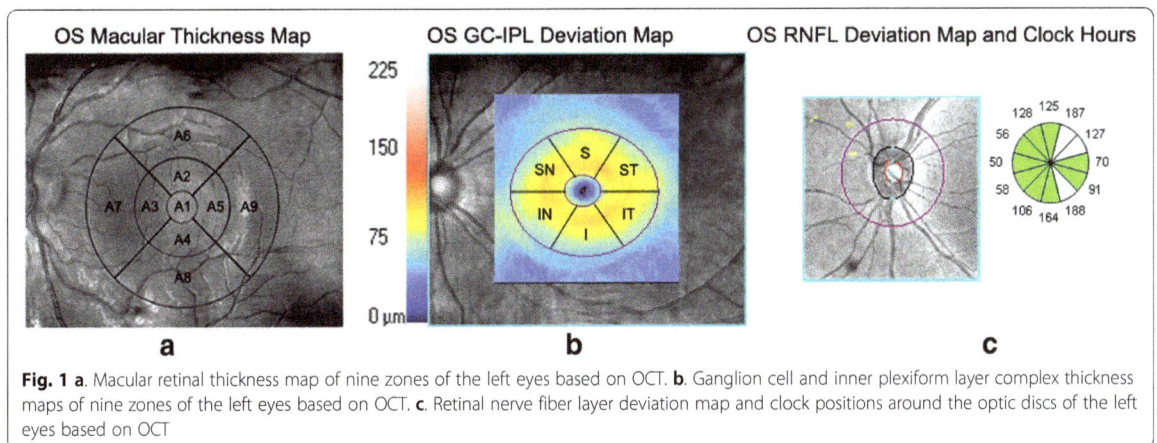

Fig. 1 a. Macular retinal thickness map of nine zones of the left eyes based on OCT. **b.** Ganglion cell and inner plexiform layer complex thickness maps of nine zones of the left eyes based on OCT. **c.** Retinal nerve fiber layer deviation map and clock positions around the optic discs of the left eyes based on OCT

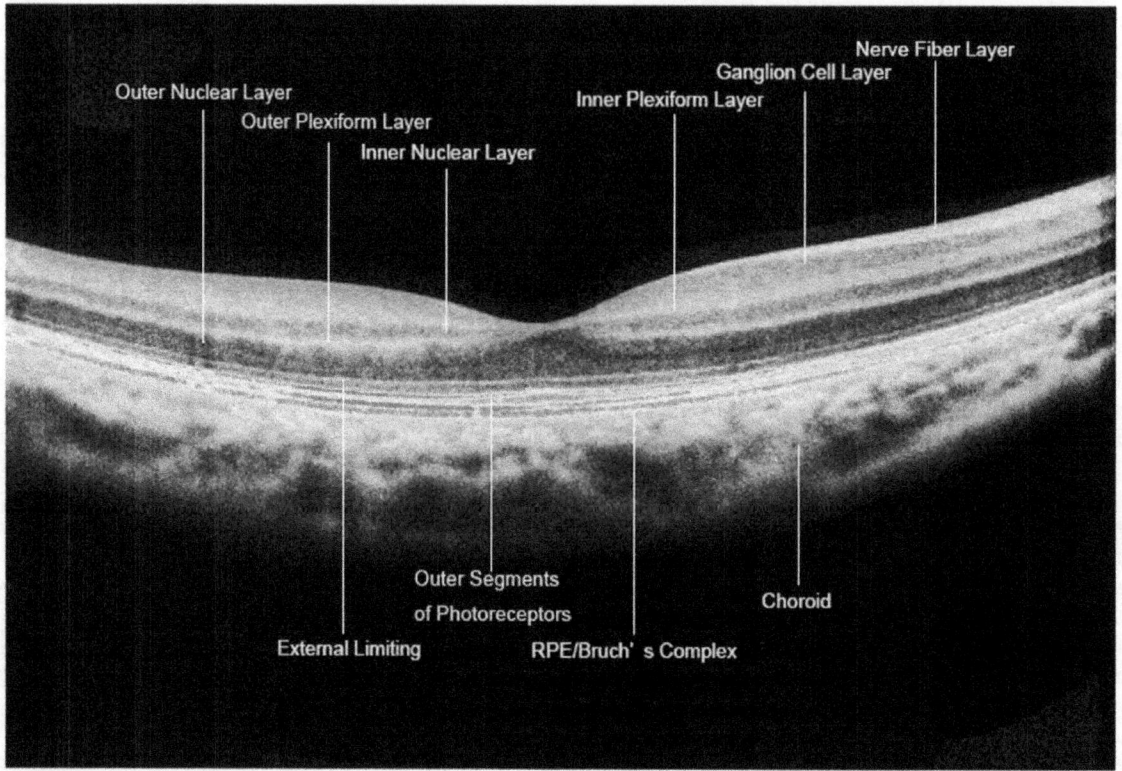

Fig. 2 Retinal layers shown in an OCT EDI pattern scan image

sectors of the GC-IPL complex in the macular zones of the T1DM patients. Additionally, among the tested points, N2.0 in the INL and N0.5, N2.0, T0.5, T1.0, and T2.0 in the ONL were found to be decreased in the patients. In the RNFL, the 9 o'clock position, i.e., the nasal section, was found to be reduced in the patients. In sharp contrast to the T1DM group, we did not observe many positive findings in the T2DM patients. No measured RT or GC-IPL complex thicknesses were found to be different between the T2DM patients and controls. However, increased thicknesses in the testing points N1.5, N2.0, T1.0, T1.5, and T2.0 in the INL and N0.5 and N1.0

in the ONL were observed. In the SFCT, we did not observe any changes in either the T1DM or T2DM patients.

To our knowledge, there were no previous ophthalmological studies of newly diagnosed T1DM patients. In the present study, the mean disease durations were 2.1 ± 3.0 years for the type 1 DM patients and 10.17 ± 6.84 years for the type 2 DM patients ($p < 0.05$). The T2DM patients exhibited no significant differences in the measures of retinal thickness or the GC-ILP complex, but these measures were decreased in the T1DM patients. Similar results have been reported in other studies [8, 9], which have detected either thickening or thinning of the

Table 3 The retinal thicknesses in nine zones in type 1 and type 2 DM patients and controls

	Type 1 DM	Control	p value	Type 2 DM	Control	p value
Superior	80.72±9.65	85.50±6.05	0.044*	82.74±8.91	85.24±6.47	0.316
Superotemporal	78.64±8.78	85.17±7.45	0.007*	81.13±8.19	82.59±6.29	0.527
Inferotemporal	80.00±7.09	85.29±5.29	0.005*	81.81±8.29	82.47±6.41	0.776
Inferior	78.28±7.01	82.35±6.34	0.041*	79.13±7.56	81.12±5.94	0.354
Inferonasal	79.96±6.49	84.63±6.61	0.016*	80.03±11.58	82.94±5.99	0.340
Superonasal	82.96±5.95	86.71±6.98	0.049*	84.19±10.49	86.59±6.54	0.399

All values are presented as the mean ± SD
*Statistically meaningful

Table 4 Thicknesses of the ganglion cell layer and inner plexiform layer in six sectors in the type 1 and type 2 DM patients and controls

	Type 1 DM	Control	p value	Type 2 DM	Control	p value
Superior	80.72±9.65	85.50±6.05	0.044*	82.74±8.91	85.24±6.47	0.316
Superotemporal	78.64±8.78	85.17±7.45	0.007*	81.13±8.19	82.59±6.29	0.527
Inferotemporal	80.00±7.09	85.29±5.29	0.005*	81.81±8.29	82.47±6.41	0.776
Inferior	78.28±7.01	82.35±6.34	0.041*	79.13±7.56	81.12±5.94	0.354
Inferonasal	79.96±6.49	84.63±6.61	0.016*	80.03±11.58	82.94±5.99	0.340
Superonasal	82.96±5.95	86.71±6.98	0.049*	84.19±10.49	86.59±6.54	0.399

All values are presented as the mean ± SD
*Statistically meaningful

retina. The majority of these reports found that the retina becomes thinner when DR is present [9, 16]. Together, all of the above-mentioned findings lead to the conclusion that the retinal and ganglion cell layer thicknesses are correlated with DM duration. In the initial few years of diabetes, the macular thickness decreases due to neural tissue loss, but as diabetes progresses, these thicknesses gradually increase due to vascular permeability in the retina [10, 11]. In patients without DR, Bronson-Castain et al. [17] found that the RT was decreased in a group of adolescent T2DM patients with a mean disease duration of 2.1 years. However, the authors of this study expressed doubt about the neural tissue theory based on the short duration of DM in their adolescent patients.

Our results indicated that the neurodegenerative effects on the retina probably occurred prior to vasculopathy in the early stages of diabetes based on the variations in the ages and disease durations of our population. Therefore, our results do not mean that there were no changes in the RTs of the T2DM patients; rather, the thickening of other layers, such as the INL and ONL, which were observed in the present study, probably masked these changes.

Due to technical limitations, we were unable to directly measure the ganglion cell layer thickness, but the newly updated OCT software provides accurate data about the GC-IPL complex for clinical studies.

Other studies have also observed ganglion cell loss in DR and nonproliferative diabetic retinopathy (NDR) patients [10], and axonal loss may lead to the thinning of the RNFL [18]. Moreover, both ganglion cells loss and axonal loss are correlated with HbAc1 and duration [19] and worsen as disease severity increases. The pericentral macular area has been found to be significantly thinner in patients with minimal DR [18, 20] and thicker in patients with preproliferative diabetic retinopathy [19], which suggests that neuronal abnormalities may precede vascular abnormalities [11].

We found that the RNFL around the optic disc was thinner in the patients than in the controls only at the 9 o'clock position, which may prove that RNFL degeneration occurs in the onset stage of diabetes [14, 21]; however, it is difficult to determine which area is the first to be affected.

In the inner nuclear layer, the pericentral and peripheral macular thicknesses were decreased in the T1DM patients compared to the controls, whereas they were thicker in the T2DM group, and the same pattern of

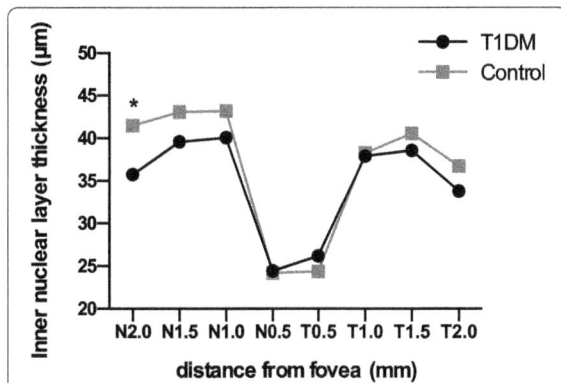

Fig. 3 Comparison of the inner nuclear layer thicknesses in the perifoveal area between the type 1 diabetes patients and the control group. *Statistically meaningful

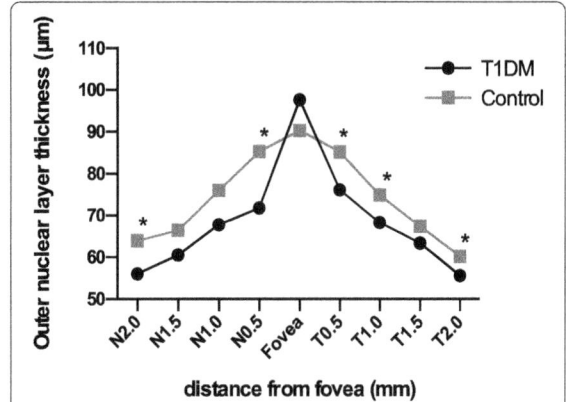

Fig. 4 Comparison of the outer nuclear layer thicknesses in the perifoveal area between the type 1 diabetes patients and controls. *Statistically meaningful

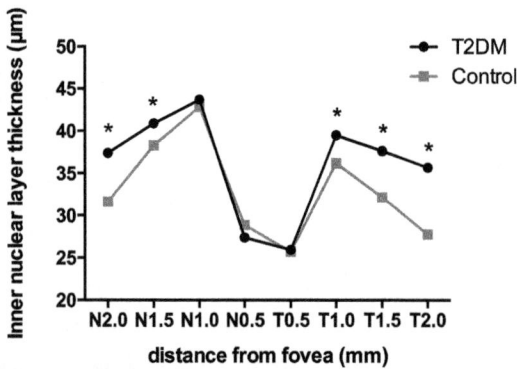

Fig. 5 Comparison of the inner nuclear layer thicknesses in the perifoveal area between the type 2 diabetes patients and controls. *Statistically meaningful

alterations was observed in the outer nuclear layer. These results confirm our speculation that neurodegeneration occurs during the early stages of disease and that the vascular permeability increases with disease duration and leads to increased retinal thickness. However, the differences were not significantly meaningful at all of the tested points; thus, we may need to increase our sample size. Only manual measurements and horizontal EDI scans were used to determine the INL and ONL thicknesses, which limited our statistical power. Continuous follow-up of these subjects is also needed for further study.

The reports regarding choroidal thickness (CT) in diabetes patients seem to be consistent in that they have all reported decreased CTs in subjects with proliferative diabetic retinopathy or diabetic macular edema and a lack of significant changes in NDR patients [22, 23] and T1DM children without DR [24]. The breakdown of the blood-retinal barrier, loss of retinal vasculature integrity

and the presence of hemodynamic abnormalities may contribute to changes in the choroidal thicknesses of diabetic eyes [25, 26]. In our study, the SFCTs of the T1DM and T2DM patients were similar to those of the controls, which may suggest that the choroid tissue is affected later than the neuroretinal layer in diabetic retinopathy.

Conclusion

We detected morphological changes in DM patients with Cirrus HD-OCT, and the remarkable results observed in the T1DM patients confirmed that the loss of neural tissue begins in the early stages of diabetes. As diabetes develops, neurodegeneration may be masked by changes in vascular permeability that cause thickening of the retinal layers.

Abbreviations
BCVA: best-corrected visual acuity; DR: diabetic retinopathy; EDI: enhanced depth imaging; GC-IPL: ganglion cell and inner plexiform layer; INL: inner nuclear layer; IOP: intraocular pressure; NDR: nonproliferative diabetic retinopathy; OCT: optical coherence tomography; ONL: outer nuclear layer; RNFL: retinal fiber layer; RT: retinal thickness; SFCT: subfoveal choroid thickness; T1DM: type 1 diabetes mellitus; T2DM: type 2 diabetes mellitus.

Competing interests
The authors declare that they have no financial competing interests.

Authors' contributions
All authors conceived of and designed the experimental protocol. XS and YY contributed to the study design and performed critical revision of the manuscript for important intellectual content. YC and JL performed the eye examinations and analyzed the data. YC wrote the paper. All authors have read and approved the final manuscript.

Acknowledgements
This work was supported by the National Nature Science Foundation of China grants 81170860 and 81470639 and the Shanghai Nature Science Foundation grant 14411968400.

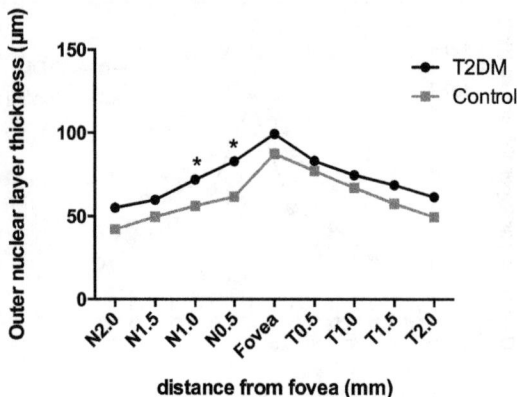

Fig. 6 Comparison of the outer nuclear layer thicknesses in the perifoveal area between the type 2 diabetes patients and controls. *Statistically meaningful

References
1. Wild S, Roglic G, Green A, Sicree R, King H. Global prevalence of diabetes: estimates for the year 2000 and projections for 2030. Diabetes Care. 2004;27(5):1047–53.
2. Kempen JH, O'Colmain BJ, Leske MC, Haffner SM, Klein R, Moss SE, et al. The prevalence of diabetic retinopathy among adults in the United States. Arch Ophthalmol. 2004;122(4):552–63. Chicago, Ill : 1960.
3. Roy MS, Klein R, O'Colmain BJ, Klein BE, Moss SE, Kempen JH. The prevalence of diabetic retinopathy among adult type 1 diabetic persons in the United States. Arch Ophthalmol. 2004;122(4):546–51. Chicago, Ill : 1960.
4. Xie XW, Xu L, Wang YX, Jonas JB. Prevalence and associated factors of diabetic retinopathy. The Beijing Eye Study 2006. Graefes Arch Clin Exp Ophthalmol. 2006;246(11):1519–26.
5. Wang FH, Liang YB, Zhang F, Wang JJ, Wei WB, Tao QS, et al. Prevalence of diabetic retinopathy in rural China: the Handan eye study. Ophthalmol. 2009;116(3):461–7.
6. Querques G, Lattanzio R, Querques L, Del Turco C, Forte R, Pierro L, et al. Enhanced depth imaging optical coherence tomography in type 2 diabetes. Invest Ophthalmol Vis Sci. 2012;53(10):6017–24.
7. Pires I, Santos AR, Nunes S, Lobo C. Macular thickness measured by stratus optical coherence tomography in patients with diabetes type 2 and mild nonproliferative retinopathy without clinical evidence of macular edema. Ophthalmologica. 2013;229(4):181–6.

8. Demir M, Oba E, Dirim B, Ozdal E, Can E. Central macular thickness in patients with type 2 diabetes mellitus without clinical retinopathy. BMC Ophthalmol. 2013;13:11.
9. van Dijk HW, Kok PH, Garvin M, Sonka M, Devries JH, Michels RP, et al. Selective loss of inner retinal layer thickness in type 1 diabetic patients with minimal diabetic retinopathy. Invest Ophthalmol Vis Sci. 2009;50(7):3404–9.
10. Araszkiewicz A, Zozulinska-Ziolkiewicz D, Meller M, Bernardczyk-Meller J, Pilacinski S, Rogowicz-Frontczak A, et al. Neurodegeneration of the retina in type 1 diabetic patients. Pol Arch Med Wewn. 2012;122(10):464–70.
11. Cabrera DeBuc D, Somfai GM. Early detection of retinal thickness changes in diabetes using Optical Coherence Tomography. Med Sci Monit. 2010;16(3):Mt15–21.
12. Villarroel M, Ciudin A, Hernandez C, Simo R. Neurodegeneration: An early event of diabetic retinopathy. World J Diabetes. 2010;1(2):57–64.
13. Antonetti DA, Klein R, Gardner TW. Diabetic retinopathy. N Engl J Med. 2012;366(13):1227–39.
14. Lecleire-Collet A, Tessier LH, Massin P, Forster V, Brasseur G, Sahel JA, et al. Advanced glycation end products can induce glial reaction and neuronal degeneration in retinal explants. Br J Ophthalmol. 2005;89(12):1631–3.
15. Barber AJ. A new view of diabetic retinopathy: a neurodegenerative disease of the eye. Prog Neuropsychopharmacol Biol Psychiatry. 2003;27(2):283–90.
16. Biallosterski C, van Velthoven ME, Michels RP, Schlingemann RO, DeVries JH, Verbraak FD. Decreased optical coherence tomography-measured pericentral retinal thickness in patients with diabetes mellitus type 1 with minimal diabetic retinopathy. Br J Ophthalmol. 2007;91(9):1135–8.
17. Bronson-Castain KW, Bearse Jr MA, Neuville J, Jonasdottir S, King-Hooper B, Barez S, et al. Adolescents with Type 2 diabetes: early indications of focal retinal neuropathy, retinal thinning, and venular dilation. Retina. 2009;29(5):618–26. Philadelphia, Pa.
18. van Dijk HW, Verbraak FD, Kok PH, Garvin MK, Sonka M, Lee K, et al. Decreased retinal ganglion cell layer thickness in patients with type 1 diabetes. Invest Ophthalmol Vis Sci. 2010;51(7):3660–5.
19. Oshitari T, Hanawa K, Adachi-Usami E. Changes of macular and RNFL thicknesses measured by Stratus OCT in patients with early stage diabetes. Eye (Lond). 2009;23(4):884–9.
20. Park HY, Kim IT, Park CK. Early diabetic changes in the nerve fibre layer at the macula detected by spectral domain optical coherence tomography. Br J Ophthalmol. 2011;95(9):1223–8.
21. Martin PM, Roon P, Van Ells TK, Ganapathy V, Smith SB. Death of retinal neurons in streptozotocin-induced diabetic mice. Invest Ophthalmol Vis Sci. 2004;45(9):3330–6.
22. Regatieri CV, Branchini L, Carmody J, Fujimoto JG, Duker JS. Choroidal thickness in patients with diabetic retinopathy analyzed by spectral-domain optical coherence tomography. Retina. 2012;32(3):563–8. Philadelphia, Pa.
23. Unsal E, Eltutar K, Zirtiloglu S, Dincer N, Ozdogan Erkul S, Gungel H. Choroidal thickness in patients with diabetic retinopathy. Clin Ophthalmol. 2014;8:637–42. Auckland, NZ.
24. Sayin N, Kara N, Pirhan D, Vural A, Ersan HB, Onal H, et al. Evaluation of subfoveal choroidal thickness in children with type 1 diabetes mellitus: an EDI-OCT study. Semin Ophthalmol. 2014;29(1):27–31.
25. Cunha-Vaz J, de Abreu JR F, Campos AJ. Early breakdown of the blood-retinal barrier in diabetes. Br J Ophthalmol. 1975;59(11):649–56.
26. Ciulla TA, Harris A, Latkany P, Piper HC, Arend O, Garzozi H, et al. Ocular perfusion abnormalities in diabetes. Acta Ophthalmol Scand. 2002;80(5):468–77.

14

Ocular pulse amplitude and retina nerve fiber layer thickness in migraine patients without aura

Semra Acer[1*], Attila Oğuzhanoğlu[2], Ebru Nevin Çetin[1], Nedim Ongun[2], Gökhan Pekel[1], Alper Kaşıkçı[1] and Ramazan Yağcı[1]

Abstract

Background: To evaluate the ocular pulse amplitude (OPA), the posterior pole asymmetry analysis (PPAA), the peripapillary retinal nerve fiber layer (RNFL) thickness, the ganglion cell layer (GCL) thickness, macular thickness and visual field testing in migraine patients without aura.

Methods: In this prospective, cross-sectional and comparative study 38 migraine patients and 44 age and sex matched controls were included. OPA was measured by dynamic contour tonometry (DCT), PPAA, RNFL, GCL and macular thickness were measured by Heidelberg Spectral Domain Optical Coherence Tomography (SD-OCT) and standard perimetry was performed using the Humphrey automated field analyzer.

Results: The difference in OPA was not statistically significant between the two groups ($p \geq 0.05$). In the PPAA there was no significant difference between two hemispheres in each eye ($p \geq 0.05$). The RNFL thickness was significantly reduced in the temporal and nasal superior sectors in the migraine group ($p \leq 0.05$). The GCL and macular thickness measurements were thinner in migraine patients but the difference between groups was not statistically significant ($p \geq 0.05$). There was no correlation between RNFL, GCL, macular thickness measurements and OPA values. There was no significant difference in the mean deviation (MD) and pattern standard deviation (PSD) between the two groups ($p \geq 0.05$).

Conclusions: Migraine patients without aura have normal OPA values, no significant asymmetry of the posterior pole and decreased peripapillary RNFL thickness in the temporal and nasal superior sectors compared with controls. These findings suggest that there is sectorial RNFL thinning in migraine patients without aura and pulsative choroidal blood flow may not be affected during the chronic course of disease.

Keywords: Cerebrovascular disease, Ocular pulse amplitude, Choroidal perfusion, Nerve fiber, Retinal imaging

Background

Migraine is a form of headache that has been regarded as a *neurovascular* disorder. The theories about its mechanism do not provide satisfactory clarification and the underlying pathophysiology still remains unclear. Recent studies declared that neural events trigger vascular dilatation, which aggravates the pain and results in further nerve activation [1]. Migraine has several ocular manifestations including visual disturbances during attacks [2],

visual field defects [3], reduction in retinal nerve fiber layer (RNFL) thickness [4, 5], and normal tension glaucoma [6]. Central retinal artery occlusion and ischemic optic neuropathy were also reported previously, which may indicate possible ocular vascular involvement as well as central vascular system in migraine [7–9]. Vasospastic events and ocular involvement were reported mostly in migraine patients with aura [1].

Ocular pulse amplitude (OPA), which is described as the difference between systolic and diastolic intraocular pressure (IOP), is accepted as an indirect indicator of choroidal perfusion [10]. It is measured by dynamic contour tonometry, which is a contact tonometry providing

* Correspondence: drsemraacer@gmail.com
[1]Department of Ophthalmology, Kinikli Kampusu, Pamukkale University, Denizli, TR 20100, Turkey
Full list of author information is available at the end of the article

intraocular pressure and OPA simultaneously and was suggested as a diagnostic tool for diseases in which choroidal perfusion changes might occur [10, 11].

The posterior pole asymmetry analysis (PPAA) is a new method determining the hemisphere asymmetry of the macula by comparing the thickness of the two hemispheres on a map, which are divided into equal cells. It is reported that PPAA could show early glaucomatous damage before it could be documented by the optic disc analysis [12]. Therefore, there is a current trend towards investigating the change in PPAA in various ocular disorders in which retinal ganglion cell or axonal damage may occur.

The majority of migraine patients (85 %) have migraine without aura [1]. Recently intracerebral vascular alterations were reported in patients without aura which may support that vascular dysregulation is an integral mechanism of the migraine pathophysiology [13]. Therefore we conducted this study to evaluate the ocular involvement in migraine patients without aura, using OPA, PPAA, peripapillary RNFL thickness, GCL thickness, macular thickness and visual field test.

Methods

This prospective observational cross sectional study was approved by the Ethical Committee of Pamukkale University and adhered to the tenets of the Declaration of Helsinki. The study was conducted in the Department of Ophthalmology and the Department of Neurology in our university. All participants provided informed written consent to participate in the study. The diagnostic criteria for migraine without aura was based on the international Classification of Headache Disorder (ICHD-II) [14];

At least five of the following criteria need to be met:

- Treated or untreated headache attacks lasting 4 to 72 h.

Headache has at least two of the following characteristics:

- Moderate or severe pain intensity.
- Pulsating quality.
- Unilateral location.
- Aggravation by physical activity or causing avoidance of routine physical activity (eg, walking).

During a headache at least one of the following:

- Photophobia and phonophobia.
- Nausea and/or vomiting.
- Symptoms not associated with another disorder.

Study population

The participants were 38 migraine patients without aura and 44 age and sex matched controls.

The exclusion criteria for both groups were;

- Age ≥ 45 (to exclude age related changing)
- Best corrected visual acuity (BCVA) with Snellen chart < 1.0 (in decimals, any level of visual impairment was excluded)
- Having spherical or cylindrical refractive error ≥ 2D
- Having any ocular disease that could affect the RNFL thickness (glaucoma etc.)
- Previous ocular inflammation or surgery
- Any systemic or neurologic disorder
- Chronic drug use including migraine prophylactic agents which could influence ocular blood flow and RNFL thickness.

Examination techniques

All patients underwent detailed ophthalmic examination including visual acuity, intraocular pressure with non contact tonometry, ocular motility, anterior and posterior segment evaluations. OCT measurements were performed first, as DCT may cause transient corneal opacifications. Visual field testing was performed on a separate day.

OPA was measured by dynamic contour tonometry (DCT, Ziemer Ophthalmic Systems, Port, Switzerland) after applying a topical anaesthetic eye drop. The DCT is attached to a slit lamp, like classic applanation tonometers, giving a medium value of 100 IOP measurements per second and determines OPA, by providing dynamic IOP measurements. The mean value of two reliable measurements (Q1, Q2, Q3, as recommended by the manufacturer) was used.

Without pupillary dilatation, the PPAA, peripapillary RNFL thickness, GCL thickness and macular thickness were analysed with the Heidelberg Spectral Domain Optical Coherence Tomography (SD-OCT, Heidelberg Engineering, Dossenheim, Germany). The images that individual retinal layers could be identified were used. Asymmetry analysis of the posterior pole was evaluated with a map which compares the superior to inferior hemispheres (hemisphere asymmetry) for each eye. See Fig. 1 for asymmetry analysis of the posterior pole. One hemisphere includes 32 cells and each cell has an equivalent in the opposite hemisphere. The difference in retinal thickness between the two equivalent cells are indicated with colors changing from white to black. A black cell means that the difference in retinal thickness is ≥30 μm. For cell to cell comparison between two hemispheres, two or more consecutive black cells were taken into consideration and recorded as asymmetry positivity. The peripapillary RNFL thickness was evaluated in six sectors including temporal inferior, temporal, temporal superior, nasal superior, nasal, nasal inferior. GCL thickness

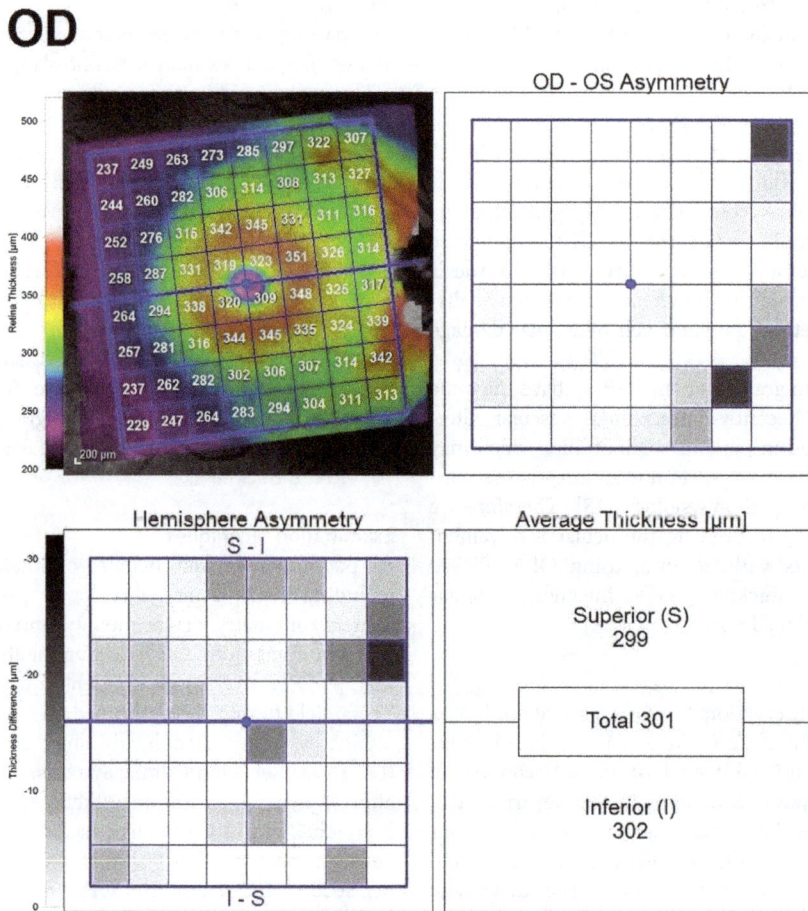

Fig. 1 Topographic measurement of PPAA. This migraine patient has a few gray cells, but no black cells and no significant hemisphere asymmetry

was measured on a central macular map which was automatically divided into ETDRS macular fields with a diameter of 1 mm (central sector),3 mm (internal sectors) and 6 mm (external sectors) in horizontal and vertical planes. The mean GCL thickness of central macular field with a diameter of 3 mm was estimated as the mean GCL thickness in each patient. See Fig. 2 for topographic measurement of GCL thickness.

Standard perimetry was performed using the central 30-2 threshold algorithm program on a Humphrey automated field analyser (HFA, CarlZeiss Inc, Dublin, California). The criteria for visual field reliability included <20 % fixation loss and < 20 % false positive and negative ratios. The test was repeated in patients with low reliability. The mean deviation (MD) and pattern standard deviation (PSD) values were recorded.

Randomly one eye of each participant was selected for the comparison of the parameters between the migraine and the control group.

Statistical analysis

Statistical analysis was performed by SPSS statistical software 17.0 (SPSS Inc., Chicago, IL). Independent samples t test, Pearson's correlation, and chi-square test were used for statistical analysis. Descriptive statistics were stated as means ± SD. A value of p ≤ 0.05 has been accepted as significant.

Results

The mean age was 30.17 ± 11.15 years in the migraine group, and 28.75 ± 7.06 years in the control group ($p = 0.42$). There were 35 females and 3 males in the migraine group and 40 females and 4 males in the control group ($p = 0.84$). The two groups were equivalent in terms of ethnicity. There was no difference in the refractive status between groups ($p = 0.77$). The mean number of migraine attacks per month was 4.30 ± 2.50. The mean length of migraine history was 3.72 ± 3.16.months.

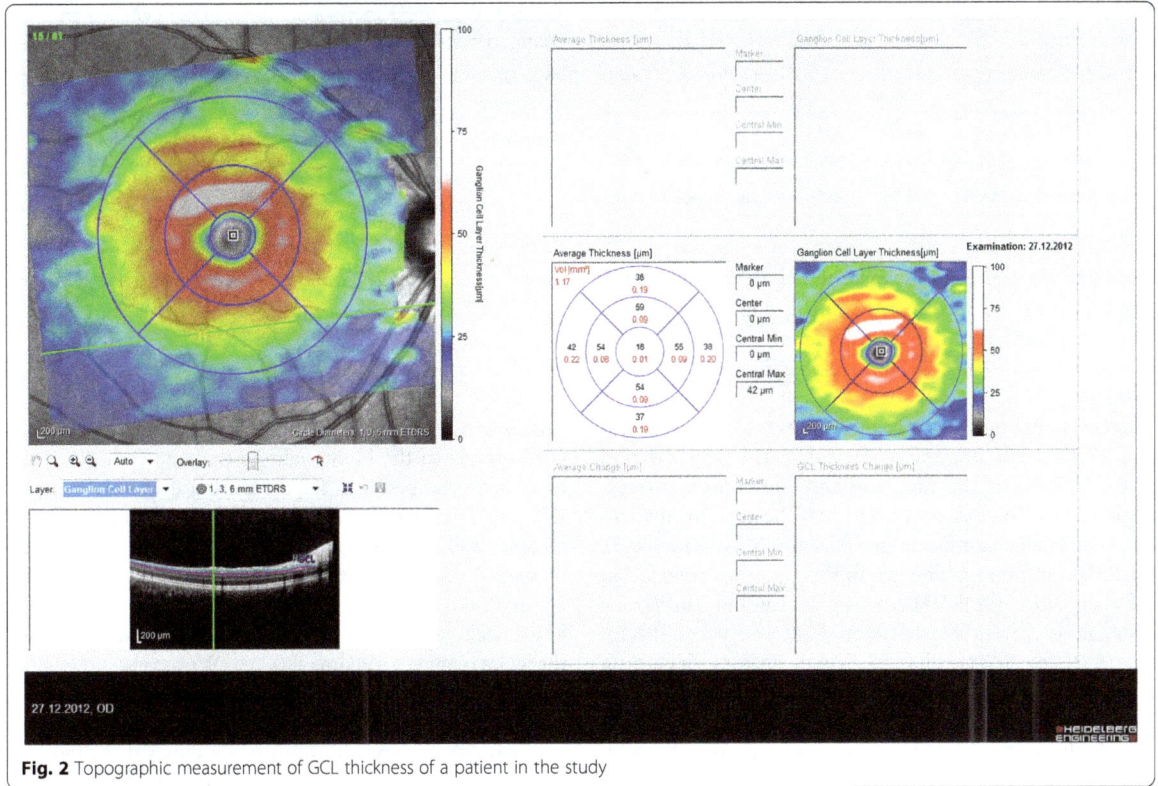

Fig. 2 Topographic measurement of GCL thickness of a patient in the study

The OPA value was 2.78 ± 1.02 mmHg and 2.61 ± 0.81 mmHg in the migraine and the control group respectively ($p = 0.48$). The correlation between OPA and the mean RNFL thickness in the migraine and the control group is shown in Fig. 3. There was no correlation between OPA and mean RNFL thickness ($r = 0.19$, $p = 0.26$), mean GCL thickness ($r = 0.06$, $p = 0.56$), macular

thickness ($r = 0.23$, $p = 0.16$), MD ($r = 0.01$, $p = 0.95$) and PSD ($r = -0.37$, $p = 0.12$) in the migraine group.

The difference in PPAA between the two groups was not statistically significant ($p = 0.83$). The PPAA of a migraine patient is shown in Fig. 2. Table 1 shows the macular thickness measurements and Table 2 shows the GCL thickness measurements in both groups. RNFL

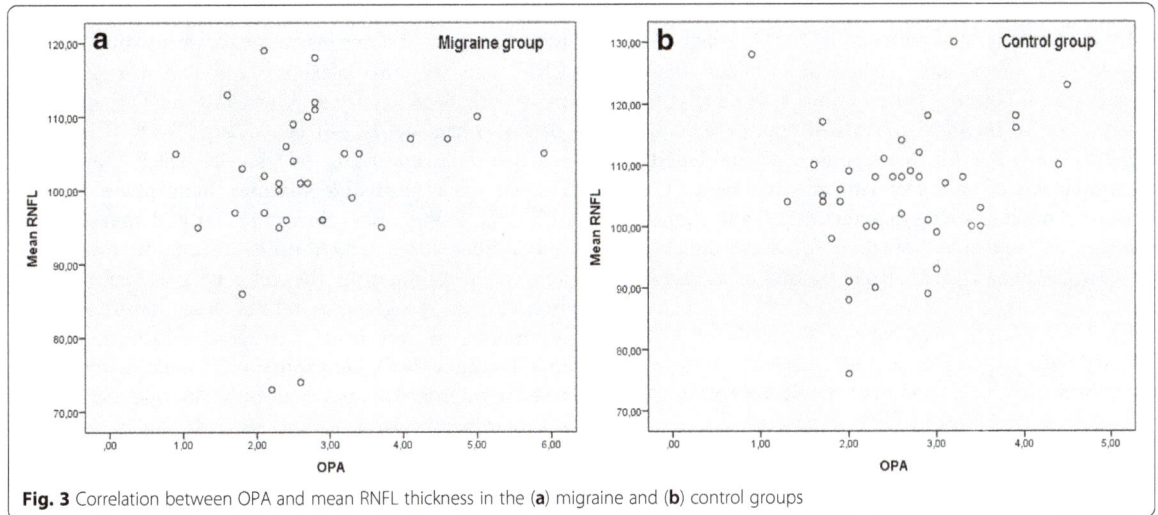

Fig. 3 Correlation between OPA and mean RNFL thickness in the (**a**) migraine and (**b**) control groups

Table 1 Macular thickness measurements in migraine and control group

Macular thickness (μm)	Migraine (n = 38)	Control (n = 44)	p value
Macular thickness	296.80 ± 12.47	299.02 ± 12.86	0.46
Superior hemifield thickness	296.83 ± 12.92	297.73 ± 13.63	0.77
Inferior hemifield thickness	297.58 ± 12.55	299.78 ± 12.90	0.47

Table 3 RNFL thickness measurements in the migraine and control groups

RNFL Thickness (μm)	Migraine (n = 38)	Control (n = 44)	p value
Mean RNFL	102.39 ± 8.91	105.63 ± 10.64	0.15
Temporal inferior	151.64 ± 17.95	157.89 ± 20.88	0.16
Temporal	71.47 ± 10.29	77.93 ± 11.34	**0.01**
Temporal superior	142.38 ± 13.50	143.27 ± 22.10	0.83
Nasal superior	103.94 ± 13.67	112.25 ± 22.02	**0.04**
Nasal	80.97 ± 13.73	76.93 ± 12.16	0.17
Nasal inferior	119.08 ± 19.68	119.48 ± 22.79	0.93

RNFL retinal nerve fiber layer
The bold p values were statically significant

thickness was significantly lower in the temporal and the nasal superior sectors in migraine group as shown in Table 3. Illness duration or frequency did not show a correlation with OPA, RNFL thickness, macular thickness, GCL thickness, MD or PSD.

In the visual field testing; the MD was -2.90 ± 1.81 dB and -2.32 ± 1.86 dB, the PSD was 2.01 ± 0.55 dB and 1.90 ± 0.73 dB in the migraine and the control groups, respectively. The difference between the two groups was not statistically significant ($p = 0.24$ for MD and $p = 0.51$ for PSD). In the migraine group there was no correlation between MD and RNFL in any sector but there was a negative correlation between PSD and mean RNFL ($p = 0.01$, $r = -0.54$) and in some sectors including temporal superior ($p = 0.03$, $r = -0.48$) nasal superior ($p = 0.04$, $r = -0.45$), nasal inferior ($p = 0.02$, $r = -0.52$). Fig. 4 shows visual field defects and sectorial RNFL thinning in a migraine patient.

Discussion

Our findings suggest that the choroidal perfusion assessed by OPA, is not significantly different between the migraine patients and the controls. Similarly, PPAA is not significantly different between the groups. However, there is significant sectoral RNFL thinning which correlates with PSD –an indicator of localized visual field defects- but not with OPA in migraine patients without aura.

Recent studies have reported choroidal and retinal involvement in migraine patients [4, 5, 15]. Using colored doppler ultrasonography, reduction of blood flow has been shown in both the central retinal artery and posterior ciliary artery in migraine patients without aura compared to healty subjects [16]. Decrease in choroidal blood flow by stimulation of choroidal sympathetic supply [17, 18], amaurosis fugax in young migraneurs [19] and pigmentary changes on fundus examination following attacks [20] were suggested as signs of affected choroidal circulation in

Table 2 GCL thickness measurements in the migraine and control groups

GCL thickness (μm)	Migraine (n = 38)	Control (n = 44)	p value
Mean GCL thickness	42.84 ± 4.14	44.53 ± 3.81	0.07
Central sector GCL thickness	12.79 ± 3.42	13.00 ± 3.04	0.78

GCL Ganglion cell layer

migraine. OPA reflects pulsatile variations in IOP which corresponds to the blood volume (mostly from the choroidal bed) pumped into the eye during each cardiac cycle [10, 11]. Therefore, OPA was suggested as an indirect indicator of choroidal blood flow and has been investigated in several disorders with vascular origin [10, 21, 22]. Decreased OPA values were reported in patients with carotid artery stenosis, uveitis, normal tension glaucoma and primary open angle glaucoma [10, 23]. We assessed the choroidal blood flow by measuring OPA and could not find a significant difference in OPA between the migraine group and controls. The result of this study shows that there is a possibility that the pulsative choroidal blood flow is not affected in patients without aura. This outcome does not rule out the involvement of choroidal perfusion but rather shows that the pulsatile choroidal blood flow is not permanently compromised in this subgroup.

If migraine might affect the peripapillary RNFL, it might also affect the GCL. The GCL is thickest at macula and the RNFL is thickest at peripapillary region [24]. Although glaucoma damages both GCL and RNFL, the peripapillary RNFL thickness has been shown to be more sensitive in the detection of glaucoma [25]. In recent years measurements of inner macular layers consisting of GCL, RNFL and the inner plexifom layer and macular asymmetry has been reported as an early predicting sign of glaucoma damage [12, 24]. Heidelberg SD-OCT has a new macular map consisting of 64 cells which may give a chance of a particular macular hemisphere analysis [12, 26]. PPAA may show the early damage of the nerve fiber layer, which usually starts in one hemisphere, by comparing the cells of two hemispheres. But in the progressive retinal fiber layer loss, an asymmetry is not usually present as advanced fiber loss includes both hemispheres [12]. Performing this test in migraneurs may not only provide data about macular nerve damage, but also may help detect an early onset of normal tension glaucoma in these patients. There was no significant difference between the two groups with cell to cell comparison. We also compared

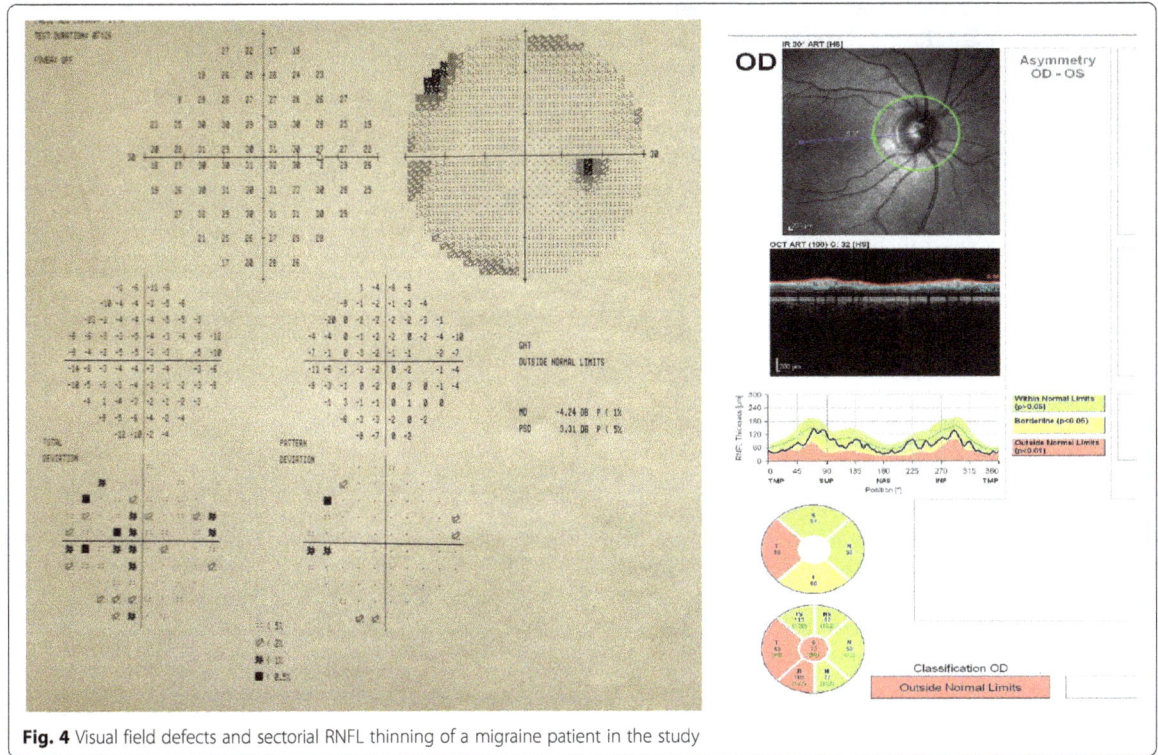

Fig. 4 Visual field defects and sectorial RNFL thinning of a migraine patient in the study

GCL and macular thickness in the two groups. Both GCL and macular thickness measurements were thinner in migraine patients but the difference was not statistically significant. Reduction in macular thickness with accompanying peripapillary RNFL thinning was documented in a migraine patient [27]. Ekinci et all reported decreased GCL thickness measurements in migraine patients and thinning in GCL was significant in migraine patients with aura [15]. Our results may reflect that nerve damage is not significant in the macular area in migraine patients without aura.

RNFL thickness was significantly lower in the temporal and nasal superior sectors. Inner retinal layers including RNFL and GCL are supplied by retinal vessels and outer retinal layers are supplied by choroidal vessels [28]. In contrast to choroidal vessels, retinal vessels have no autonomic innervations [29]. During an acute attack, the neural events result in dilation of blood vessels that cause nerve activation and vasoactive peptides being released into the extracerebral circulation. The vasoactive substances initiate a neurogenic inflammation and these neurovascular events are assumed to be the cause of pain [1]. These vasoactive substances may also reduce the ocular blood flow and adequate oxygen may not be provided to the retinal neural cells, which may result in cell deterioration. Ekinci et al showed that RNFL thickness was thinner in migraine patients with aura,

compared with patients without aura and healthy controls [15]. Gipponi and Martinez reported a reduction in RNFL thickness in migraine patients with and without aura [4, 5]. In this study we reported decreased RNFL thickness in patients without aura which may suggest that the neurovascular pathway underlying the migraine may play a role in reducing RNFL thickness independent of aura. Previous studies have reported segmental thinning of the temporal and superior RNFL which is consistent with our results [4, 5]. Finding RNFL thinning in similar sectors may be accidental or may be specific for migraine disease. There was no correlation between RNFL thinning and illness duration or frequency, however to exclude patients with anti-migraine drug use, we had to include patients who had newly diagnosed migraine or had short illness duration. Therefore, a long term follow-up is needed to observe the course of thinning.

In the visual field testing, both MD and PSD were worse in the migraine group, but the difference was not statistically significant and no correlation was found between MD, PSD and illness duration or frequency. Unexpectedly, MD was -2.32 ± 1.86 dB in controls, which might be a result of the practice and learning effect. Migraine patients had localized superior and inferior hemifield visual field losses (25 %), most of which correlated with the thinning of the corresponding RNFL quadrants. There was no correlation between MD and RNFL in any sector, but there was a negative correlation between PSD and the mean RNFL, temporal superior, nasal superior and nasal inferior sectors. General reduction of sensitivity was present in 10 % of migraine patients. Different forms of visual field defects, most of which were present in the midperipheral field have been reported in migraneurs, reflecting a precortical region [30, 31]. Cortical visual field defects are not common in migraine patients [32]. Because of the relationship between normal tension glaucoma and migraine, migraine patients who have RNFL thinning and visual field defects, even though they have no glaucomatous cupping, should be carefully monitored, in terms of glaucoma.

Our study has several limitations. Firstly; OPA measurements could not be obtained during migraine attacks because most of the patients were not able to show up during their attacks. Secondly; choroidal thickness with enhanced deep imaging OCT should have been measured and the results should have been compared between groups. Lastly; It would be better to evaluate the choroidal doppler ultrasound and correlate it with OPA findings.

Conclusions

In migraine patients without aura, the pulsative choroidal blood flow is not affected, at least between attacks. There is significant sectorial RNFL thinning which correlates with localized visual field defects. This finding may indicate an axonal insult and the necessity of monitoring RNFL and visual field testing in migraine patients without aura.

Abbreviations

BCVA: best corrected visual acuity; DCT: dynamic contour tonometry; GCL: Ganglion cell layer; ICHD: international classification of headache disorder; MD: mean deviation; OCT: optical coherence tomography; OPA: ocular pulse amplitude; PPAA: posterior pole asymmetry analysis; PSD: pattern standard deviation; RNFL: retinal nerve fiber layer.

Competing interests

The authors declare that they have no competing interests.

Authors' contributions

SA conceived of the study, participated in its design and coordination, participated in the sequence alignment and drafted the manuscript. AO conceived of the study, participated in its design. ENÇ conceived of the study, participated in its design and coordination. NO collected the data and drafted the manuscript. GP participated in the design of the study and performed the statistical analysis. AK collected the data and carried out the OPA measurements. RY conceived of the study, participated in the sequence alignment and drafted the manuscript. All authors read and approved the final manuscript.

Acknowledgments

No financial support was received for this submission. A part of this study was presented at 14th Euretina Congress which took place in London between 11-14 September 2014. The authors thank to Deniz Elena Newman for language revision.

Author details

[1]Department of Ophthalmology, Kinikli Kampusu, Pamukkale University, Denizli, TR 20100, Turkey. [2]Department of Neurology, Kinikli Kampusu, Pamukkale University, Denizli, Turkey.

References

1. Goadsby PJ. Pathophysiology of migraine. Neurol Clin. 2009;27:335–60.
2. Lepore FE. Effects of visual pathway lesions on the visual aura of migraine. Cephalalgia. 2009;29:430–5.
3. Dersu II, Thostenson J, Durcan FJ, Hamilton SM, Digre KB. Optic disc and visual test findings in patients with migraine. J Clin Neurosci. 2013;20:72–4.
4. Gipponi S, Scaroni N, Venturelli E, Forbice E, Rao R, Liberini P, et al. Reduction in retinal nerve fiber layer thickness in migraine patients. Neurol Sci. 2013;34(6):841–5.
5. Martinez A, Proupim N, Sanchez M. Retinal nerve fibre layer thickness measurements using optical coherence tomography in migraine patients. Br J Ophthalmol. 2008;92:1069–75.
6. Phelps CD, Corbett JJ. Migraine and low-tension glaucoma. A case-control study. Invest Ophthalmol Vis Sci. 1985;26:1105–8.
7. Sacco S, Ricci S, Carolei A. Migraine and vascular diseases: a review of the evidence and potential implications for management. Cephalalgia. 2012;32:785–95.
8. Tzourio C, Iglesias S, Hubert JB, Visy JM, Alpérovitch A, Tehindrazanarivelo A, et al. Migraine and risk of ischaemic stroke: a case-control study. BMJ. 1993;307(6899):289–92.
9. Katz B. Migrainous central retinal artery occlusion. J Clin Neuroophthalmol. 1986;6:69–75.
10. Schwenn O, Troost R, Vogel A, Grus F, Beck S, Pfeiffer N. Ocular pulse amplitude in patients with open angle glaucoma, normal tension glaucoma, and ocular hypertension. Br J Ophthalmol. 2002;86:981–4.
11. Knecht PB, Menghini M, Bachmann LM, Baumgartner RW, Landau K. The ocular pulse amplitude as a noninvasive parameter for carotid artery stenosis screening: a test accuracy study. Ophthalmology. 2012;119(6):1244–9.
12. Um TW, Sung KR, Wollstein G, Yun SC, Na JH, Schuman JS. Asymmetry in hemifield macular thickness as an early indicator of glaucomatous change. Invest Ophthalmol Vis Sci. 2012;53:1139–44.
13. Asghar MS, Hansen AE, Amin FM, van der Geest RJ, Koning P, Larsson HB, et al. Evidence for a vascular factor in migraine. Ann Neurol. 2011;69:635–45.
14. Olesen J. The international classification of headache disorders. 2nd edition (ICHD-II). Rev Neurol (Paris). 2005;161:689–91.
15. Ekinci M, Ceylan E, Cağatay HH, Keleş S, Hüseyinoğlu N, Tanyildiz B, et al. Retinal nerve fibre layer, ganglion cell layer and choroid thinning in migraine with aura. BMC Ophthalmol. 2014;14:75.
16. Kara SA, Erdemoğlu AK, Karadeniz MY, Altinok D. Color Doppler sonography of orbital and vertebral arteries in migraineurs without aura. J Clin Ultrasound. 2003;31(6):308–14.
17. Ruskell GL. Facial parasympathetic innervation of the choroidal blood vessels in monkeys. Exp Eye Res. 1971;12:166–72.
18. Bill A. Blood circulation and fluid dynamics in the eye. Physiol Rev. 1975;55:383–417.
19. O'Sullivan F, Rossor M, Elston JS. Amaurosis fugax in young people. Br J Ophthalmol. 1992;76:660–2.
20. Connor RC. Complicated migraine. A study of permanent neurological and visual defects caused by migraine. Lancet. 1962;2:1072–5.
21. McKee HD, Saldana M, Ahad MA. Increased ocular pulse amplitude revealing aortic regurgitation. Am J Ophthalmol. 2004;138:503.
22. Golnik KC, Miller NR. Diagnosis of cavernous sinus arteriovenous fistula by measurement of ocular pulse amplitude. Ophthalmology. 1992;99:1146–52.
23. Cetin EN, Bulgu Y, Taslı L, Cobankara V, Yildırım C. Ocular pulse amplitude in Behçet disease. Ocul Immunol Inflamm. 2011;19:376–8.
24. Tan O, Chopra V, Lu AT, Schuman JS, Ishikawa H, Wollstein G, et al. Detection of macular ganglion cell loss in glaucoma by Fourier-domain opticalcoherence tomography. Ophthalmology. 2009;116(12):2305-14.
25. Sung KR, Kim JS, Wollstein G, Folio L, Kook MS, Schuman JS. Imaging of the retinal nerve fibre layer with spectral domain optical coherence tomography for glaucoma diagnosis. Br J Ophthalmol. 2011;95:909–14.
26. Seo JH, Kim TW, Weinreb RN, Park KH, Kim SH, Kim DM. Detection of localized retinal nerve fiber layer defects with posterior pole asymmetry analysis of spectral domain optical coherence tomography. Invest Ophthalmol Vis Sci. 2012;53:4347–53.
27. Cunha LP, Vessani RM, Monteiro ML. Localized neural loss detected by macular thickness reduction using optical coherence tomography: case report. Arq Bras Oftalmol. 2008;71:743–6.

28. Linsenmeier RA, Braun RD. Oxygen distribution and consumption in the cat retina during normoxia and hypoxemia. J Gen Physiol. 1992;99(2):177–97.
29. Riva CE, Grunwald JE, Petrig BL. Retinal vessels lack a functional sympathetic innervation. "Autoregulation of human retinal blood flow. An investigation with laser Doppler velocimetry". Invest Ophthalmol Vis Sci. 1986;27:1706–12.
30. McKendrick AM, Vingrys AJ, Badcock DR, Heywood JT. Visual field losses in subjects with migraine headaches. Invest Ophthalmol Vis Sci. 2000;41: 1239–47.
31. Lewis RA, Vijayan N, Watson C, Keltner J, Johnson CA. Visual field loss in migraine. Ophthalmology. 1989;96:321–6.
32. Wakakura M, Ichibe Y. Permanent homonymous hemianopias following migraine. J Clin Neuro-ophthalmol. 1992;12:198–202.

15

Strategies to estimate the characteristics of 24-hour IOP curves of treated glaucoma patients during office hours

Leonardo Colombo*, Paolo Fogagnolo, Giovanni Montesano, Stefano De Cillà, Nicola Orzalesi and Luca Rossetti

Abstract

Background: It is known that office-hour measurements might not adequately estimate IOP mean, peaks and fluctuations in healthy subjects. The purpose of the present study is to verify whether office-hour measurements in patients in different body positions can estimate the characteristics of 24-hour intraocular pressure (IOP) in treated POAG patients.

Methods: The 24-hour IOP curves of 70 eyes of 70 caucasian patients with treated glaucoma were analyzed. Measurements were taken at 9 AM; 12, 3, 6, and 9 PM; and 12, 3, and 6 AM, both in the supine (TonoPen XL) and sitting (Goldmann tonometer) positions. The ability of five strategies to estimate IOP mean, peak and fluctuation was evaluated. Each method was analyzed both with regression of the estimate error on the real value and with "hit or miss" analysis.

Results: The least biased estimate of the Peak IOP was obtained using measurements from both supine and sitting positions, also yielding the highest rate of correct predictions (which was significantly different from 3 of the remaining 4 strategies proposed, $p < 0.05$). Strategies obtained from the combination of supine, sitting and peak measurements resulted to be least biased for the Mean IOP and the IOP Fluctuation estimate, but all strategies were not found significantly different in terms of correct prediction rate (the only significant difference being between the two strategies based on sitting or supine measurements only, with the former being the one with the highest correct prediction rate).

Conclusions: The results of this study remark the concept that IOP is a dynamic parameter and that intensive measurement is helpful in determining its characteristics. All office-hour strategies showed a very poor performance of in correctly predicting the considered parameters within the thresholds used in this paper, all scoring a correct prediction rate below 52 %.

Keywords: Glaucoma, 24-hour IOP, Office-hour IOP, IOP peak and fluctuation, Timolol, Latanoprost, Brimonidine, Fixed combination timolol dorzolamide

Background

Intraocular pressure (IOP) is the main risk factor for the development and progression of glaucoma [1–4] and the only treatable one. IOP parameters (mean, peak and fluctuation) should be measured at diagnosis and strictly monitored in order to address the efficacy of IOP-lowering interventions. Mean IOP has been consistently recognized as a major risk factor for glaucoma and its progression [1, 2, 4] whereas the role of peak [5, 6] and fluctuation [7–12] as independent risk factors is still controversial.

Many studies report that mean IOP is not significantly different when measured during office-hour and 24-hour [13–16], but that office-hour data may significantly underestimate IOP peak and fluctuation: the majority of glaucoma patients had their IOP peaks outside office hours, most frequently occurring in night hours [14, 16–19].

* Correspondence: leonardo.colombo.82@gmail.com
Eye Clinic, San Paolo Hospital, University of Milan, Via A. Di Rudinì 8, 20142 Milan, Italy

In addiction to that supine office hour IOP measurements were described to better estimate IOP peaks than sitting measurements alone [16].

The most precise procedure to investigate IOP characteristics is 24-hour phasing [13–16, 20, 21] though it is unpractical, expensive and can be performed in a small subgroup of patients in few institutions. In addiction to that, due to the unavailability of IOP-measuring techniques that can be used while the patient sleeps, nighttime evaluations require awakening of patients, potentially causing artifacts related to stress.

In 2009 the group of Leonardi developed a disposable contact lens sensor (CLS) that allows continous IOP monitoring (Sensimed AG, Lausanne, Switzerland) [22]. Nowadays the major limitation of this technology is the fact that the results of IOP evaluations are not provided in the habitual mmHg units but in an arbitrary unit and a direct comparison between the two methods cannot be performed yet [23].

The difficulty in obtaining 24-hour curves and the possible discrepancies between 24-hour and office-hour data led our [14] and other groups [16, 18, 19] to develop strategies to estimate 24-hour parameters by office-hour data. We showed that the collection of supine and sitting office-hour measurements may enhance the correct identification of 24-hour IOP characteristics in both healthy subjects and untreated POAG [14].

The purpose of the present study was to verify whether office-hour measurements taken in different body positions can estimate the characteristics of 24-hour IOP in POAG patients using different IOP-lowering treatments.

Methods

This study was a retrospective analysis of 24-hour IOP curves of POAG treated patients, collected in the context of clinical trials investigating the circadian effect of antiglaucoma drugs. It was conducted at the Eye Clinic of San Paolo Hospital, University of Milan, Italy, after approval by the local Ethics Committee of San Paolo Hospital in Milan, and according to the tenets of the Declaration of Helsinki and national laws for the protection of personal data. Written informed consent was obtained from all the study participants.

Study population

Seventy caucasian patients were enrolled (39 men and 31 women): 19 of them were treated with timolol (twice a day), 29 with latanoprost (once a day), ten with brimonidine (twice a day) and 12 with the fixed combination dorzolamide/timolol (FCDT, twice a day). These treatments options were part of their standard care.

To be included in the study, patients had to have glaucomatous visual fields (abnormal mean defect and corrected pattern standard deviation on at least two consecutive, reliable Humphrey 30–2 full-threshold tests), optic nerve head (ONH) changes (presence of concentric enlargement of the optic cup, localized notching, or both, as evaluated by means of color stereophotographs), and/or retinal nerve fiber layer (RNFL) defects (presence of focal or diffuse neuroretinal rim thinning, as evaluated by means of a scanning laser ophthalmoscope). Patients with ocular hypertension were excluded. Patients with untreated POAG were not included in this study.

Exclusion criteria included angle-closure glaucoma, secondary glaucomas, corneal abnormalities preventing reliable IOP measurement, previous filtration surgery, having one eye, pregnancy, significant disturbances of wake-sleep rhythms, and/or the regular use of hypnotic drugs reported by the patients. Eligibility was verified by means of a complete ophthalmic assessment.

Twenty-four-Hour IOP evaluation

The methodology to assess 24-hour IOP is described in previous papers [14, 24] and summarized in Fig. 1.

The patients were hospitalized in the morning at 7 AM and stayed for the following 24 h. The awake period lasted from approximately 6:30 AM to 11:00 PM. IOP was measured at 9 AM; 12,3,6, and 9 PM; and 12, 3 and 6 AM both in the supine and sitting positions.

For the daytime measurements (9 AM–9 PM), patients were asked to go to bed and relax for approximately 15 min, after which supine IOP was measured in both eyes. After approximately 10 min, a second IOP value was measured at the slit lamp. During the night, the patients were awakened approximately 10 min before each measurement to prevent a sudden increase in IOP. The IOP supine measurements were taken with a handheld electronic tonometer (TonoPen XL; Bio-Rad, Glendale, CA); the IOP sitting measurements on the other hand were taken with Goldmann applanation tonometer at the slit lamp. Every measurement by TonoPen XL consisted of a variable number of readings until the coefficient of variation was less than 5 %. All measurements were taken at each time point by two well-trained glaucoma specialists who had obtained good accordance between their measurements ($\kappa = 0.82$ with both tonometers). If the measurements differed by >2 mm Hg, a third measurement was taken; the mean of two or the median of three recordings was used for the analysis.

Peak IOP estimator strategies

Five parameters were tested in their ability of extrapolating peak IOP from office-hour readings:

1. The highest value obtained from the office-hour curve in the sitting position.

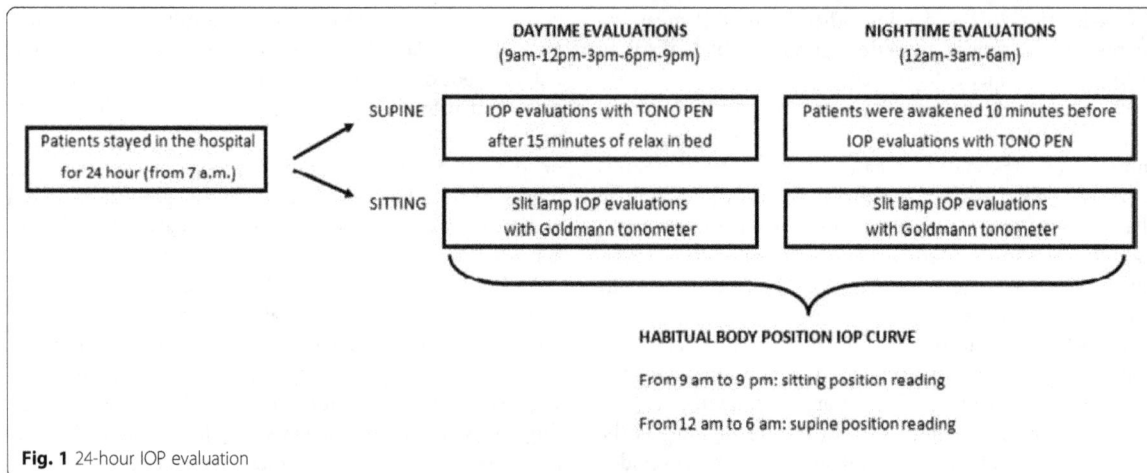

Fig. 1 24-hour IOP evaluation

2. The formula proposed by Mosaed et al. 21 based on office-hour supine IOP (peak IOP = 5.98 + 0.771 + average office-hour supine IOP).
3. The formula proposed by Mosaed et al. 21 based on office-hour sitting IOP (peak IOP = 12.04 + 0.616 + average office-hour sitting IOP).
4. The mean of values obtained with the previous two formulas.
5. The highest value obtained from the office-hour curve in both supine and sitting positions.

Mean IOP and IOP fluctuations estimator strategies

The 24-hour mean IOP and IOP fluctuations in habitual body position were compared to those calculated from:

1. Office-hour readings only in the sitting position (four measurements).
2. Office-hour readings only in the supine position (four measurements).
3. Office-hour sitting readings (four measurements) + the peak IOP, as estimated with the better of the previous formulas.
4. A combination of sitting and supine office-hour readings (four + four measurements).
5. A combination of sitting and supine office-hour readings (four + four measurements) + the estimated peak IOP.

Statistical analysis

We considered the 24-hour curves obtained in habitual body position—that is sitting readings during waking time (from 9 AM to 9 PM) and supine readings during night time (from 12 to 6 AM). These curves were compared to the readings of the same 24-hour curves obtained during office hours (from 9 AM to 6 PM) in both

supine and sitting positions in order to evaluate the ability of off-h readings to predict 24-h characteristics.

The following parameters were calculated: mean and range of the difference between estimate and 24-hour IOP parameter (expressed as absolute values, i.e., both an underestimation of –4 mm Hg and an overestimation of +4 mm Hg counting as 4 mm Hg. Linear models and generalized linear models were used to assess the quality of the analyzed estimators. First, we analyzed the relation between the real value to be estimated and the estimate error (specifically the difference between the estimate and the real value). For most of the cases, a linear regression approach properly modeled the relation between the real value and the estimate. For two strategies (Strategy 1 for the peak value and Strategy 1 for the fluctuations) a Zero Inflated Compound Poisson Model (ZICP) was used to model the estimate error dependency on the real value due its peculiar skewed distribution and high zero counts. A ZICP model can be broken down in two parts: the first part uses a binomial distribution to model the zero/non zero outcome of the Estimate Error, while the second part models the distribution of the continuous Estimate Error value when not zero.

Next, we adopted a "hit or miss" approach to assess the error rate of each strategy, considering an estimate error within ± 2 mmHg as a correct prediction for the Peak IOP and Mean IOP, ± 1 mmHg for IOP Fluctuations. In this context, a multinomial logit model was used on the various strategies to assess the odds of overestimation, underestimation and correct prediction. For the two strategies for which the ZICP was used, a completely correct prediction odds (0 mmHg error) was also derived from the binomial part of the model.

All numeric predictors (i.e. the real values) were mean centered, so the intercept corresponds to the estimates for the mean predictor value.

Then, an analysis by treatment groups was conducted to assess differences in estimation. In this case a classical ANOVA approach was chosen and a post-hoc correction (Tukey-Kramer) was used for multiple comparisons.

Finally, an overall comparison of the strategies was performed fitting a logit model for each feature considered (Mean, Peak and Fluctuation) with the Strategy as the predictor (where each strategy represented a level) and "Hit" or "Miss" as the response variable, according to the above classification of hits or misses. A Subject random effect was included to account for the fact that each strategy estimated the same real value for each subject. Then a post hoc analysis (Tukey-Kramer) was performed to compare the various strategies in terms of odds of hits or misses.

All calculations were made in R scripting environment.

Results

The mean age was 73.1 ± 9.09 years. 24-hour IOP data in habitual body position are shown in Table 1.

Mean and peak IOP were lower in patients treated with latanoprost than in patients treated with timolol (respectively $P = 0.03$ and 0.05); significant differences were not found among the other groups. Differences in fluctuation between groups were negligible.

IOP peaked outside office hours in 65 % of all patients (timolol, 58 %; latanoprost, 76 %; brimonidine, 60 %; FCDT, 58 %).

The analysis focused on the accuracy of predictions from the various methods tested. Each method was analyzed both with regression of the estimate error (*estimated value – real value*) on the real value and with "hit or miss" analysis. For each of the three variables analyzed (Mean, Peak and Fluctuation) no significant differences were found among the treatment groups (*p*-values all greater than 0.13, ANOVA).

Regression analysis

Peak estimate

The five strategies presented above were analyzed, in terms of difference of the estimated value from the corresponding real value (Estimate Error). Strategies from 2 to 5 were analyzed using simple regression with Gaussian error distribution using the real Peak IOP value as a

predictor of the Estimate Error. The results are reported in Table 2. All strategies showed a significant dependency of the Estimate Error on the real Peak value with a negative slope, i.e. overestimation was more likely for smaller values and underestimation for larger values. Strategy 5 showed the smallest slope, yielding the least biased estimate of the Peak value.

Strategy 1 required a detailed analysis due to its peculiar Estimate Error distribution: only underestimation errors were allowed with a relatively high rate of correct prediction (zero Estimate Error). To properly model such negatively skewed distribution with high zero counts we reversed the sign of the Error and used a ZICP model. This allowed accurate modeling of the odds of correct predictions and of the skewed negative errors. Particularly, the odds of correct prediction did not depend on the peak value (*p*-value = 0.3) and was significantly different from 1 (odds = 0.52, probability of correct prediction = 0.34, *p*-value < 0.01). The mean prediction for non zero errors was significantly dependent on the real peak IOP value (*p* < 0.001) in a non linear fashion, as depicted in Fig. 2.

Mean estimate

Five strategies for estimating the Mean IOP value were analyzed as for the Peak strategies. In this case only linear regression analysis was necessary. Results are presented in Table 3. Strategies 3 and 4 showed a non significant dependency on the real Mean IOP value and a global mean non significantly different from zero (*p*-values > 0.05). Strategy 1 and 5 showed a non significant dependency of the Estimate Error on the Real Mean IOP but had a significant offset (negative for Strategy 1, positive for Strategy 5).

Fluctuation estimate

As for the Peak Value, Strategies from 2 to 5 were analyzed using simple regression with Gaussian error distribution using the real value as a predictor of the estimate error. The results are reported in Table 4.

As in the Peak estimate, one of the Strategies, specifically Strategy 1, showed a limiting effect to overestimation, yielding a relatively high rate (although much lower than for Strategy 1 for the Peak value) of correct

Table 1 The 24-hour IOP data in Habitual Body Position

	Mean ± SD (Range)	Peak ± SD (Range)	Fluctuation ± SD (Range)	Timing of peaks During office hours	Outside office hours
All patients	18.1 ± 3.4 (11.8–28.9)	22.5 ± 4.1 (15–33)	8.7 ± 2.9 (4–17)	35 %	65 %
Timolol	19.4 ± 3.5 (15.5–28.9)	24 ± 4 (19–33)	9 ± 2.7 (6–16)	42 %	58 %
Latanoprost	17.2 ± 3 (11.8–25.4)	21.7 ± 3.4 (16–29)	8.5 ± 2.7 (4–15)	24 %	76 %
Brimonidine	18.7 ± 3 (15.4–24)	22.5 ± 3,3 (19–28)	8.1 ± 2.2 (4–12)	40 %	60 %
DTFC	17.6 ± 3.9 (13.4–26.2)	22.2 ± 5.7 (15–32)	9 ± 4,3 (4–17)	42 %	58 %

Table 2 Estimated regression coefficients of the Estimate Error on the real IOP Peak value. In brackets, the standard errors of the coefficient estimates

| | Estimate Error | | | |
	Strategy 2	Strategy 3	Strategy 4	Strategy 5
IOP Peak Coefficient	−0.561***	−0.559***	−0.560***	−0.225**
	(0.056)	(0.045)	(0.045)	(0.089)
Global Mean	−1.858***	0.389**	−0.734***	0.229
	(0.228)	(0.181)	(0.182)	(0.361)
Observations	70	70	70	70
R^2	0.594	0.696	0.696	0.086
Adjusted R^2	0.588	0.691	0.692	0.072
Residual Std. Error (df = 68)	1.905	1.518	1.520	3.024
F Statistic (df = 1; 68)	99.566***	155.494***	155.859***	6.376**

Asterisks represent the significance level according to the legend in the footnotes
Note: *$p < 0.1$; **$p < 0.05$; ***$p < 0.01$

predictions (zero error) and a negatively skewed error distribution. Again, this was modeled using a ZICP model and the odds of correct prediction did not depend on the real fluctuation value (p-value = 0.60) and was significantly different from 1 (odds = 0.13, probability of correct prediction = 0.11, p-value < 0.01). The mean prediction for non zero errors was significantly dependent on the real IOP fluctuation value ($p < 0.001$) in a non linear fashion, as depicted in Fig. 3.

Hit or miss analysis

A second step of the analysis was aimed at the characterization, for each strategy, of the probability of yielding clinically reliable estimates of the quantities of interest. To test this, we chose a rage of clinical tolerance (±2 mmHg for the IOP Peak estimate and the Mean IOP estimate, ± 1 for the IOP Fluctuation

estimate). Errors within the tolerance range were considered as "Hit", errors outside the range were counted as "Miss" (subdivided in overestimates, "Over" and underestimates, "Under"). Then, a multinomial logit model was used for each strategy to model the "hit or miss". This approach had the advantage of allowing a comparison the different strategies independent of the error distribution. Hits were used as the reference category, so the model summary tables (see below) present the logit coefficients of "Over" versus "Hit" and "Under" versus "Hit".

Peak strategies

Table 5 shows the results for the multinomial logit model for IOP Peak strategies. Each model compares the selected strategy in terms of odds of overestimation or underestimation with respect to correct hits (within ±2 mmHg). The first Strategy had no "Over"

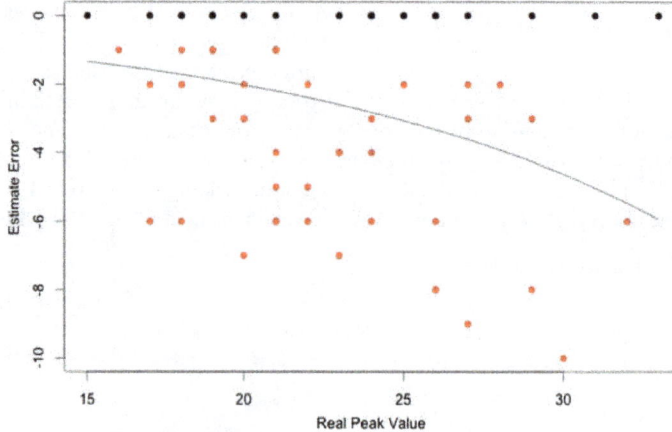

Fig. 2 Scatterplot for Estimate Error of Strategy 1. *Black dots* represent the correct estimates (zero error), red dots the incorrect estimates. The *black line* represents the prediction from the ZICP model showing the non linear dependency of the non zero error on the real peak value. Note the skewed distribution around the mean

Table 3 Estimated regression coefficients of the dependent variable (Estimate Error) on the real Mean IOP value

	Estimate Error:				
	Strategy 1	Strategy 2	Strategy 3	Strategy 4	Strategy 5
Mean IOP Coefficient	0.036	−0.226***	0.034	−0.095*	−0.082
	(0.052)	(0.076)	(0.049)	(0.052)	(0.050)
Global Mean	−0.412**	0.978***	0.288*	0.281	0.593***
	(0.175)	(0.255)	(0.166)	(0.175)	(0.168)
Observations	70	70	70	70	70
R^2	0.007	0.116	0.007	0.047	0.038
Adjusted R^2	−0.007	0.103	−0.008	0.033	0.024
Residual Std. Error (df = 68)	1.467	2.134	1.389	1.465	1.406
F Statistic (df = 1; 68)	0.487	8.925***	0.475	3.376*	2.708

In brackets, the standard errors of the coefficient estimates. Asterisks represent the significance level according to the legend in the footnotes
Note: *$p < 0.1$; **$p < 0.05$; ***$p < 0.01$

since it never overestimated the Peak Value. Strategy 5 resulted to be the most balanced in terms of over and underestimate and showed no significant ($p > 0.05$) relation with the true Peak IOP value (i.e. almost constant error rate) although, as for all the proposed strategies, overestimate tended to cluster at low peak values and underestimate at high peak values. Figure 4 shows scatter plots of the estimated values versus the real values, with misses highlighted in red.

Mean strategies

Table 6 shows the results for the multinomial logit model for Mean IOP strategies. Each model compares the selected strategy in terms of odds of overestimation or underestimation with respect to correct hits (within ±2 mmHg). Strategy 2 showed the highest rate of Overestimates, being even higher that correct Hits. Strategy 1 showed the highest Hit rate and no correlation of errors with the true Mean IOP value. All strategies except for Strategy 2 showed no significant correlation with the

Table 4 Estimated regression coefficients of the dependent variable (Estimate Error) on the real IOP Fluctuation value

	Estimate Error			
	(2)	(3)	(4)	(5)
IOP Fluctuation Coefficient	−1.010***	−0.720***	−0.759***	−0.759***
	(0.132)	(0.097)	(0.124)	(0.124)
Global Mean	−2.100***	−2.714***	−0.200	−0.200
	(0.383)	(0.281)	(0.360)	(0.360)
Observations	70	70	70	70
R^2	0.462	0.448	0.356	0.356
Adjusted R^2	0.454	0.440	0.346	0.346
Residual Std. Error (df = 68)	3.206	2.354	3.008	3.008
F Statistic (df = 1; 68)	58.480***	55.171***	37.562***	37.562***

In brackets, the standard errors of the coefficient estimates. Asterisks represent the significance level according to the legend in the footnotes
Note: *$p < 0.1$; **$p < 0.05$; ***$p < 0.01$

true Mean IOP value. Figure 5 shows scatter plots of the estimated values versus the real values, with misses highlighted in red.

Fluctuation strategies

Table 7 shows the results for the multinomial logit model for IOP Fluctuation strategies. Each model compares the selected strategy in terms of odds of overestimation or underestimation with respect to correct hits (within ± mmHg). The strategies with the highest Hit rate and more balanced Over/Underestimation rate were Strategy 4 and 5 (which yielded the exact same estimates for all subjects), although showing a strong correlation with the real IOP fluctuations, especially for the odds of underestimations, being more likely for higher Fluctuation value. Figure 6 shows scatter plots of the estimated values versus the real values, with misses highlighted in red.

Treatment group analysis

In general, no significant differences were found among the treatment groups. The only exceptions were for Strategy 1 for the Peak IOP, where a significant difference in the Estimate Error was found between the Brimonidine and the Latanoprost group (Latanoprost Mean Error = −3.01, Brimonidine Mean Error = −1.4, $p = 0.0105$), for Strategy 1 for the IOP Fluctuations, where a significant difference in the Estimate Error was found between the Timolol and the Latanoprost group (Latanoprost Mean Error = −4.41, Timolol Mean Error = −3.37, $p = 0.0045$) and for Strategy 3 for the IOP Fluctuations, where a significant difference in the Estimate Error was found between the Cosopt and the Latanoprost group (Latanoprost Mean Error = −1.52, Cosopt Mean Error = −4.33, $p = 0.0095$). A logit regression model was also calculated for each Strategy to test differences in Hit/Miss rate among the treatment groups, but no significant

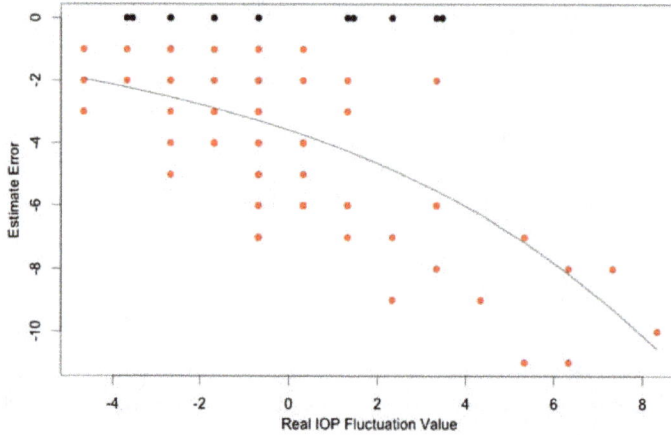

Fig. 3 Scatterplot for Estimate Error of Strategy 1. *Black dots* represent the correct estimates (zero error), red dots the incorrect estimates. The *black line* represents the prediction from the ZICP model showing the non linear dependency of the non zero error on the real peak value

difference among treatment groups could be detected for all strategies.

Hit rate comparison of the strategies

For each considered feature (Peak, Mean and Fluctuations) all strategies were compared in terms of Hits using a logit model corrected for repeated measures with a Subject random effect and a post hoc analysis. For the Peak strategies Strategy 5 yielded the highest Hit count (37/70) and resulted to be significantly different from Strategies 2, 3 and 4 (corrected $p < 0.05$). Strategy 1 resulted to be significantly different from Strategy 2 ($p = 0.0079$) with a higher Hit count, but not from Strategy 3, 4 and 5 (although the comparisons with strategies 3 and 4 had low p-

values, respectively 0.11 and 0.07). For the Mean IOP, only Strategy 1 resulted to be significantly different from Strategy 2 ($p = 0.031$) but any other difference was not significant, with Strategy 1 being the one with the highest Hit count (36/70). No significant differences could be found between the Strategies for the IOP Fluctuations, Strategy 4 and 5 being the ones with the highest Hit count (36/70).

Discussion

The results of this study on glaucoma patients treated with different IOP lowering eye drops remark the concept that IOP is a dynamic parameter and that intensive measurement is helpful in determining its characteristics.

Table 5 Estimated logit coefficients from the multinomial logit model (coefficients and standard errors in brackets)

	Over/Underestimate logit				
	Strategy 1	Strategy 2	Strategy 3	Strategy 4	Strategy 5
"Over" at average Peak IOP		−1.395	−0.618	−2.117**	−0.737**
		(0.882)	(0.451)	(0.844)	(0.292)
"Under" at average Peak IOP	0.060	1.486***	−1.441**	0.075	−0.984***
	(0.242)	(0.475)	(0.592)	(0.339)	(0.324)
"Over" True Value Coefficient		−0.295	−0.629***	−0.781***	−0.030
		(0.218)	(0.176)	(0.253)	(0.076)
"Under" True Value Coefficient	0.077	0.611***	0.559***	0.387***	0.122
	(0.061)	(0.171)	(0.180)	(0.123)	(0.076)
Hits	34/70	16/70	21/70	20/70	37/70
Overestimates	0/70	11/70	30/70	19/70	18/70
Underestimates	36/70	43/70	19/70	31/70	15/70

The first two rows report the odds of Overestimates (first row) an Underestimate (second row) with respect to the Hits at the average Peak value. The third and fourth rows report the logit coefficients for Over and Underestimate for the Peak Value (i.e. how the odds vary with the real Peak value). Asterisks represent the significance level according to the legend in the footnotes. The second half of the table reports the actual Hits, Over and Underestimate counts for each strategy
Note: *$p < 0.1$; **$p < 0.05$; ***$p < 0.01$

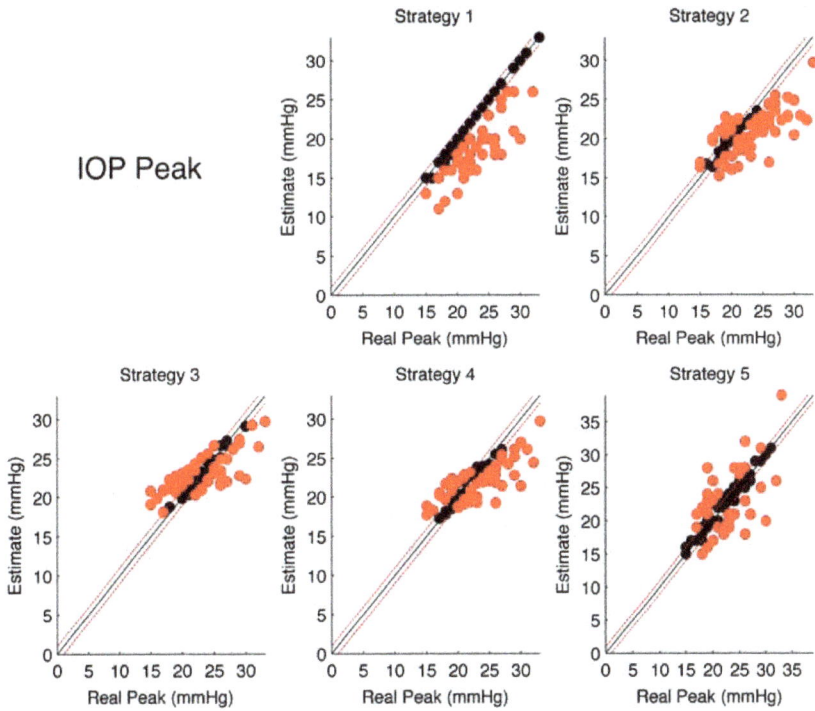

Fig. 4 Scatter plots of the estimated IOP Peak for each stratgy versus the real IOP Peak. The *black line* represents the the ideal line of correct predictions, i.e. estimates exactly equal to the real value. *Dashed red lines* represents the range of clinical tolerance (±2 mmHg). *Black dots* represent the "Hits", while *red dots* represent the "Misses"

Table 6 Estimated logit coefficients from the multinomial logit model (coefficients and standard errors in brackets)

	Over/Underestimate logit				
	Strategy 1	Strategy 2	Strategy 3	Strategy 4	Strategy 5
"Over" at average Mean IOP	−1.141***	0.648**	−0.408	−0.441	−0.167
	(0.346)	(0.285)	(0.279)	(0.282)	(0.258)
"Under" at average Mean IOP	−0.483*	−0.926**	−0.776**	−0.821***	−1.361***
	(0.272)	(0.452)	(0.313)	(0.318)	(0.393)
"Over" True Value Coefficient	0.137	0.080	0.104	−0.096	−0.011
	(0.095)	(0.100)	(0.083)	(0.092)	(0.079)
"Under" True Value Coefficient	0.052	0.355***	0.070	0.063	0.113
	(0.083)	(0.126)	(0.095)	(0.087)	(0.102)
Hits	36/70	21/70	33/70	33/70	33/70
Overestimates	12/70	38/70	22/70	22/70	28/70
Underestimates	22/70	11/70	15/70	15/70	9/70

The first two rows report the odds of Overestimates (first row) an Underestimate (second row) with respect to the Hits at the average Mean IOP value. The third and fourth rows report the logit coefficients for Over and Underestimate for the Mean IOP Value (i.e. how the odds vary with the real Mean IOP value). Asterisks represent the significance level according to the legend in the footnotes. The second half of the table reports the actual Hits, Over and Underestimate counts for each strategy

Note: *$p < 0.1$; **$p < 0.05$; ***$p < 0.01$

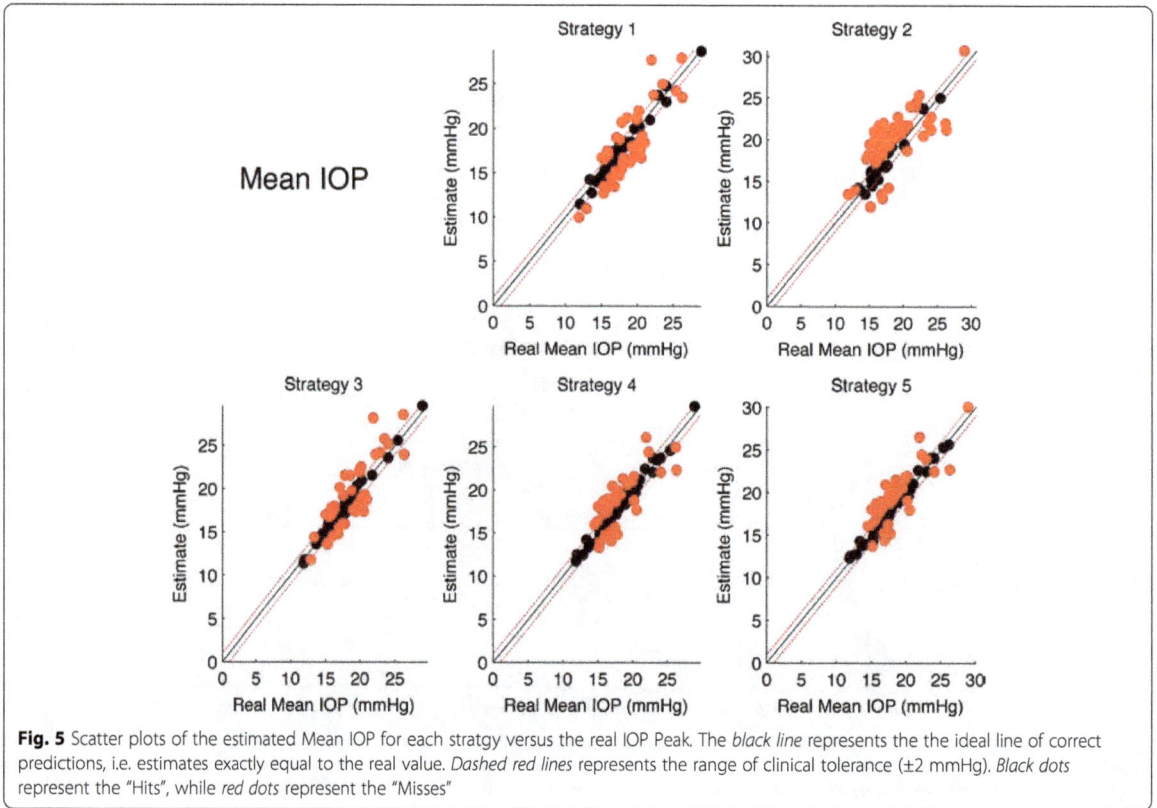

Fig. 5 Scatter plots of the estimated Mean IOP for each stratgy versus the real IOP Peak. The *black line* represents the the ideal line of correct predictions, i.e. estimates exactly equal to the real value. *Dashed red lines* represents the range of clinical tolerance (±2 mmHg). *Black dots* represent the "Hits", while *red dots* represent the "Misses"

Table 7 Estimated logit coefficients from the multinomial logit model (coefficients and standard errors in brackets)

	Over/Underestimate logit				
	Strategy 1	Strategy 2	Strategy 3	Strategy 4	Strategy 5
"Over" at average IOP Fluctuation		−2.040***	−3.218***	−0.870**	−0.870**
		(0.641)	(1.098)	(0.343)	(0.343)
"Under" at average IOP Fluctuation	0.700**	−0.214	0.089	−1.329***	−1.329***
	(0.277)	(0.296)	(0.258)	(0.426)	(0.426)
"Over" True Value Coefficient		−0.438*	−0.460	−0.109	−0.109
		(0.235)	(0.356)	(0.147)	(0.147)
"Under" True Value Coefficient	0.294**	0.470***	0.248**	0.634***	0.634***
	(0.115)	(0.141)	(0.102)	(0.174)	(0.174)
Hits	25/70	32/70	32/70	36/70	36/70
Overestimates	0/70	9/70	3/70	17/70	17/70
Underestimates	45/70	29/70	35/70	17/70	17/70

The first two rows report the odds of Overestimates (first row) an Underestimate (second row) with respect to the Hits at the average Mean IOP value. The third and fourth rows report the logit coefficients for Over and Underestimate for the Mean IOP Fluctuation value (i.e. how the odds vary with the real IOP Fluctuation value). Asterisks represent the significance level according to the legend in the footnotes. The second half of the table reports the actual Hits, Over and Underestimate counts for each strategy
Note: *$p < 0.1$; **$p < 0.05$; ***$p < 0.01$

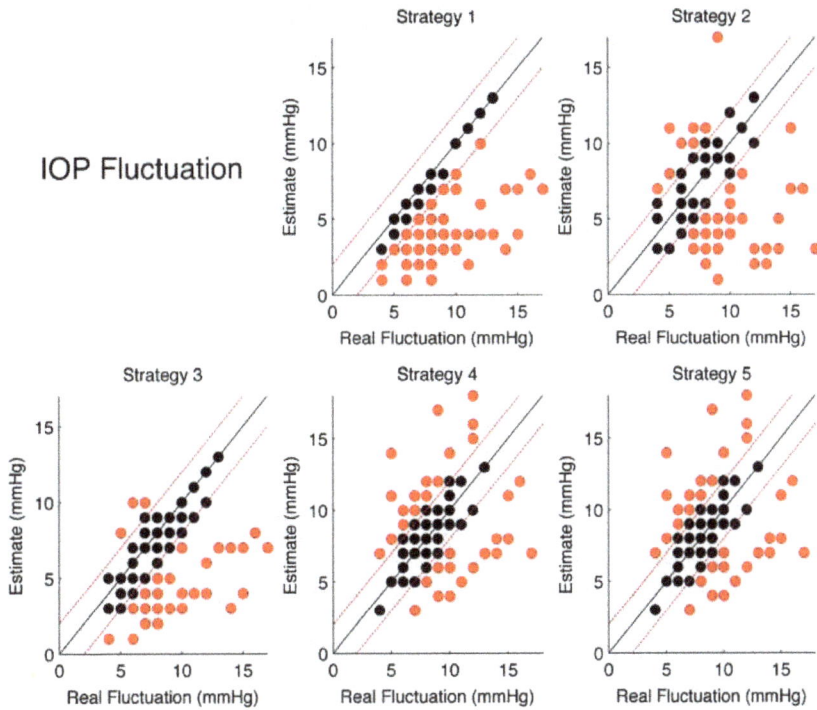

Fig. 6 Scatter plots of the estimated IOP Fluctuations for each stratgy versus the real IOP Peak. The *black line* represents the the ideal line of correct predictions, i.e. estimates exactly equal to the real value. *Dashed red lines* represents the range of clinical tolerance (±1 mmHg). *Black dots* represent the "Hits", while *red dots* represent the "Misses"

Our dataset confirms the critical role of IOP variations during night hours in glaucoma: IOP peaked outside office-hour in 65 %, which is similar to 52–66 % of other studies [13, 19, 25]. This remarks the importance of considering the 24-hour characteristics of IOP, at least in critical patients, in order to better tailor treatments to individual IOP patterns [15].

Different strategies to predict the 24-hour rhythm of IOP have been reported in literature [14, 16, 18, 19]. In general, supine IOP is higher than sitting IOP due to increased episcleral venous pressure, and the concept that supine measurement may be used to predict 24-hour IOP peak dates 1975 [26].

Correction formulas to predict peak from both sitting [16] and supine [14, 16] measurements have also been suggested. Water drinking test [27] and ibopamine [28] have also been suggested to predict peak IOP. The strategy used in this study (a combination of office-hour supine and sitting measurements) had been previously used on untreated subjects [14], and we clearly showed that the relevant 24-hour IOP characteristics that can be missed by routine examination (ie office-hour sitting measurements) can be frequently detected when sitting and supine readings are associated.

When compared to our previous report, this study seems to suggest that, in general, office hour measurements are not adequate to correctly estimate peak, mean and fluctuations values within the acceptance thresholds considered in this paper in treated glaucoma patients.

The best office-hour strategy to estimate the peak IOP was the combination of sitting and supine office hour measurements (strategy 5). The error in this strategy was the least correlated with the real IOP value when compared with other strategies. In addition it was not affected by a significant mean offset (i.e. yelding the overall least biased estimate).

Strategy 1 and 5 were similar in terms of number of correct peak predictions and resulted not to be significantly different upon the correct prediction analysis. It is important to notice, although, that strategy 1 was greatly affected by the highly negatively skewed distribution (i.e. allowed only underestimations) which were not counterbalanced by the zero error predictions (34 %). From a clinical point of view this is of particular importance, showing that sitting office hour measurements tend to underestimate the correct peak value. This error is not only significantly correlated with the real Peak IOP value, but its non linear relation with the real Peak IOP is difficult to model and to compensate for.

All office-hour strategies for the Mean IOP estimate, except Strategy 2, showed similar features. The best strategy in terms of number of correct predictions was sitting office hour measurments alone (strategy 1), although the odds of correct predictions were not significantly different from strategies 3, 4 and 5. Strategies 1, 3 and 4 could be considered equal since no correlation of the errors with the real values or significant mean offset (i.e. no systematic bias) could be found; they performed equally in terms of correct predictions (about 50 %) and the wrong prediction rate was not correlated with the real Mean IOP values. Strategy 5 had a significant mean offset (0.6 mmHg) but this did not affect the correct prediction rate significantly. Strategy 2 was the worst both in terms of correct predictions and in terms of significant systematic bias (especially, exhibited a strong correlation of the errors with the real Mean IOP value).

The IOP Fluctuation strategies were affected by several flaws. Strategy 1 performed very poorly in terms of correct predictions and, as for Strategy 1 for the Peak IOP, suffered from a non linear strong correlation of the error rate with the real IOP value and a skewed error distribution, allowing only underestimates. The best in terms of correct predictions were strategies 4 and 5 (which yielded the same estimates for all subjects) although they were not significantly different from the other strategies. All strategies showed a strong correlation of the error with the real IOP Fluctuation value, underestimating higher values.

As shown in Table 8 using sitting office-hour measurements, a correct identification of all parameters (peak, mean and fluctuation) was achieved in 24 % of cases,

which was very similar to untreated patients (20 %) [14], with a slight increased percentage of cases fully characterized adding supine office-hour values (27 %).

The analyses of this study may be prone to a number of possible limitations that have been previously described and discussed in details [14]. The accuracy of 24-hour data may be affected by a number of factors, including hospitalization, disturbed sleep, sudden waking and exposure to light at night [29, 30]. The use of two tonometers could also be a specific limit of this paper [31, 32]. Still, this 24-hour procedure is strictly standardized and controlled, and it has been largely used in our center for nearly two decades [14, 24, 33–36]. Different characteristics of the study groups (in particular, baseline IOP) may largely influence our findings. In fact, we found that mean 24-hour IOP was higher with timolol than with others glaucoma medications, thus confirming previous findings, showing a substantial effect of timolol during the day, but no measurable effect at night [24]. Also the choice of timepoints was critical in determining the results: in particular, latanoprost patients received their medication after the 9-pm-measurement, a fact that could explain the high percentage of IOP peaks outside office-hours. Adherence to treatment was not a concern, as medications were administered by study personnel during the study period.

Conclusions

The results of this study remark the concept that IOP is a dynamic parameter and that intensive measurement is helpful in determining its characteristics. The methods of this study have been previously used for untreated subjects, for whom we clearly showed that relevant 24-hour IOP characteristics may be missed by routine examination (ie office-hour sitting measurements), whereas a combination of office-hour sitting and supine measurements can provide more accurate information.

The results of this study on treated glaucoma patients show a very poor performance of all office-hour strategies in correctly predicting the considered parameters within the thresholds used in this paper, all scoring a correct prediction rate below 52 %. Some strategies allowed a simple linear modeling. In these cases a model to correct for the systematic bias could be theoretically applicable, but a much larger sample size would be required for precise parameter estimation. In all cases, however, the residual standard error was relatively high (ranging from 1.4 to 3.2) so that a model correction (i.e. zero mean error) would hardly succeed in obtaining reliable estimates.

Table 8 The Clinical Impact: Improvement in the Characterization of the 24-Hour Curve Using Different Criteria

	All patients
Fully characterized by sitting office-hour estimates	24
Fully characterized by sitting + supine office-hour estimates	27
Fully characterized by sitting office-hour estimates + peak estimation	22
Supine + sitting office hour strategy at least partially improves office-hour sitting estimates	66
Supine office-hour estimates + peak estimation strategy* at least partially improves office-hour sitting estimates	30
Fully uncharacterized	9

Data are percentages
Full characterization: mean IOP, peak, and fluctuations, respectively, within 1, 1, 2 mm Hg from the 24-hour value
Full absence of characterization: mean IOP, peak, and fluctuations, respectively, outside 1, 1, 2 mm Hg from the 24-hour value

Abbreviations
IOP: intraocular pressure; POAG: primary open angle glaucoma; FCDT: fixed combination dorzolamide timolol.

Competing interests
The authors declare that they have no competing interests.

Authors' contributions
LC: participated in the interpretation of data, drafted the manuscript; PF: conceived of the study, and participated in its design and coordination, critically revised the manuscript; GM: performed the statistical analysis, participated in the interpretation of data and helped to draft the manuscript; SDC: critically revised the manuscript; NO: critically revised the manuscript; LR: conceived of the study, and participated in its design and coordination, critically revised the manuscript; All authors read and approved the final manuscript.

Acknowledgement
Presented in part at the annual meeting of the Association for Research in Vision and Ophthalmology (ARVO), Fort Lauderdale, Florida, May 2010.

References
1. AGIS Investigators. Advanced Glaucoma Intervention Study(AGIS), 7: the relationship between control of intraocular pressure and visual field deterioration. Am J Ophthalmol. 2000;130:429–40.
2. Higginbotham EJ, Gordon MO, Beiser JA, Drake MV, Bennet GR, Wilson MR, et al. The Ocular Hypertension Treatment Study: topical medication delays or prevents primary open-angle glaucoma in African American individuals. Arch Ophthalmol. 2004;122:813–20.
3. Leske MC, Heijl A, Hussein M, Bengtsson B, Hyman L, Komaroff E, et al. Factors for glaucoma progression and the effect of treatment: the early manifest glaucoma trial. Arch Ophthalmol. 2003;121:48–56.
4. Lichter PR, Musch DC, Gillespie BW, Guire KE, Janz NK, Wren PA, et al. Interim clinical outcomes in the Collaborative Initial Glaucoma Treatment Study comparing initial treatment randomized to medications or surgery. Ophthalmology. 2001;108:1943–53.
5. Konstas AG, Quaranta L, Mikropoulos DG, Nasr MB, Russo A, Jaffee HA, et al. Peak intraocular pressure and glaucomatous progression in primary open-angle glaucoma. J Ocul Pharmacol Ther. 2012;28(1):26–32.
6. Hara T, Hara T, Tsuru T. Increase of peak intraocular pressure during sleep in reproduced diurnal changes by posture. Arch Ophthalmol. 2006;124:165–8.
7. Asrani S, Zeimer R, Wilensky J, Gieser D, Vitale S, Lindenmuth K. Large diurnal fluctuations in intraocular pressure are an independent risk factor in patients with glaucoma. J Glaucoma. 2000;9:134–42.
8. Bengtsson B, Leske MC, Hyman L, Heijl A, Early Manifest Glaucoma Trial Group. Fluctuation of intraocular pressure and glaucoma progression in the Early Manifest Glaucoma Trial. Ophthalmology. 2007;114:205–9.
9. Caprioli J, Coleman AL. Intraocular pressure fluctuation: a risk factor for visual field progression at low intraocular pressures in the advanced glaucoma intervention study. Ophthalmology. 2008;115:1123–9.
10. Medeiros FA, Weinreb RN, Zangwill LM, Alencar LM, Sample PA, Vasile C, et al. Long-term intraocular pressure fluctuations and risk of conversion from ocular hypertension to glaucoma. Ophthalmology. 2008;115:934–40.
11. Caprioli J. Intraocular pressure fluctuation: an independent risk factor for glaucoma? Arch Ophthalmol. 2007;125:1124–5.
12. Fogagnolo P, Orzalesi N, Centofanti M, Oddone F, Manni G, Rossetti L. Short- and Long-Term Phasing of Intraocular Pressure in Stable and Progressive Glaucoma. Ophthalmologica. 2013;230:87–92.
13. Hughes E, Spry P, Diamond J. 24-Hour monitoring of intraocular pressure in glaucoma management: a retrospective review. J Glaucoma. 2003;12:232–6.
14. Fogagnolo P, Orzalesi N, Ferreras A, Rossetti L. The Circadian Curve of Intraocular Pressure: Can We Estimate Its Characteristics during Office Hours? Invest Ophthalmol Vis Sci. 2009;50:2209–15.
15. Barkana Y, Anis S, Liebmann J, Tello C, Ritch R. Clinical utility of intraocular pressure monitoring outside of normal office hours in patients with glaucoma. Arch Ophthalmol. 2006;124:793–7.
16. Mosaed S, Liu JH, Weinreb RN. Correlation between office and peak nocturnal intraocular pressures in healthy subjects and glaucoma patients. Am J Ophthalmol. 2005;139:320–4.
17. Drance SM. Diurnal variation of intraocular pressure in treated glaucoma: significance in patients with chronic simple glaucoma. Arch Ophthalmol. 1963;70:302–11.
18. Liu JH, Bouligny RP, Kripke DF, et al. Nocturnal elevation of intraocular pressure is detectable in the sitting position. Invest Ophthalmol Vis Sci. 2003;44:4439–42.
19. Nakakura S, Nomura Y, Ataka S, Shiraki K. Relation between office intraocular pressure and 24-hour intraocular pressure in patients with primary open-angle glaucoma treated with a combination of topical antiglaucoma eye drops. J Glaucoma. 2007;16:201–4.
20. Liu JHK, Kripke DE, Twa MD, Hoffman RE, Mansberger SL, Rex KM, et al. Twenty-four-hour pattern of intraocular pressure in the aging population. Invest Ophthalmol Vis Sci. 1999;40:2912–7.
21. Liu JHK, Zhang X, Kripke DF, Weinreb RN. Twenty-four-hour intraocular pressure pattern associated with early glaucomatous changes. Invest Ophthalmol Vis Sci. 2003;44:1586–90.
22. Leonardi M, Pitchon EM, Bertsch A, Renaud P, Mermoud A. Wireless contact lens sensor for intraocular pressure monitoring: assessment on enucleated pig eyes. Acta Ophthalmol. 2009;87:433–7.
23. Mansouri K, Medeiros FA, Tafreshi A, Weinreb RN. Continuous 24-hour monitoring of intraocular pressure patterns with a contact lens sensor: safety, tolerability, and reproducibility in patients with glaucoma. Arch Ophthalmol. 2012;130:1534–9.
24. Orzalesi N, Rossetti L, Invernizzi T, Bottoli A, Autelitano A. Effect of timolol, latanoprost, and dorzolamide on circadian IOP in glaucoma or ocular hypertension. Invest Ophthalmol Vis Sci. 2000;41:2566–73.
25. Tajunisah I, Reddy SC, Fathilah J. Diurnal variation of intraocular pressure in suspected glaucoma patients and their outcome. Graefes Arch Clin Exp Ophthalmol. 2007;245:1851–7.
26. Krieglstein G, Langham ME. Influence of body position on the intraocular pressure of normal and glaucomatous eyes. Ophthalmologica. 1975; 171(2):132–45.
27. Kumar RS, de Guzman MH, Ong PY, Goldberg I. Does peak intraocular pressure measured by water drinking test reflect peak circadian levels? A pilot study. Clin Experiment Ophthalmol. 2008;36(4):312–5.
28. Magacho L, Costa ML, Reis R, Rios N, de Avila MP. Correlation between the ibopamine provocative test and the diurnal tension curve in glaucoma patients. Arq Bras Oftalmol. 2006;69(4):477–80.
29. Liu JHK, Kripke DF, Hoffman RE, Twa MD, Loving RT, Rex KM, et al. Nocturnal elevation of intraocular pressure in young adults. Invest Ophthalmol Vis Sci. 1998;39:2707–12.
30. Weinreb RN. Nocturnal rhythms of intraocular pressure. Arch Ophthalmol. 2006;124:269–70.
31. Abrams LS, Vitale S, Jampel HD. Comparison of three tonometers for measuring intraocular pressure in rabbits. Invest Ophthalmol Vis Sci. 1996;37:940–4.
32. Horowitz GS, Byles J, Lee J, D'Este C. Comparison of the Tono-Pen and Goldmann tonometer for measuring intraocular pressure in patients with glaucoma. Clin Experiment Ophthalmol. 2004;32:584–9.
33. Orzalesi N, Rossetti L, Bottoli A, Fumagalli E, Fogagnolo P. The effect of latanoprost, brimonidine, and a fixed combination of timolol and dorzolamide on circadian intraocular pressure in patients with glaucoma or ocular hypertension. Arch Ophthalmol. 2003;121:453–7.
34. Orzalesi N, Rossetti L, Bottoli A, Fogagnolo P. Comparison of the effects of latanoprost, travoprost, and bimatoprost on circadian intraocular pressure in patients with glaucoma or ocular hypertension. Ophthalmology. 2006; 113:239–46.
35. Fogagnolo P, Rossetti L, Mazzolani F, Orzalesi N. Circadian variations in central corneal thickness and intraocular pressure in patients with glaucoma. Br J Ophthalmol. 2006;90:24–8.
36. Fogagnolo P, Capizzi F, Orzalesi N, Figus M, Ferreras A, Rossetti L. Can mean central corneal thickness and its 24-hour fluctuation influence fluctuation of intraocular pressure? J Glaucoma. 2010;19:418–23.

16

Multiplex cytokine levels of aqueous humor in acute primary angle-closure patients: fellow eye comparison

Shaolin Du[1,2], Wenbin Huang[1], Xiulan Zhang[1*†], Jiawei Wang[1], Wei Wang[1] and Dennis S. C. Lam[1*†]

Abstract

Background: The existing literature contains no information regarding inflammatory cytokine expression in unilateral acute primary angle-closure (APAC) affected eyes and fellow eyes with primary angle closure suspect (PACS). To measure levels of various inflammatory cytokines in the aqueous humor (AH) of APAC affected eyes and fellow eyes with a diagnosis of PACS (18 unilateral APAC eyes and 18 fellow eyes with PACS), and determine the underlying correlation between them.

Methods: The total levels of 12 cytokines including granulocyte colony-stimulating factor (G-CSF), interleukin (IL)-6, IL-8, monocyte chemotactic protein (MCP)-1, MCP-3, macrophage-derived chemokine (MDC), macrophage inflammatory protein (MIP)-1β, and vascular endothelial growth factor (VEGF) etc. were assessed using the multiplex bead immunoassay technique. The level of cytokines in different groups was analyzed by a 2-related-samples nonparametric test. Data on patient demographics, preoperative intraocular pressure (IOP), number of glaucoma medications, as well as several ocular biological parameters were also collected for correlation analysis.

Results: The APAC patients had significantly higher levels of G-CSF, IL-6, IL-8, MCP-1, MCP-3, MDC, MIP-1β, and VEGF in the AH samples from unilateral APAC affected eyes than in fellow eyes with PACS (all $P < 0.05$). The cytokines showed positive correlations between each other ($P < 0.0071$).

Conclusions: Cytokine networks in the AH may have critical roles in the progression of APAC. Thus, different cytokine expression in both eyes of the same patient may help us to understand the different pathology in APAC and PACS.

Keywords: Cytokines, Angle-closure, Aqueous humor

Background

Acute primary angle-closure (APAC) presents with typical symptoms and clinical signs such as sudden onset of ocular discomfort or pain, subjective blurring of vision, and suddenly excessive increases in intraocular pressure (IOP). In APAC, the position of the iris causes the normally open anterior chamber angle to close. Aqueous humor (AH) that should normally drain out of the anterior chamber is then trapped inside the eye, increasing the IOP [1].

The AH plays an important role in the pathogenesis of glaucoma [2]. Furthermore, AH has the task of protecting and supplying nutrients and antioxidants to the cornea, lens, and trabecular meshwork (TM) [3, 4]. A number of cytokines, including transforming growth factor (TGF-β2), interleukin (IL-6, and IL-8), have been detected in the AH [5, 6]. Several studies that measured cytokine concentrations in AH samples have revealed significantly high levels in primary open angle glaucoma, exfoliation glaucoma [7], and primary angle closure glaucoma [8].

By 2020, it is estimated almost 80 million persons will have glaucoma worldwide. Particularly in Asian countries, angle closure glaucoma accounts for no less than half of the blindness arising from glaucoma. Therefore,

* Correspondence: zhangxl2@mail.sysu.edu.cn; dlam.sklo.sysu.cn@gmail.com
†Equal contributors
[1]Zhongshan Ophthalmic Center, State Key Laboratory of Ophthalmology, Sun Yat-Sen University, Guangzhou, China
Full list of author information is available at the end of the article

more attention needs to be paid to APAC in China. In our previous report, compared with the cataract group, APAC showed clear and significantly elevated concentrations of IL-6, IL-8, granulocyte colony-stimulating factor (G-CSF), monocyte chemotactic protein (MCP)-1, MCP-3, and vascular endothelial growth factor (VEGF) [9]. However, the existing literature contains no information regarding inflammatory cytokine expression in unilateral APAC affected eyes and fellow eyes with primary angle-closure suspect (PACS).

In this study, we want to exlore whether some different inflammation-related cytokines expressed in APAC compared with fellow eyes with PACS and whether there are novel findings different from those previously published by Huang et al. [9]. Huang's previous report have measured levels of various inflammation-related cytokines in the aqueous humor of patients with acute primary angle-closure (APAC) and senile cataract. The present study want to explore different inflammatory cytokine expression in unilateral acute primary angle-closure (APAC) affected eyes and fellow eyes with primary angle closure suspect (PACS). The design of fellow eye comparison may help us to find novel things. Our finding may expand the understanding of asymmetric glaucoma pathophysiology.

Methods

Subjects and enrollment criteria

Participants in this study were selected as a convenience sample of patients at the Glaucoma Department, Zhongshan Ophthalmic Center. Both eyes of each subject were included. All enrolled glaucoma patients fulfilled the following criteria: Subjects were > 18 years old. APAC was defined according to the following criteria: [10] ① Presence of at least two of the following symptoms: ocular or periocular pain, nausea and/or vomiting, and an antecedent history of intermittent blurring of vision with halos; ② IOP of at least 22 mm Hg (as measured by Goldmann applanation tonometry); ③ presence of at least three of the following signs of conjunctival injection: corneal epithelial edema, mid-dilated unreactive pupil, and a shallow anterior chamber; and ④ presence of an occluded angle in the affected eye, verified by gonioscopy. Ultrasound biomicroscopy (UBM) examination confirmed that a narrow-angle pupillary block component existed in all eyes. PACS fulfilled the following criteria: ①narrow angles (defined as eyes in which at least 180°of the posterior pigmented trabecular meshwork was not visible on gonioscopy in the primary position of gaze without indentation); ② IOP less than or equal to 21 mmHg ③ healthy optic disc; ④ without primary angle closure [11].

The AH collection was performed under sterile conditions via an anterior chamber paracentesis or peripheral iridectomy, or before commencement of surgery for all trabeculectomy-required patients, and their fellow PACS eyes were scheduled for prophylactic surgical peripheral iridectomy according to agreements of the patients and the requirements of the Chinese medical association. These management recommendations are decided according to the American Academy of Ophthalmology Preferred Practice Pattern guidelines on primary angle closure (http://www.aao.org) and individual situations.

The antiglaucomatous medication treatment for APAC was standardized as follows: topical pilocarpine 1 % four times daily; topical beta-blocker (timolol 0.5 %) twice daily and/or brinzolamide (Azopt; Alcon Laboratories, Elkridge, MD), and/or topical alpha-2 agonists (Alphagan; Allergan, Inc., Irvine, CA); topical steroids; oral acetazolamide 250 mg three times daily and intravenous mannitol 20 % at 1 to 2 g/kg 4 h after the initiation of the treatment in cases where the IOP was not reduced by 20 % from the initial IOP, excluding contraindicated by systemic disease (e.g., congestive heart failure).

Patients who met any of the following criteria were excluded: a secondary acute attack because of lens subluxation, uveitis, iris neovascularization, trauma, tumor, or any obvious cataract leading to an intumescent lens; a known systemic inflammatory, autoimmune, or immunosuppressive disease; a pre-existing ocular disease (retinal vein occlusion, retinal artery occlusion, diabetic retinopathy, age-related macular degeneration); or a history of previous ocular surgery.

All eyes of the subjects underwent a thorough ophthalmic evaluation, including slit-lamp biomicroscopy, IOP measurement (Goldmann applanation tonometry), gonioscopy, fundus examination, UBM, and B-scanning. IOP was measured preoperatively, mainly in the afternoon on the day before the AH sampling for all studied eyes. We believe that this minimized the influences of diurnal variation of IOP and closely reflected the IOP at the time of AH sampling.

Aqueous humor collection

The AH samples (50–100 µL) were collected by a procedure described in our previous study [12]. Two AH samples of APAC eyes were collected during an anterior chamber paracentesis procedure, and 16 samples were collected at the beginning of peripheral iridectomy or trabeculectomy. The AH samples of PACS eyes were collected at the beginning of peripheral iridectomy. All samples were obtained prior to any conjunctival or intraocular manipulation to avoid breakdown of the blood–aqueous barrier associated with surgical trauma. All samples were immediately frozen and stored at −80 °C until the analyses were performed.

Cytokine analysis

Cytokine concentrations were analyzed using a multiplex bead immunoassay system (Milliplex Human Cytokine®

kit; Millipore Corp., Billerica, MA). The assays were performed according to the manufacturer's instructions and analyzed using the Bio-Plex suspension array system (Bio-plex200, Bio-Rad, Hercules, CA). Cytokines related to the inflammatory process [G-CSF, IL-6, IL-8, MCP-1, MCP-3, macrophage-derived chemokine (MDC), MIP-1β, VEGF, GM-CSF (granulocyte-macrophage, colony-stimulating factor), IFN-γ (interferon-gamma), IL-1βand TNF-β (tumor necrosis factor-beta)] were analyzed in a 25 μl volume of AH sample for each reaction. Based on the information provided by the manufacturer, the multiplex assay kit can quantitatively measure multiple cytokines from as little as 25 μL of body fluids. The detection limit for any analyte was 1 pg/ml, with a dynamic range up to 10000 pg/ml (according to the manufacturer).

Statistical analysis

The data were processed and analyzed statistically using SPSS (Version 13.0; SPSS, Chicago, IL). The level of cytokines in different groups was analyzed by a 2-related-samples nonparametric test. Statistical significance was accepted at $P < 0.05$. Correlations among cytokines and correlations between cytokine concentrations and subjects' demographic data (including age, IOP and anterior chamber depth (ACD), lens thickness (LT) and vitreous chamber depth (VCD) in the macular region) were calculated using Spearman's correlation test. For the correction of multi-group comparisons, P values of 0.0071 for Spearman's correlation test were considered statistically significant, with significance levels of 0.05 based on Bonferroni's methods.

Ethics

This study was approved by the Ethical Review Committee of Zhongshan Ophthalmic Center and adhered to the provisions of the Declaration of Helsinki for research involving human subjects. All subjects participating in this study were given a detailed explanation about the study and signed an informed consent form. Participants were recruited prospectively and consecutively for this study, between January 2013 and May 2014. All subjects were from a Chinese Han population.

Results

Patients' demographic data

Eighteen APAC patients (18 unilateral APAC affected eyes and 18 fellow eyes with PACS) who fulfilled the inclusion criteria were included in the study.

The demographic data of the subjects, including age, sex, number, and details of glaucoma medication use, are summarized in Table 1. Biological parameters of APAC eyes and PACS eyes are summarized in Table 2. The mean age of the APAC patients was 63.80 ± 6.76 (mean ± standard

Table 1 Demographic and baseline characteristics of patients

Characteristics	Subjects of study
No. of patients (No. of eyes)	18 (36)
Age, y (mean [SD])	63.80 (6.76)
Sex (male/female)	5/13
Laterality of affected eye, right/left	7/11
Duration of experienced attack, d (median [IQ])	5.50 (8.25)
No. of glaucoma medications in APAC eyes, n (median [IQ])	1.00 (1.00)

SD standard deviation, *IQ* inter-quartile

deviation) years. Data for duration of experienced attack, number of glaucoma medications, IOP at the day of surgery, Axial Length (AL), ACD, LT and VCD are expressed as the median [IQ]. IOP on the day of surgery was higher in the APAC eyes than in PACS eyes as determined by a 2-related-samples nonparametric test ($P = 0.008$).

The comparison of cytokines between APAC eyes and PACS eyes

GM-CSF, IFN-γ, IL-1β, and TNF-β were detected in less than 50 % of samples in both control and glaucoma groups and therefore were not included in further analysis. The concentrations of the remaining eight cytokines analyzed are shown in Table 3. All measurements were performed successfully. In the APAC patients, the levels of G-CSF ($P = 0.001$), IL-6 ($P = 0.000$), IL-8 ($P = 0.000$), MCP-1 ($P = 0.000$), MCP-3 ($P = 0.008$), MDC ($P = 0.009$), MIP-1β ($P = 0.001$), and VEGF ($P = 0.035$) in AH samples from unilateral APAC affected eyes were significantly higher than those from fellow eyes with PACS (Fig. 1).

The correlations among different cytokine concentrations

The correlations among the different cytokine concentrations are shown in Table 4. Among seven cytokines (G-CSF, IL-6, IL-8, MCP-1, MCP-3, MDC, and macrophage inflammatory protein (MIP-1β) positive correlations were found between each other ($P < 0.0071$).

Table 2 Characteristics of Acute Primary Angle-Closure Eyes and Primary Angle-Closure Suspect Eyes

Characteristics	Affected eyes, APAC	Fellow eyes, PACS	P value
IOP at the day of surgery, mmHg	19.5 (20.68)	13.5 (6.0)	0.008*
Axial Length (AL), mm	22.42 (1.50)	22.25 (1.26)	0.138
Anterior Chamber Depth (ACD), mm	2.24 (0.21)	2.22 (0.28)	0.236
Lens Thickness (LT), mm	5.17 (0.61)	5.29 (0.67)	0.244
Vitreous Chamber Depth (VCD), mm	14.96 (1.35)	14.91 (1.32)	0.206

Data are expressed as the median (IQ). *P*-values were obtained from 2-related-samples nonparametric test. * *P*-value < 0.05 was considered to be significant

Table 3 Level of cytokines in aqueous humor from APAC eyes and fellow eyes with PACS

	Affected eyes, APAC (pg/ml)	Fellow eyes, PACS (pg/ml)	P value
G-CSF	1608.42 (13.71; 0.00, 17420.00)	1.11 (0.00; 0.00, 13.58)	0.001*
IL-6	520.24 (14.62; 0.00, 3470.00)	0.35 (0.00; 0.00, 1.82)	0.000*
IL-8	160.37 (23.28; 0.00, 1043.00)	2.96 (1.09; 0.00, 13.64)	0.000*
MCP-1	2537.39 (1507.50; 696.75, 7384.00)	641.71 (661.50; 281.49, 1051.00)	0.000*
MCP-3	9.30 (6.45; 0.00, 50.90)	2.34 (0.49; 0.00, 7.35)	0.008*
MDC	38.80 (5.60; 0.00, 268.00)	10.98 (3.61; 0.00, 50.00)	0.009*
MIP-1β	23.67 (21.21; 0.00, 63.10)	3.95 (0.16; 0.00, 21.07)	0.001*
VEGF	701.60 (120.43; 0.00, 5162.00)	93.87 (91.01; 0.00, 182.00)	0.035*

APAC acute primary angle-closure; *PACS* primary angle-closure suspect. Granulocyte colony-stimulating factor (G-CSF), interleukin (IL)-6, IL-8, monocyte chemotactic protein (MCP)-1, MCP-3, macrophage-derived chemokine (MDC), macrophage inflammatory protein (MIP)-1β, and vascular endothelial growth factor (VEGF). Data are expressed as the mean (median; range). *P*-values were obtained from 2-related-samples nonparametric test.* *P*-value <0.05 was considered to be significant

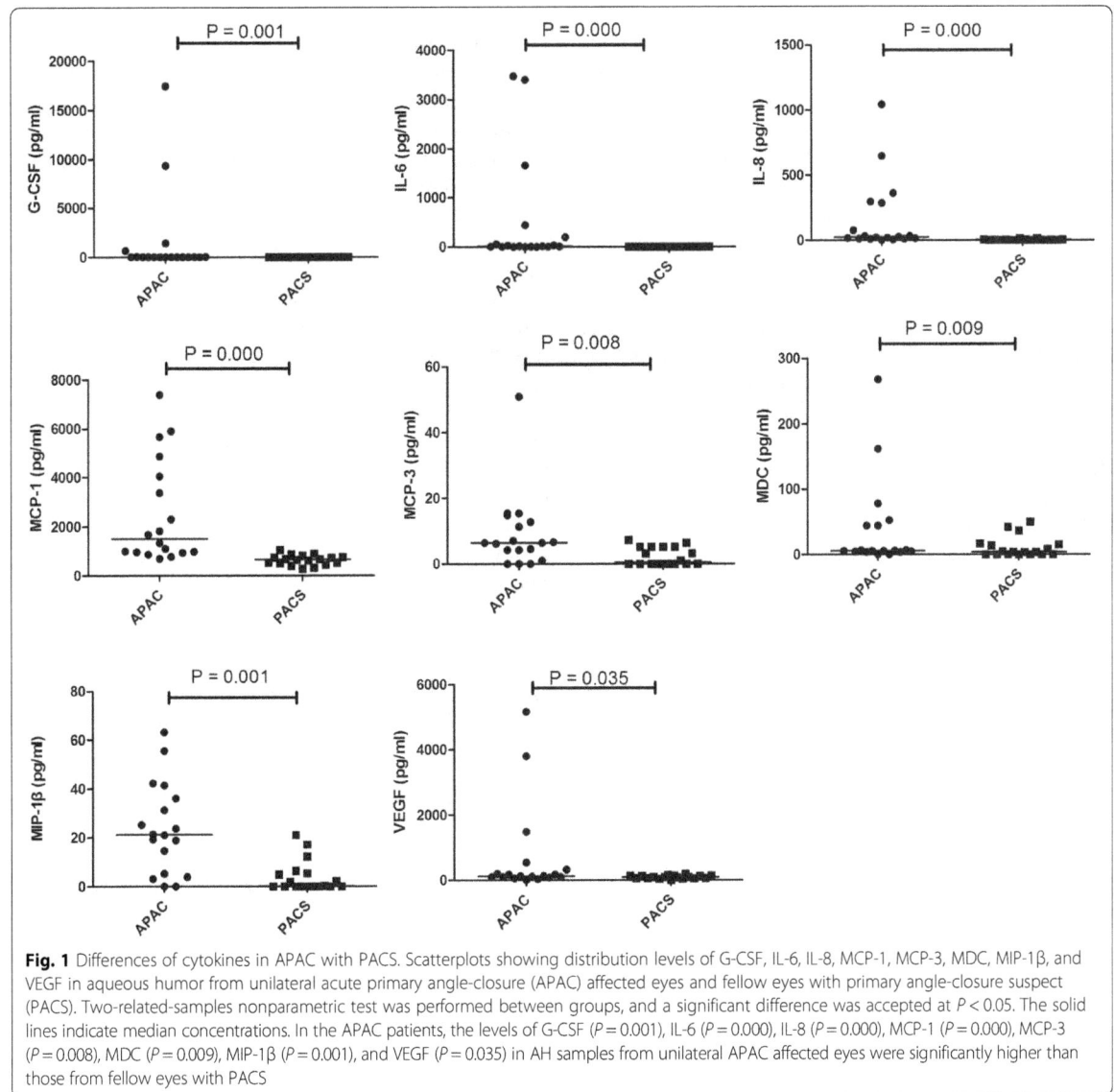

Fig. 1 Differences of cytokines in APAC with PACS. Scatterplots showing distribution levels of G-CSF, IL-6, IL-8, MCP-1, MCP-3, MDC, MIP-1β, and VEGF in aqueous humor from unilateral acute primary angle-closure (APAC) affected eyes and fellow eyes with primary angle-closure suspect (PACS). Two-related-samples nonparametric test was performed between groups, and a significant difference was accepted at $P < 0.05$. The solid lines indicate median concentrations. In the APAC patients, the levels of G-CSF ($P = 0.001$), IL-6 ($P = 0.000$), IL-8 ($P = 0.000$), MCP-1 ($P = 0.000$), MCP-3 ($P = 0.008$), MDC ($P = 0.009$), MIP-1β ($P = 0.001$), and VEGF ($P = 0.035$) in AH samples from unilateral APAC affected eyes were significantly higher than those from fellow eyes with PACS

Table 4 Correlations among cytokines

ρ/P value	G-CSF	IL-6	IL-8	MCP-1	MCP-3	MDC	MIP-1β	VEGF
G-CSF	—	0.829	0.726	0.696	0.785	0.547	0.608	0.307
IL-6	0.000*	—	0.811	0.886	0.703	0.549	0.647	0.480
IL-8	0.000*	0.000*	—	0.785	0.715	0.647	0.841	0.512
MCP-1	0.000*	0.000*	0.000*	—	0.649	0.461	0.631	0.515
MCP-3	0.000*	0.000*	0.000*	0.000*	—	0.500	0.607	0.434
MDC	0.001*	0.001*	0.000*	0.005*	0.002*	—	0.461	0.250
MIP-1β	0.000*	0.000*	0.000*	0.000*	0.000*	0.005*	—	0.472
VEGF	0.068	0.003*	0.001*	0.001*	0.008	0.141	0.004*	—

Granulocyte colony-stimulating factor (G-CSF), interleukin (IL)-6, IL-8, monocyte chemotactic protein (MCP)-1, MCP-3, macrophage-derived chemokine (MDC), macrophage inflammatory protein (MIP)-1β, and vascular endothelial growth factor (VEGF)
Correlation coefficient (ρ) and P values are calculated by Spearman's correlation
*Significance level at 5 % ($P < 0.0071$) by Bonferroni correction for multiple comparisons

Negative correlations were found between VEGF and G-CSF ($\rho = 0.307$; $P = 0.068$), VEGF and MCP-3 ($\rho = 0.434$; $P = 0.008$), and VEGF and MDC ($\rho = 0.250$; $P = 0.141$).

The correlations between each cytokine and age, IOP, the number of glaucoma medications, and some ocular biological parameters in APAC patients
The correlations between each cytokine and age, IOP, number of Glaucoma Medications, AL, ACD, LT, and VCD in APAC patients are shown in Table 5. Positive correlations existed between IOP and G-CSF ($\rho = 0.506$; $P = 0.002$). The number of glaucoma medications was positively correlated with G-CSF ($\rho = 0.464$; $P = 0.004$), IL-6 ($\rho = 0.443$; $P = 0.007$), and IL-8 ($\rho = 0.439$; $P = 0.007$).

Discussion
The bead immunoassay revealed that the levels of G-CSF, IL-6, IL-8, MCP-1, MCP-3, MDC, MIP-1β, and VEGF were significantly higher in AH samples from unilateral APAC affected eyes than from fellow eyes with

PACS. Clear elevations of cytokines related to an immune reaction or inflammation existed in AH samples from APAC eyes. This is one of the earliest studies to report successful detection of multiple cytokines with the method of the multiplex bead immunoassay in AH samples from APAC and PACS eyes. A previous study showed that normal TME cells constitutively secreted chemotactic cytokines like IL-8 and MCP-1. Secretion of these chemokines was augmented by treatment with the pro-inflammatory cytokines or other stimulations [13].

IL-8, also called chemokine (C-X-C motif) ligand-8 (CXCL8), is a member of the CXC family of chemokines and is known to have both immune and vascular functions [14, 15]. Multiple studies have demonstrated an elevation of IL-8 under suboptimal oxygenation conditions, which suggests a possible mechanism for the increased IL-8 found in our study of APAC patients [5, 16]. The concentration of the inflammatory cytokine IL-8 was significantly elevated in the AH of primary open angle glaucoma (POAG) patients, supporting the

Table 5 Correlations between Cytokines and relevant factors in APAC patients

	Age		IOP		Number of Glaucoma Medications		AL		ACD		LT		VCD	
	ρ	P value	ρ	P value	ρ	P value	ρ	P value	ρ	P value	ρ	P value	ρ	P value
G-CSF	−0.232	0.173	0.506	0.002*	0.464	0.004*	−0.060	0.729	−0.074	0.670	0.121	0.482	−0.097	0.572
IL-6	−0.115	0.503	0.424	0.010	0.443	0.007*	−0.089	0.605	0.031	0.860	0.040	0.815	−0.132	0.444
IL-8	−0.143	0.406	0.375	0.024	0.439	0.007*	−0.198	0.246	0.056	0.743	0.004	0.980	−0.201	0.239
MCP-1	−0.097	0.573	0.291	0.085	0.285	0.092	−0.110	0.523	0.040	0.817	−0.002	0.989	−0.140	0.414
MCP-3	−0.127	0.460	0.420	0.011	0.347	0.038	−0.040	0.816	0.005	0.977	0.177	0.300	−0.108	0.531
MDC	−0.261	0.125	0.201	0.240	0.131	0.445	−0.411	0.013	0.193	0.259	−0.182	0.288	−0.364	0.029
MIP-1β	−0.166	0.335	0.387	0.020	0.395	0.017	−0.130	0.450	0.003	0.985	0.029	0.865	−0.126	0.463
VEGF	0.013	0.941	0.318	0.058	0.198	0.247	−0.051	0.769	−0.091	0.597	0.300	0.075	−0.185	0.280

Relevant factors: Age, intraocular pressure (IOP), Number of Glaucoma Medications, Axial Length (AL), Anterior Chamber Depth (ACD), Lens Thickness (LT), Vitreous Chamber Depth (VCD) and Choroidal Thickness in the Macular Region (CT)
Granulocyte colony-stimulating factor (G-CSF), interleukin (IL)-6, IL-8, monocyte chemotactic protein (MCP)-1, MCP-3, macrophage-derived chemokine (MDC), macrophage inflammatory protein (MIP)-1β, and vascular endothelial growth factor (VEGF)
Correlation coefficient (ρ) and P values are calculated by Spearman's correlation
*Significance level at 5 % ($P < 0.0071$) by Bonferroni correction for multiple comparisons

hypothesis that immune activation occurs during glaucoma [5, 7]. A study by Kuchtey et al. also demonstrated a significantly higher IL-8 concentration in the more severely affected eyes of the patients with asymmetric glaucoma [5]. The present study showed that IL-8 was higher in the APAC eyes than the fellow eyes with PACS. In an acute attack of glaucoma immunological activation probably has nothing to do. It is evident that if the iris touches the trabecular meshwork occurs inflammation, but then it is possible that this will stimulate the production of this cytokine because the outflow is hampered. In fact, IL-8 modulates the permeability of the Schlemm's canal endothelial cells reported by Alvarado et al. [17]. Therefore, it is more plausible that the IL-8 presence in APAC eyes is due to the attempt by the trabecular meshwork to increase the outflow is hampered [18].

Furthermore, monocytes, presumably under the influence of chemotactic signals, circulate through the trabecular meshwork in the normal state and also that cytokines regulate the permeability of Schlemm's canal endothelial cells [19]. Therefore, the increase of MCP-1 should be viewed in the same way or to attempt to do work better than the outflow of the trabecular meshwork. Also the granulocyte colony-stimulating factor is produced by the TM endothelial cells and probably works as a reminder for the stem cells of the TM, because in an acute attack of glaucoma occurs severe suffering of the TM endothelial cells.

VEGF was another important cytokine investigated in this study, and its level was significantly higher in APAC eyes. Previous studies have detected VEGF protein in AH from eyes with POAG, angle closure glaucoma, and exfoliation glaucoma (EXG) [20]. Although the study by Takai et al. reported a mean difference in the level of VEGF that did not reach significance, the level was higher in the EXG group [7]. Another study reported a significant association between VEGF and the final IOP in patients with POAG [21]. The study by Kim et al. reported that the level of VEGF in the AH was significantly higher in the failure group after the Ahmed glaucoma implantation compared with the success group, implying that VEGF may play a role in determining surgical success after Ahmed valve implantation in patients with neovascular glaucoma (NVG) [22]. VEGF expression can be induced by subjecting cells to hypoxia or hypoglycemia [23]. In this present study, our findings for VEGF suggest that an anoxic environment possibly plays a key role in the pathogenesis of glaucoma and in surgical success.

The present study also indicated significant differences in the levels of IL-6, MDC, and MIP-1β between APAC eyes and PACS eyes. Some past studies found no significant correlations for IL-6 levels in AH from POAG

patients [7, 24]. Interleukin-6 (IL-6) is a multi-functional cytokine that regulates immune responses, acute phase reactions, and hematopoiesis, and may play a central role in host defense mechanisms. MDC is produced by both immune and nonimmune cells, usually in response to inflammatory stimuli or tissue damage. The study by Yin et al. suggested that macrophage-derived factors stimulate optic nerve regeneration [25]. MIP-1β, which induces both chemotaxis and adhesion of T cells [26], may play a key role in an immune reaction in the APAC eyes.

The significant correlations among the cytokines (G-CSF, IL-6, IL-8, MCP-1, MCP-3, MDC and MIP-1β) suggested that the cytokine networks play important roles in inflammation and IOP elevations in APAC, although the exact mechanism of the interactions among these cytokines are unclear. Therefore, evaluation of the AH composition of various inflammatory cytokines may expand the understanding of APAC pathophysiology.

Other parameters, such as axial length of the eye, age, and gender, may also affect the measured cytokine data [27]. In the present study, the data for age, IOP, number of glaucoma medications, AL, ACD, LT and VCD were analyzed for correlations and statistically significant differences were noted between G-CSF and IOP, G-CSF and number of glaucoma medications, IL-6 and number of glaucoma medications, and IL-8 and number of glaucoma medications.

Although the exact mechanism of this interaction is unclear, the IOP levels suggested a strong correlation between G-CSF and IOP elevation. Recently, Freedman and Iserovich [28] have reported that IOP is a potential stimulus for cytokine production. Huang's report [9] suggests that the IOP itself may be responsible for the production of cytokines. However, in this study the finding was only G-CSF was correlated with IOP. That's different with the findings by Huang et al. who have found that IL-8, MCP-3, and VEGF also correlated with IOP besides G-CSF. Lots of reports suggest that the relationship between IOP and inflammation is complex. IOP elevation may cause disruption of the blood–aqueous barrier, thereby resulting in production of cytokines in aqueous humor [29]. The inflammatory cells and proteins can result in the formation of posterior synechiae leading to peripheral anterior synechiae and even IOP elevation [30]. To analyze the deep reasons for the differences with previous studies, the main reason maybe the high-efficiency of statistical method. It's obvious that fellow eye comparison can test the results more effectively than other way. The present study may suggest PACS eyes G-CSF has played more important role than other cytokines in APAC eyes, and other influencing factors may also play important roles.

Previous studies have revealed that conjunctival inflammation can be developed in eyes treated with topical antiglaucoma medication [31]. Particularly, conjunctival inflammatory infiltrates may be caused by high cumulative antiglaucoma treatments [32, 33]. Similar histopathological effects of antiglaucomatous drugs may also happened in the trabecular meshwork [34]. What about the effects of topical glaucoma medications on inflammatory cytokine expression? Engel et al's reported that preoperative IOP-lowering eye drops did not significantly alter the anterior chamber milieu in POAG [35]. The number of glaucoma medications was positively correlated with G-CSF, IL-6, and IL-8. Topical glaucoma medications may take more important effects on conjunctival inflammation than the inflammation in aqueous humor.

Lastly, in a study such as the present one, which involve the simultaneous analysis of multiple factors from each sample, some factors such as sample size and method of data analysis may affect the outcome. The Bonferroni correction was applied in the present case. This is a conservative statistical adjustment used for the verification of data observations but it may mask potential changes in exploratory studies. Some potential limitations in our study should also be mentioned. Use of topical anti-glaucoma medications may influence the aqueous immune milieu [7]. Another limit of the study is the sample size: the number of patients enrolled into our study was relatively low. Nevertheless, the results were statistically significant, so the relatively small number of patients may serve to strengthen the results and conclusions of the study.

Conclusions
In conclusion, the present study showed that APAC is associated with changes in the AH cytokine profile. These findings may support the hypothesis that inflammation and hypoxia may play a key role in the pathogenesis of glaucoma. Thus, different cytokine expression in both eyes of the same patient may help us to understand the different pathology in APAC and PACS. However, we can not explain why PACS do not develop into APAC at the same time or some PACS eyes do not develop into APAC forever. Further studies will be necessary to resolve these issues.

Abbreviations
APAC: Acute primary angle-closure; IOP: Intraocular pressure; AH: Aqueous humor; TM: Trabecular meshwork; TGF-β2: Transforming growth factor; IL: Interleukin; G-CSF: Granulocyte colony-stimulating factor; MCP: Monocyte chemotactic protein; VEGF: Vascular endothelial growth factor; PACS: Primary angle closure suspect; UBM: Ultrasound biomicroscopy; TNF-β: Tumor necrosis factor-beta; ACD: Anterior chamber depth; LT: Lens thickness; VCD: Vitreous chamber depth; AL: Axial length; MDC: Macrophage-derived chemokine; MIP: Macrophage inflammatory protein; CXCL: Chemokine (C-X-C motif) ligand; POAG: Primary open angle glaucoma; NVG: Neovascular glaucoma.

Competing interests
The authors declare that they have no competing interests.

Authors' contributions
All authors conceived of and designed the experimental protocol. SLD and WBH collected the data. All authors were involved in the analysis and interpretation of the data. SLD wrote the first draft of the manuscript. WBH, XLZ, JWW, WW and DL reviewed and revised the manuscript and produced the final version. All authors read and approved the final manuscript.

Acknowledgements
We thank Xinbo Gao for providing technical help in the study and also wish to thank all participants in the study.

Funding
This research was supported by the National Natural Science Foundation of China (81170849, 81371008), and Dongguan medical science and technology project (2015105101008).

Author details
[1]Zhongshan Ophthalmic Center, State Key Laboratory of Ophthalmology, Sun Yat-Sen University, Guangzhou, China. [2]Tungwah Hospital of Sun Yat-Sen University, Dongguan, China.

References
1. Pokhrel PK, Loftus SA. Ocular emergencies. Am Fam Physician. 2007;76(6):829–36.
2. Saccà SC, Izzotti A, Rossi P, Traverso C. Glaucomatous outflow pathway and oxidative stress. Exp Eye Res. 2007;84(3):389–99.
3. Izzotti A, Bagnis A, Saccà SC. The role of oxidative stress in glaucoma. Mutat Res. 2006;612(2):105–14.
4. Fuchshofer R, Tamm ER. Modulation of extracellular matrix turnover in the trabecular meshwork. Exp Eye Res. 2009;88(4):683–8.
5. Kuchtey J, Rezaei KA, Jaru-Ampornpan P, Sternberg Jr P, Kuchtey RW. Multiplex cytokine analysis reveals elevated concentration of interleukin-8 in glaucomatous aqueous humor. Invest Ophthalmol Vis Sci. 2010;51(12):6441–7.
6. Zenkel M, Lewczuk P, Jünemann A, Kruse FE, Naumann GO, Schlötzer-Schrehardt U. Proinflammatory cytokines are involved in the initiation of the abnormal matrix process in pseudoexfoliation syndrome/glaucoma. Am J Pathol. 2010;176(6):2868–79.
7. Takai Y, Tanito M, Ohira A. Multiplex cytokine analysis of aqueous humor in eyes with primary open-angle glaucoma, exfoliation glaucoma, and cataract. Invest Ophthalmol Vis Sci. 2012;53(1):241–7.
8. Chua J, Vania M, Cheung CM, Ang M, Chee SP, Yang H, et al. Expression profile of inflammatory cytokines in aqueous from glaucomatous eyes. Mol Vis. 2012;18:431–8.
9. Huang W, Chen S, Gao X, Yang M, Zhang J, Li X, et al. Inflammation-related cytokines of aqueous humor in acute primary angle-closure eyes. Invest Ophthalmol Vis Sci. 2014;55(2):1088–94.
10. Ang LP, Aung T, Chew PT. Acute primary angle closure in an Asian population: long-term outcome of the fellow eye after prophylactic laser peripheral iridotomy. Ophthalmology. 2000;107(11):2092–6.
11. Guzman CP, Gong T, Nongpiur ME, Perera SA, How AC, Lee HK, et al. Anterior segment optical coherence tomography parameters in subtypes of primary angle closure. Invest Ophthalmol Vis Sci. 2013;54(8):5281–6.
12. Zhang X, Li A, Ge J, Reigada D, Laties AM, Mitchell CH. Acute increase of intraocular pressure releases ATP into the anterior chamber. Exp Eye Res. 2007;85(5):637–43.
13. Shifera AS, Trivedi S, Chau P, Bonnemaison LH, Iguchi R, Alvarado JA. Constitutive secretion of chemokines by cultured human trabecular meshwork cells. Exp Eye Res. 2010;91(1):42–7.
14. Charo IF, Ransohoff RM. The many roles of chemokines and chemokine receptors in inflammation. N Engl J Med. 2006;354(6):610–21.
15. Keeley EC, Mehrad B, Strieter RM. Chemokines as mediators of neovascularization. Arterioscler Thromb Vasc Biol. 2008;28(11):1928–36.

16. Patel N, Gonsalves CS, Malik P, Kalra VK. Placenta growth factor augments endothelin-1 and endothelin-B receptor expression via hypoxia-inducible factor-1 alpha. Blood. 2008;112(3):856–65.
17. Alvarado JA, Alvarado RG, Yeh RF, Franse-Carman L, Marcellino GR, Brownstein MJ. A new insight into the cellular regulation of aqueous outflow: how trabecular meshwork endothelial cells drive a mechanism that regulates the permeability of Schlemm's canal endothelial cells. Br J Ophthalmol. 2005;89(11):1500–5.
18. Saccà SC, Pulliero A, Izzotti A. The dysfunction of the trabecular meshwork during glaucoma course. J Cell Physiol. 2015;230(3):510–25.
19. Alvarado JA, Yeh RF, Franse-Carman L, Marcellino G, Brownstein MJ. Interactions between endothelia of the trabecular meshwork and of Schlemm's canal: a new insight into the regulation of aqueous outflow in the eye. Trans Am Ophthalmol Soc. 2005;103:148–62.
20. Hu DN, Ritch R, Liebmann J, Liu Y, Cheng B, Hu MS. Vascular endothelial growth factor is increased in aqueous humor of glaucomatous eyes. J Glaucoma. 2002;11(5):406–10.
21. Lopilly Park HY, Kim JH, Ahn MD, Park CK. Level of vascular endothelial growth factor in tenon tissue and results of glaucoma surgery. Arch Ophthalmol. 2012;130(6):685–9.
22. Kim YG, Hong S, Lee CS, Kang SY, Seong GJ, Ma KT, et al. Level of vascular endothelial growth factor in aqueous humor and surgical results of ahmed glaucoma valve implantation in patients with neovascular glaucoma. J Glaucoma. 2009;18(6):443–7.
23. Stein I, Neeman M, Shweiki D, Itin A, Keshet E. Stabilization of vascular endothelial growth factor mRNA by hypoxia and hypoglycemia and coregulation with other ischemia-induced genes. Mol Cell Biol. 1995;15(10):5363–8.
24. Sorkhabi R, Ghorbanihaghjo A, Javadzadeh A, Motlagh BF, Ahari SS. Aqueous humor hepcidin prohormone levels in patients with primary open angle glaucoma. Mol Vis. 2010;16:1832–6.
25. Yin Y, Cui Q, Li Y, Irwin N, Fischer D, Harvey AR, et al. Macrophage-derived factors stimulate optic nerve regeneration. J Neurosci. 2003;23(6):2284–93.
26. Tanaka Y, Adams DH, Hubscher S, Hirano H, Siebenlist U, Shaw S. T-cell adhesion induced by proteoglycan-immobilized cytokine MIP-Iβ. Nature. 1993;361(6407):79–82.
27. Yamamoto N, Itonaga K, Marunouchi T, Majima K. Concentration of transforming growth factor beta2 in aqueous humor. Ophthalmic Res. 2005;37(1):29–3.
28. Freedman J, Iserovich P. Pro-inflammatory cytokines in glaucomatous aqueous and encysted Molteno implant blebs and their relationship to pressure. Invest Ophthalmol Vis Sci. 2013;54(7):4851–5.
29. Freddo TF, Patterson MM, Scott DR, Epstein DL. Influence of mercurial sulfhydryl agents on aqueous outflow pathways in enucleated eyes. Invest Ophthalmol Vis Sci. 1984;25(3):278–85.
30. Bodh SA, Kumar V, Raina UK, Ghosh B, Thakar M. Inflammatory glaucoma. Oman J Ophthalmol. 2011;4(1):3–9.
31. Broadway DC, Grierson I, O'Brien C, Hitchings RA. Adverse effects of topical antiglaucoma medication. II. The outcome of filtration surgery. Arch Ophthalmol. 1994;112(11):1446–54.
32. Sherwood MB, Grierson I, Millar L, Hitchings RA. Long-term morphologic effects of antiglaucoma drugs on the conjunctiva and Tenon's capsule in glaucomatous patients. Ophthalmology. 1989;96(3):327–35.
33. Nuzzi R, Vercelli A, Finazzo C, Cracco C. Conjunctival and subconjunctival tissue in primary open-angle glaucoma after longterm topical treatment: an immunohistochemical and ultrastructural study. Graefes Arch Clin Exp Ophthalmol. 1995;233(3):154–62.
34. Baudouin C, Pisella PJ, Fillacier K, Goldschild M, Becquet F, De Saint JM, et al. Ocular surface inflammatory changes induced by topical antiglaucoma drugs: human and animal studies. Ophthalmology. 1999;106(3):556–63.
35. Engel LA, Muether PS, Fauser S, Hueber A. The effect of previous surgery and topical eye drops for primary open-angle glaucoma on cytokine expression in aqueous humor. Graefes Arch Clin Exp Ophthalmol. 2014;252(5):791–9.

17

Biodegradable collagen matrix implant versus mitomycin-C in trabeculectomy: five-year follow-up

Salvatore Cillino[1*], Alessandra Casuccio[2], Francesco Di Pace[1], Carlo Cagini[3], Lucia Lee Ferraro[1] and Giovanni Cillino[1]

Abstract

Background: Clinical studies comparing trabeculectomy augmented with Ologen implant (OLO) versus trabeculectomy plus mitomycin-C (MMC) show contradictory results. To obtain long-term data, we report an extended 5-year follow-up trial evaluating the safety and efficacy of OLO as adjuvant compared to low-dosage MMC in trabeculectomy.

Methods: Forty glaucoma patients (40 eyes) assigned to trabeculectomy with MMC or Ologen. Primary outcome: target IOP at ≤21, ≤17 and ≤15 mmHg; complete and qualified success endpoint rates. Secondary outcomes: visual acuity (VA), mean deviation (MD), bleb evaluation, according to Moorfields Bleb Grading System (MBGS); spectral domain OCT (SD-OCT) bleb examination; number of glaucoma medications; frequency of postoperative complications.

Results: The mean preoperative IOP was 26.7(±5.2) in MMC and 27.3(±6.0) in OLO eyes. Mean 60-month percentage reduction in IOP was significant in both groups [40.9 (±14.2) and 42.1(±13.3) $P = 0.01$], with an endpoint value of 15.2 (±3.2) and 15.8 (±2.3) mmHg in MMC and OLO, respectively. Complete success rates at ≤ 21 mmHg target IOP were 65 % and 70 %, at ≤17 mm Hg 60 % and 55 %, and at the ≤15 mm Hg target IOP 35 % and 45 % in MMC and OLO, respectively.
The Kaplan–Meier curves did not differ both for complete and qualified success at any target IOP, with no significant endpoint intergroup difference at ≤ 15 mm Hg (log-rank $P = 0.595$).The intergroup MBGS scores differed due to reduced central and peripheral vascularity in MMC group ($P = 0.027$; $P = 0.041$).
SD-OCT analysis denied differences in bleb height between MMC vs OLO (140.5 ± 20.3 μ vs 129.2 ± 19.3 μ respectively; $P = 0.079$).
Mean antiglaucoma medications were significantly reduced ($P < 0.0005$) from 2.5 (±0.3) to 1.2 (±0.4) in MMC and from 2.6 (±0.2) to 1.4 (±0.3) in OLO group, with no intergroup differences ($P = 0.08$).
Six (30 %) cystic thin avascular blebs without oozing were recorded in the MMC group and 2 (10 %) in the OLO group, without intergroup difference ($P = 0.235$).

Conclusions: Our extended follow-up results confirm that Ologen implant yields efficacy and long-term success rates quite similar to MMC, with at least equivalent safety.

Keywords: Mitomycin-C, Ologen, Trabeculectomy, Extended 5-yrs follow-up

* Correspondence: salvatore.cillino@unipa.it
[1]Department of Experimental Biomedicine and Clinical Neuroscience, Ophthalmology Section, University of Palermo (Italy), via Liborio Giuffrè, 13, 90127 Palermo, Italy
Full list of author information is available at the end of the article

Background

Trabeculectomy with mitomycin-C (MMC) today is still regarded as the gold-standard in glaucoma surgery. Yet, in many studies MMC-related complications such as prolonged wound leaks, hypotony with choroidal effusions and maculopathy, thin avascular blebs, and/or bleb leaks with late infection are frequently reported [1–9].

A biodegradable collagen-glycosaminoglycan copolymer matrix implant (Ologen®) has been proposed as an alternative adjuvant, used as a spacer to mechanically separate the sub conjunctival and episcleral tissues to preventing fibrosis, and also helps in reorganizing the subconjunctival scar formation.

In fact, it should induce fibroblasts and myofibroblasts to grow randomly into its porous structure and secrete a loose connectival matrix, reducing the scarring degree. The implant is recommended to be placed subconjunctivally over the scleral flap posteriorly and possibly a small portion covering the scleral flap, else the ologen disc would act as a mechanical tamponade and prevent fluid outflow from the sub scleral space.

In 2010, a medium-term RCT did not show any intraocular pressure-lowering advantage of the Ologen-augmented trabeculectomy vs trabeculectomy alone, with a higher yet not significant incidence of complications with the collagen implant [10]. In the same year another randomized study of MMC-augmented trabeculectomy vs trabeculectomy using Ologen showed a lower complete success rate but a lower bleb-associated complication rate in Ologen group [11].

In 2011, we published the results of a 24-month, randomized prospective clinical trial on Ologen implant vs MMC in trabeculectomy [12]. The intraocular pressure (IOP) reduction was significant at endpoint in all groups ($P = 0.01$). The rates and Kaplan–Meier curves did not differ for both complete and qualified success at any target IOP. The bleb height in the Ologen-treated group was higher than in the MMC one ($P < 0.05$). No adverse reaction to Ologen was noted.

In the past three years, a number of clinical studies have compared the efficacy and tolerability of trabeculectomy augmented with Ologen versus trabeculectomy plus MMC, with somehow contradictory results [13–20].

To obtain more data on the long-term IOP lowering effect of the Ologen implant compared to MMC as adjuvant in trabeculectomy, we extended to five years the follow-up on the same cohort of subjects of our abovesaid study. The parameters measured included IOP, bleb morphology, and frequency of complications.

Methods

This study is an extended, 60-month follow-up data. The protocol of the randomized study had been approved by the Ethical Committee of the University Hospital of Palermo (Italy) on December 2007 and registered under the number 08/07 (12 September 2007) .We reviewed the records of 40 patients who had been randomly assigned to undergo a trabeculectomy with MMC (MMC group) or a trabeculectomy with Ologen implant (OLO group) for primary open-angle (POAG) or pseudoexfoliative glaucoma (PEXG) at the Department of Ophthalmology of the University of Palermo. The data used to generate the 5-year life table analysis were collected over the interval between enrollment in the study and 60 months following surgery.

In the previous prospective randomized clinical trial [12] a sample size of 40 patients (20 eyes in each group) had been chosen to achieve a power of 90 % for detecting a 3-mmHg difference in IOP between treatment procedures, assuming a standard deviation of three mmHg and a two-sided α error of 5 %.

In accord with tenets of Declaration of Helsinki a written informed consent has been obtained from all patients, also covering approval to publish images. We screened for uncontrolled glaucoma 65 consecutive Caucasian patients at the Glaucoma Center of the Department of Ophthalmology between January and December 2008. Sealed envelope technique from surgical chart number was used to ensure randomization just before surgery. Skilled ophthalmologists and optometrists masked to randomization collected the clinical data and the outcomes. Inclusion criteria were age 18 or older, diagnosis of POAG or PEXG with mild to moderate visual field damage [21], IOP above 21 mm Hg or visual field deterioration on maximum-tolerated medical therapy.

Exclusion criteria were advanced glaucoma or split fixation on visual field, normal-tension glaucoma, use of medications for acute or chronic disease that could affect the outcomes (eg, immunodeficiency, connective tissue disease, and diabetes), clinically significant cataract, previous ocular trauma or surgery. Included preoperative data consisted of age, gender, type of glaucoma, type and number of antiglaucoma medications; the ophthalmic examination included Goldmann applanation tonometry, biomicroscopy; Snellen visual acuity and computerized Humphrey visual field testing (Humphrey Visual Field Analyzer; HFA; Carl Zeiss Meditec. Inc.).

The primary outcome was IOP evaluated at three different IOP target levels: ≤ 21, ≤17, and ≤15 mmHg. Complete and qualified success were defined as usual, i.e. without medications in the first case and regardless of medications in the second one. Secondary outcome measures included visual acuity (VA), mean deviation (MD) change by Humphrey 24-2 full threshold testing, bleb evaluation according to Moorfields Bleb Grading System (MBGS), and bleb SD-OCT analysis. Number of glaucoma medications and frequency of postoperative adjunctive procedures and complications were also evaluated.

Surgical technique and follow-up

The technique has been described in detail in the previous study [12]. All operations, carried out by one experienced surgeon (SC), included a superior fornix-based conjunctival/tenons flap, with a rectangular scleral flap at the 12-o'clock position, fashioned according to the 'Moorfields Safer Surgery System' procedure [22, 23]. When MMC (Kyowa S.r.l., Milan, Italy) was the randomized adjunctive therapy, Weck-cell sponge pieces soaked with 0.2 mg/ml MMC were simultaneously placed under the dissected conjunctiva/tenon surrounding the scleral flap [22, 23], and on the scleral bed, underneath the scleral flap, for a total time of 2 min [24]. After thorough irrigation, trabeculectomy was performed with a Crozafon-De Laage punch. A peripheral iridectomy was performed, the anterior chamber was filled with viscoelastic device, and the scleral flap was closed with two minimally tensed 10-0 nylon sutures -one at each corner- in MMC cases and with one long and loose stitch in OLO cases. A cylindrical Ologen implant (model number 830601, Aeon Astron Europe BV), 2.0 ± 0.3 mm in height x 6.0 ± 0.5 mm in diameter was then centered over the top of scleral flap and underneath the conjunctiva in the latter leaving the limbal end of the stitch partially uncovered. The implants used in this cohort of patients consisted of porcine based lyophilized crosslinked type I atelocollagen (≥ 90 %) and glycosaminoglycans (≤ 10 %). Degradation time of this type was around 180 days. A newer version with exactly the same composition but with a bit shorter degradation time is now available.

The conjunctival flap was secured to the limbus with a tight 10-0 nylon running suture with buried knots.

Postoperatively, all eyes were treated with tapering doses of topical tobramycin 0.3 % and dexamethasone drops 0.1 % for 2 months. The 'intensified postoperative care' (IPC) protocol [25] was followed in all cases and included more frequent topical steroid administration if corkscrew bleb vessels were present. Instillation of 1 % atropine drops during the first few days was based on the hypotony degree. Adjunctive procedures included the Carlo Traverso maneuver [26], laser suture lysis or bleb needling of encapsulated blebs (without antimetabolites).

If postoperative IOP measurements were >21 mmHg after topical steroid withdrawal, IOP-lowering medication was added.

When, during the extended follow-up, a patient developed a clinically significant cataract in the operated eye, a standard sutureless cataract surgery was performed through a temporal 2.5-mm near-clear corneal tunnel incision with a precalibrated knife (Clearcut, Alcon Italia

S.P.A., Milan, Italy). Phacoemulsification was performed with the Alcon Infiniti Vision System (Alcon Italia S.P.A.), using the Ozil torsional handpiece in the majority of cases, avoiding any contact with the bleb area. The implantation of acrylic hydrophobic foldable intraocular lenses (IOLs) was performed using an Unfolder Emerald injector system (AMO Italy, Rome, Italy) or a Monarch II injector (Alcon Italia S.P.A.). The surgical wound was closed by stromal hydration. All patients received topical ofloxacin (Exocin, Allergan SpA, Rome, Italy) for 3 days preoperatively and tobramycin and dexamethasone ophthalmic suspension (Tobradex, Alcon Italia S.P.A.) for one week postoperatively, followed by nepafenac ophthalmic suspension (Nevanac, Alcon Italia S.P.A.) or bromfenac ophthalmic solution (Yellox, Bausch Lomb, Italia), for 3 weeks. In case of topical antiglaucomatous therapy use, this was continued even throughout the cataract surgery period. Even in cataract surgery cases, if postoperative IOP measurements were >21 mmHg after topical steroid withdrawal, IOP-lowering medication was added.

Expanded follow-up implied six-monthly examinations till the 60th month. All patients were thoroughly informed about the importance of a periodical examination, and were regularly visited by the same staff to create a relationship of empathy. We were lucky to be able to follow all patients for 5 years. We report data collected at 36, 48 and 60-month observation times (Additional file 1).

Follow-up visits included assessment of VA, IOP, biomicroscopic findings, number of antiglaucomatous medications, and postoperative complications. Signs of inflammation, such as cells and flare, were graded from 0 to 4. The MBGS [27] -using recorded photographs- was used for bleb grading by a single observer (GC) at each follow-up visit. Cystic or avascular blebs were noted.

Spectral domain optical coherence tomography (SD-OCT; Topcon 3DOCT-1000, Topcon Corporation, Tokyo, Japan), already performed at the previous study end point (24 month), was repeated at the 60-month observation time for bleb evaluation by ophthalmologists masked to clinical data (CG and LLF). A bleb was identified as successful or failed based on the presence or absence of bleb wall thickening and microcystic or hyporeflective intrableb wall structures (with respect to a ≤ 17 mmHg target IOP level [28, 29]). Thereafter, we add measurements of some bleb parameters, performed with calipers using the device's built-in software in a masked fashion. Bleb wall thickness was defined as the distance between the first reflective signal from the conjunctiva to the top of the sub-Tenon fluid space. Because the bleb wall thickness may vary along the scan, we analyzed only the maximum and minimum distances [30].

The whole bleb height was defined as the maximum vertical length from the outer margin of the bleb wall and the highly reflective margin of the scleral surface in the cross-sectional image.

Statistical analysis

Statistical analysis of quantitative and qualitative data, including descriptive statistics, was performed for all items. The independent Student t-test and the Mann–Whitney U statistic test were used for parametric and non-parametric analysis, respectively. Discrete variables were analyzed using the chi square test and Fisher exact test, as needed. Intragroup parametric and non-parametric analysis were carried on by using the paired-samples Student t-test and paired Wilcoxon signed-rank test respectively. Success was evaluated on the basis of Kaplan–Meier cumulative probability (log-rank test). To assess intraobserver reproducibility and consistency, an internal quality control system was established before the study onset by using three consecutive independent interpretations of the same SD-OCT scan, together with the unweighted Cohen kappa (k) test [31]. Data were analyzed by the Epi Info software (version 6.0, Centers for Disease Control and Prevention, Atlanta, GA, USA) and IBM SPSS Software 21.0 version (SPSS, Inc., Chicago, Ill, US). All P-values were two-sided and P-values less than 0.05 were considered statistically significant.

Results

Patients in the two treatment groups did not significantly differ in any of the preoperative parameters. Two women with early-onset glaucoma, aged 36 and 38 years,

were included, the former in the MMC group and the latter in the OLO one.

As above said, all 40 patients completed the 60-month follow-up. During the 3rd to 4th year of follow-up, 3 cases (15 %) in the MMC group and 2 cases (10 %) in the OLO group developed a clinically significant cataract with VA decrease in the operated eye, and therefore underwent cataract surgery with IOL implantation (Table 1).

Mean Snellen acuity and visual field test MD at the 5-years end point did not differ from the baseline in both groups (Table 1). The mean preoperative IOP (±SD) was 26.5 (±5.2) in MMC eyes and 27.3 (±6.0) in OLO eyes, without significant intergroup difference. One-day postoperatively, the IOP dropped to 5.2 (±3.5) and 9.2 (±5.5) mmHg, respectively ($P = 0.009$). No intergroup difference was present at any scheduled postoperative time interval. The postoperative IOP reduction was significant at the 24-month endpoint in both groups ($P = 0.01$). At the extended 36-month time interval, the mean IOP was 15.6 (±2.6) in the MMC group and 15.9 (±2.5) mmHg in the OLO group ($P = 0.706$), while at the 48th month the IOP values were 15.9 (±2.6) and 15.3 (±3.4) respectively ($P = 0.563$) Finally, at the 60th month the IOP values were 15.2 (±3.2) and 15.8 (±2.3) respectively ($P = 0.579$). The endpoint percentage IOP reduction from baseline was 40.9 (±14.2) and 42.1(±13.3), respectively ($P = 0.827$) (Table 2 and Fig. 1). The two cases of early-onset glaucoma exhibited an IOP within the low teens without medications.

In the cases who underwent cataract phacoemulsification, the mean pre-operative IOP was 16.9 (±2.3) in MMC eyes and 17.0 (±2.9) in OLO ones, whilst the endpoint IOP was 17.2 (±2.5) and 16.5 (±2.7) respectively

Table 1 Preoperative characteristics of patients who underwent trabeculectomy, Snellen acuity and MD change, and 3rd to 4th year follow-up cataract surgery cases

	MMC group	OLO group	P
Gender (M/F), N°	11/9	12/8	1.0[a]
Age, yrs. (mean ± SD)	63.2(7.2)	65.8(6.4)	0.234[b]
Right/left eyes, N°	7/13	11/9	0.340[a]
Type of glaucoma (POAG/PEXG), N°	12/8	13/7	1.0[a]
Preoperative IOP,mmHg (mean ± SD)	26.7(5.2)	27.3(6.0)	0.736[b]
Baseline CDVA, decimal notation	0.8 (±0.33)	0.75 (±0.31)	0.624
Endpoint CDVA, decimal notation	0.8 (±0.40)	0.8 (±0.35)	1.0
Baseline MD,dB (mean ± SD)	-7.80(4.57)	-7.41(5.35)	0.805[b]
Endpoint MD,dB (mean ± SD)	-7.60(4.3)	-7.50(5.6)	0.949[b]
Preoperative medications,N° (mean ± SD)	2.5(0.3)	2.6(0.2)	0.222[b]
Duration of preoperative antiglaucoma therapy,yrs. (mean ± SD)	5.7(1.8)	6.3(1.4)	0.246[b]
Cataract surgery cases	3 (15 %)	2 (10 %)	1.0

[a]Chi square test or Fisher exact test, as needed; [b]independent Student t test;
MMC = Mitomycin-C; OLO = Ologen; SD = standard deviation;
POAG = primary open angle glaucoma; PEXG = pseudoexfoliation glaucoma; CDVA = Corrected Distance Visual Acuity; MD = Humphrey Visual Field Analyzer Mean deviation.

Table 2 Postoperative IOP (mmHg) in the surgical groups. Mean (±SD; 95%CI); % change in IOP from baseline

	MMC group	OLO group	P^a
3rd month	14.7(3.9; 12.9-16.4)	15.0(3.8; 13.3-16.7)	0.806
	44.5 %	45.1 %	
6th month	14.7(4.3; 12.7-16.6)	14.1(3.1; 12.6-15.4)	0.615
	44.5 %	48.4 %	
12th month	15.0(3.0; 13.6-16.4)	15.2(2.8; 13.8-16.4)	0.828
	43.4 %	44.3 %	
24th month	16.0(2.9; 14.6-17.4)	16.5(2.1; 15.5-17.4)	0.536
	39.6 %	39.5 %	
36th month	15.6 (2.6; 14.3-16.9)	15.9 (2.5; 14.6-17.2)	0.706
	39.8 %	40.2 %	
48th month	15.9 (2.6; 14.5-17.2)	15.3 (3.4; 13.4-17.1)	0.563
	38.8 %	42.3 %	
60th month	15.2 (3.2; 13.4-16.9)	15.8 (±2.3; 14.4-17.1)	0.579
	41.0 %	42.1 %	

[a] Independent Student t test; MMC = Mitomycin-C; OLO = Ologen; SD = standard deviation

($P = 0.885$, and $P = 0.875$, respectively). The number of antiglaucoma medications, 0.7 (0.6) in MMC and 0.5 (0.7) in OLO cases did no change after cataract surgery. All cataract patients experienced a post-operative VA increase of at least 2 lines.

Table 3 reports the success rates in the study groups. At the 60-month endpoint follow-up, the values regarding complete success at ≤ 21 mmHg target IOP were 65 % and 70 % respectively for the MMC and the OLO group, with a qualified success of over 85 % in both. At the ≤17 mm Hg target IOP, complete success percentages were 60 % and 55 %, and qualified ones 70 % and 75 % respectively. At the ≤15 mm Hg target IOP level complete success was recorded in 35 % and 45 % of cases, and qualified one in 40 % and 50 % of patients respectively with no significant difference at any follow-up time.

At 24-month follow-up, the Kaplan–Meier cumulative survival curves relating either the ≤21, ≤17, or ≤15 mmHg target IOP had not showed significant intergroup differences for complete or qualified success rates. Figure 2, indicates the same parameter behavior relating complete success rates at ≤ 15 mm Hg target IOP up to the 60th month end point, with no significant intergroup difference (log-rank $P = 0.595$).

The area, height and vascularity MBGS scores did not generally differ on an intragroup and intergroup basis, maintaining stability till the 24th month. One exception was height, whose mean score was higher in OLO group at the third month (2.0 ± 0.8 vs 1.3 ± 0.7; $P = 0.009$; Mann–Whitney U statistic test), maintaining a higher yet not significant value till the first 24th month end point.

No significant difference was found between the 24-month and the 60-month values, either with respect to central area ($P = 0.729$ in MMC and $P = 0.231$ in OLO group), maximal area ($P = 0.769$ and $P = 0.395$, respectively) and height ($P = 0.408$ and $P = 0.478$, respectively). The 60-month mean MBGS score values in MMC vs OLO group were 2.7 ± 0.7 vs 2.3 ± 0.9 ($P = 0.191$) relating

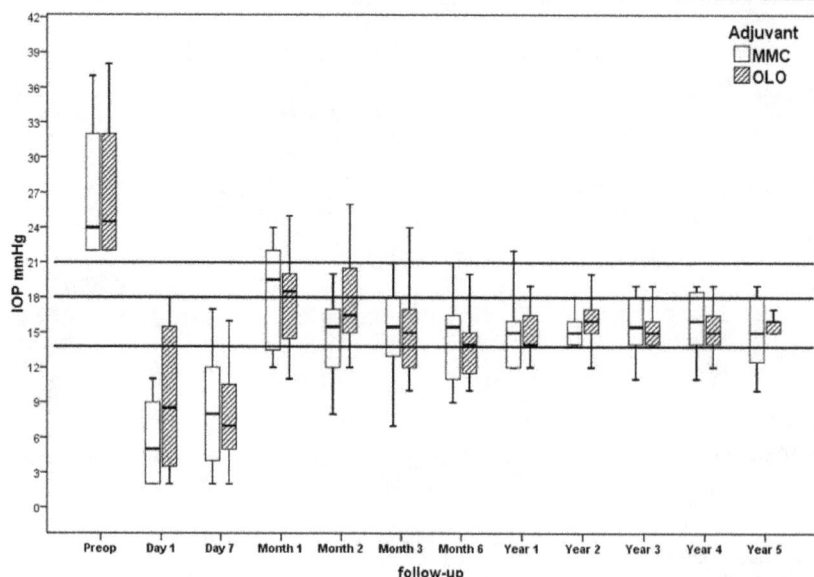

Fig. 1 Box-plot representation of IOP values over 60-months follow-up: median values (dark lines), error standard (T-bars)

Table 3 Success rates (%) at the 60-month follow-up study endpoint in the surgical groups at three target IOP levels

	MMC group	OLO group	P^a
≤21 mmHg			
Complete success	13(65 %)	14(70 %)	1.0
Qualified success	17(85 %)	18(90 %)	1.0
≤17 mmHg			
Complete success	12(60 %)	11(55 %)	1.0
Qualified success	14(70 %)	15(75 %)	1.0
≤15 mmHg			
Complete success	7(35 %)	9(45 %)	0.747
Qualified success	8(40 %)	10(50 %)	0.751

[a]Fisher exact test; MMC = Mitomycin-C; OLO = Ologen

central area, 2.9 ± 0.8 vs 2.6 ± 1.0 ($P = 0.378$) relating maximal area, and 1.2 ± 0.5 vs 1.2 ± 0.8 ($P = 0.722$) relating height, without intergroup difference. At the same time interval, central, peripheral, and non-bleb vascularity mean score values in MMC vs OLO group were 0.6 ± 0.3 vs 0.9 ± 0.5, 1.3 ± 0.3 vs 1.1 ± 0.3, and 1.6 ± 1.0 vs 1.4 ± 1.0, with intergroup difference ($P = 0.027$; $P = 0.041$; $P = 0.531$), respectively, relating the central and peripheral score. Figure 3 shows two cases with diffuse bleb, one from MMC and the other from OLO group, with a central avascular/cystic area in the former and almost normal vascularity in the latter.

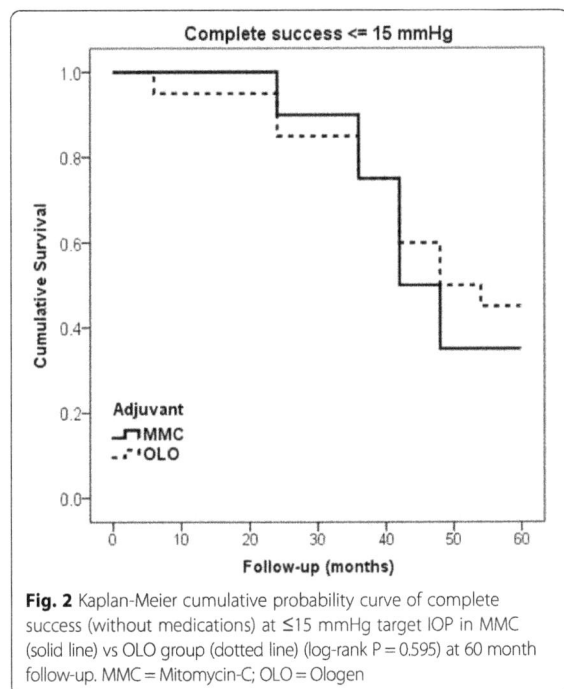

Fig. 2 Kaplan-Meier cumulative probability curve of complete success (without medications) at ≤15 mmHg target IOP in MMC (solid line) vs OLO group (dotted line) (log-rank P = 0.595) at 60 month follow-up. MMC = Mitomycin-C; OLO = Ologen

There was high intraobserver reproducibility for SD-OCT analysis (k = 0.7403, 95 % CI: 0.70–0.86). Table 4 reports the successful bleb frequencies, with respect to a ≤17 mmHg target IOP level, at 5-year follow-up.

Figure 4 displays examples of bleb thickness parameters obtained using the SD-OCT built-in software at the 60-month end point. Eight eyes, 6 in the MMC and 2 in the OLO group, with a cystic thin bleb, exhibited minimum bleb wall thickness mean values significantly smaller (54.5 ± 14.9 μ) than the remaining eyes (134.2 ± 17.3 μ) ($P = 0.004$), in agreement with the clinical appearance. No differences were found in terms of whole bleb height between groups (140.5 ± 20.3 μ vs 129.2 ± 19.3 μ respectively; $P = 0.079$).

The mean number of antiglaucoma medications was significantly reduced at end point in both groups ($P < 0.0005$ in both cases): from 2.5 (±0.3) to 1.2 (±0.4) and from 2.6 (±0.2) to 1.4 (±0.3) in the MMC and OLO groups, respectively, without significant intergroup differences ($P = 0.08$).

The Carlo Traverso maneuver was employed in two patients in each group between the 1st and the 14th postoperative day. Four cases (20 %) in the MMC group and three cases (15 %) in the OLO group -without intergroup difference- underwent Laser suture lysis between the first and the second postoperative week. Bleb needling was performed from one to four times in seven (35 %) and six (30 %) patients respectively, again without intergroup difference.

The frequency of early postoperative complication did not significantly differ between the two groups, even if a tendency toward more frequent early bleb leakage was noted in the OLO group, and toward more frequent early hypotony, defined as an intraocular pressure (IOP) equal to or less than 6 mmHg at the first postoperative day, and choroidal detachment in MMC one. No adverse reaction to the Ologen implant, matrix extrusion, or conjunctival erosion was present in OLO group. At the 60-month endpoint, three more cases of clinically significant cataract with VA decrease, 2 in the MMC and 1 in the OLO group, were found, to a total of 5 and 3 cases respectively during the whole follow-up. Five (25 %) patients in the MMC group and 4 (20 %) in the OLO one experienced > 1 line VA loss due to cataract or to age-related macular degeneration (AMD). Six (30 %) cystic thin avascular blebs without oozing, as above said, were recorded in the MMC group and 2 (10 %) in the OLO group, without intergroup difference ($P = 0.235$) (Table 5).

Discussion

Both early and long-term complications are still reported in MMC-augmented trabeculectomy: As pointed out in our previous study [12], factors such as flaps fashioning, suturing technique and prolonged fibroblast inhibition

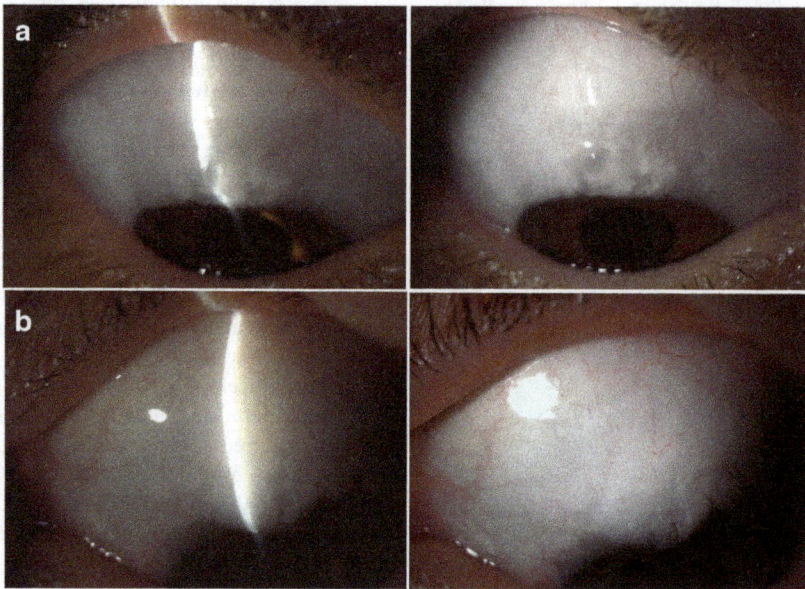

Fig. 3 Slit light and diffuser photographs of two cases. Patient **a** (top): 38 yrs-old woman from MMC group. **a** diffuse bleb with central avascular/cystic area can be seen. Patient **b** (bottom): 52 yrs-old man from OLO group. A diffuse bleb with almost normal vascularity is present

-with thin bleb leaking- are responsible for these problems [8, 9, 22, 23, 32].

In our previous study, the early postoperative hypotony rate is really quite high in both groups, probably due to the loose stitches without fashioning releasable sutures: the latter technique could avoid this complication [12]. Anyway, the reduced tendency to first postoperative day's hypotony in the OLO cases, when compared with the MMC ones, can be explained as a mechanical Ologen-induced aqueous outflow modulation.

The extended 5-year results indicate that the postoperative IOP behavior is quite similar in both groups, with a highly significant and stable IOP reduction, stable VA and MD, and reduced administration of antiglaucoma medications throughout the 60-month follow-up, without intergroup differences. The equivalence in efficacy of

Table 4 60th month bleb success rates(%) at ≤17 mmHg target IOP in the surgical groups according to the SD-OCT analysis

	MMC group60th mo	OLO group60th mo	P60th mo
Successful bleb / eyes with complete success	10/12	9/11	1.0[a]
Failed bleb / eyes without complete success	6/8	7/9	1.0[a]
SD-OCT sensitivity	83 %	82 %	0.627[b]
SD-OCT specificity	75 %	78 %	0.669[b]

[a]Fisher exact test; [b]Chi-square test for the comparison of two proportions (from independent samples), expressed as a percentage;
MMC = Mitomycin-C; OLO = Ologen

OLO vs MMC is further confirmed by their endpoint success rates at the three different target IOP levels. Even if it is well known that phacoemulsification leads to an increased risk of bleb failure of approximately 33 %, with changes in bleb morphology and elevation in IOP of 2-3 mmHg [33], in our cases the temporal access phaco did not show any effect until the endpoint. The exiguous number of cases could explain this finding.

The sample size power was calculated for the IOP endpoint. Therefore, no conclusions can be drawn from the secondary endpoints, e.g. bleb morphology, number of postoperative medications and frequency of complications. We judge anyway that our results imply some interesting observations. Testifying to the persistence of the implant, the bleb height score was higher in the OLO than in MMC group at the 3rd month. Indeed, the residual implant volume added to the fluid-filled bleb spaces could justify this finding (since its biodegradation -according to the manufacturer- can last a 6-month period as above said). It is possible that a larger sample could have confirmed this difference in height for a longer period.

In studies using either morphologic grading scale evaluation or experimental 3D anterior segment SD-OCT, bleb height is one of the parameters correlated with a lower IOP [28, 34–36]. Whether at 24-months or 60-months follow-up, our sample shows that the outer bleb morphology by SD-OCT was quite similar between groups. These findings imply that outer layers of a functioning bleb are not modified by the OLO implant on a

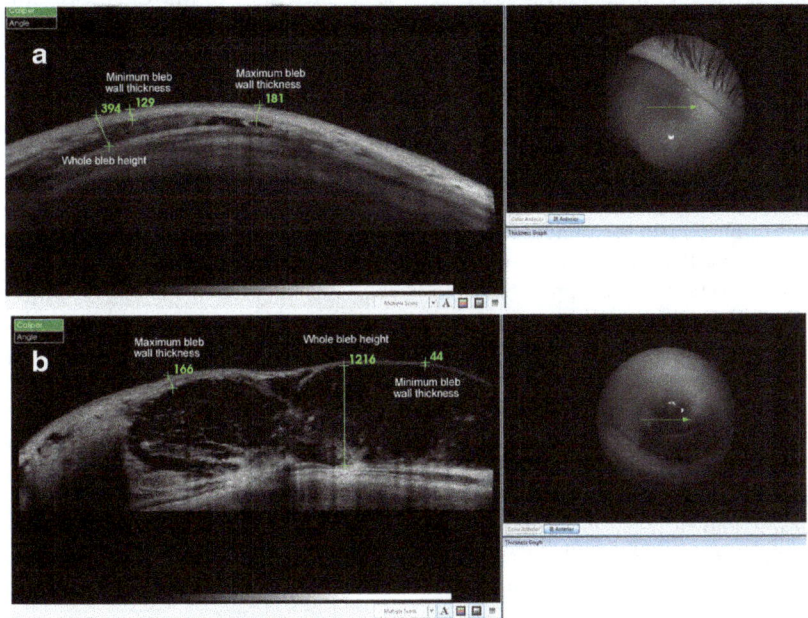

Fig. 4 SD-OCT imaging of blebs at the 60-month end point with complete success based on ≤ 15 mmHg target IOP. (**a**): Thick bleb from OLO group. (**b**): Thin bleb from MMC group. The bleb (**a**), from the OLO group, exhibited a more diffuse pattern

long term basis. In summary, the OCT bleb data indicate that bleb morphology is disappointingly not strongly correlated with function. A larger sample size could perhaps reveal that the SD-OCT pattern of a successful bleb, represents a prognostic factor for longer-term success. The end point bleb wall SD-OCT analysis confirms the critically reduced thickness of cystic thin blebs in both groups. The similarity of the whole bleb height in both groups, as measured by SD OCT, is in agreement with the above said clinical judgment by MBGS criteria.

The two groups did not differ with respect to adjunctive postoperative procedures. This could once more confirm similarity between the adjuvants.

Similar rates of early complications in the two groups further corroborate the equivalence of the effect of the two adjuvants during this postoperative period. The above said tendency to 1st day greater hypotony in MMC eyes did not reach significance in our sample. The

low complication rate with low-dosage MMC within 2 years is in agreement with our previous studies [24, 37–39]. The cataract and AMD incidence could be ascribed both to aging and to glaucoma surgery in our cases. As previously noted, late thin avascular blebs are relatively common with MMC use. In our sample, after 5 years MMC cases exhibit a reduced vascularity together with a trend toward more frequent thin blebs, confirming the long-term effect from fibroblast mitosis inhibition [40]. It is surprising that, besides vascularity, in our sample there is no difference in end point bleb morphology of MMC cases when compared to the OLO ones, especially taking into account the diffuse area of application of MMC in the former and the limited surface of the 6x2 mm Ologen implant in the latter (see Fig. 3). The Ologen volume could hypothetically lift the surrounding conjunctiva from the scleral bed for a while, allowing a diffuse bleb, and/or, our sample size could imply some biased results, as above stated.

Earlier short to medium term retrospective or prospective randomized clinical trials denied our good results with Ologen. In fact, drawbacks such as lower bleb height and higher vascularity in OLO group, with a lower success rate, or higher complication rate of the Ologen-augmented trabeculectomy with respect to the simple one, or lower complete success rate even though a lower bleb-associated complication rate in Ologen vs MMC groups, are reported [10, 11, 41]. Variations in surgical procedure could justify these different outcomes. For instance, a non running suture with only two

Table 5 Frequency (%) of 60-month postoperative complications in the surgical groups

	MMC group	OLO group	p^a
Cataract	5(25 %)	3(15 %)	0.694
Age-related macular degeneration	2(10 %)	2(10 %)	1.0
Loss > 1 line VA	5(25 %)	4(20 %)	1.0
Thin avascular bleb	6(30 %)	2(10 %)	0.235

^{a}Fisher exact test; MMC = Mitomycin-C; OLO = Ologen

10-0 nylon at the flap extremities likely lead to a higher rate of positive Seidel test with flat anterior chamber. Also, it could have reduced the role of the implant in bleb development in one study [10]. Additionally, the same study included 1-month topical steroid administration, vs 2 months with variable regimen based on IPC criteria in our study. This difference could have freed the vascular reaction in OLO eyes as aforementioned, resulting in an excess of fibroblasts surrounding the implant with higher end point IOP [10]. Finally, we note that small sample sizes, techniques of application and concentration of MMC, postoperative therapeutic regimen as well as variations in composition and different manufacturers of Ologen implants over the years could also be important factors to take into consideration [11, 12, 19, 41]. On the other hand, the difference between our results and those obtained by other centers in Germany, Singapore and India, could derive from the long-time known racial difference in the response to trabeculectomy, with white Caucasian performing better than Hispanic, East-Asian or Black population. The fibroblasts response to the Ologen implant could well follow this behavior [42, 43].

A one-year prospective interventional multicenter study including 30 eyes undergone trabeculectomy with MMC (0.2 mg/mL, 0.1 mL)-soaked Ologen, concludes that the procedure does not seem to exert any synergistic effect in terms of IOP reduction [20]. We note that, besides the lack of a control group, the MMC soaked Ologen can be by itself the cause of "ring of steel" bleb, due to the prolonged MMC localized effect with excessive surrounding fibroblast proliferation [23].

Conversely, the results of our study are in agreement, relating efficacy and safety, with recent shorter term studies comparing Ologen-augmented vs MMC-augmented trabeculectomy [14–18].

In particular, Johnson et al [17] in a 12-month retrospective review find that Ologen allows for similar success rates as MMC comparing respectively 49 vs 50 eyes of mainly POAG patients undergoing a filtering procedure using an Ex-PRESS (Alcon, Fort Worth, TX) mini glaucoma device.

A recent systematic review and meta-analysis indicates that trabeculectomy with Ologen is a safe and effective procedure in patients with glaucoma, and is comparable with MMC in IOP-lowering efficacy, even if does not seem to offer any significant advantages compared with trabeculectomy plus MMC [13].

Under this respect, especially considering the additional cost to the Ologen implant when compared to MMC, much larger trials are required to confirm possible advantages in terms of reduced incidence of early hypotony and late avascular-thin blebs. Once these requirements are met, the Ologen could be recommended

as an alternative to MMC, at least in those cases where a target IOP in low teens is unnecessary. In the latter instance, an association between both adjuvants could be interesting.

Conclusions

Our long-term study confirms that the OLO implant demonstrates efficacy in terms of IOP reduction, with a success rate quite similar to MMC, and at least equivalent safety. Moreover, outpatient surgery could benefit from this adjuvant if the lack of early significant hypotony will be confirmed by larger trials. Limits related to the small sample size must be overcome by further larger randomized trials to confirm the efficacy and safety of this device, and to accurately estimate any reduced risk for avascular and thin blebs with respect to MMC.

Additional file

Additional file 1: Consort flow chart. (DOCX 48 kb)

Abbreviations

OLO: Ologen®; MMC: mitomycin-C; VA: visual acuity; MD: Mean deviation; MBGS: Moorfields Bleb Grading System; SD-OCT: spectral domain optic coherence tomography; IOP: intraocular pressure; POAG: primary open angle glaucoma; PEXG: pseudoexfoliative glaucoma; IPC: intensified postoperative care; IOL: intraocular lens; SD: standard deviation; AMD: age-related macular degeneration.

Competing interests

The authors declare that they have no competing interests.

Authors' contributions

SC conceived of the study and participated in its design and coordination. AC participated in the design of the study and performed the statistical analysis. FDP participated in the design and drafted the manuscript. CG and LLF participated in the acquisition of data, and helped to draft the manuscript. GC participated in the design of the study and helped to draft the manuscript. All authors read and approved the final manuscript.

Acknowledgements

No funding was obtained by any of the authors for this study.

Author details

¹Department of Experimental Biomedicine and Clinical Neuroscience, Ophthalmology Section, University of Palermo (Italy), via Liborio Giuffrè, 13, 90127 Palermo, Italy. ²Department of Sciences for Health Promotion and Mother-Child Care "G. D'Alessandro", University of Palermo, Via del Vespro 127, I, 90127 Palermo, Italy. ³Department of Surgical and Biomedical Sciences, Section of Ophthalmology, University of Perugia, Piazza Menghini 1. S. Andrea delle Fratte, 06156 Perugia, Italy.

References

1. Kitazawa Y, Kawase K, Matsushita H, Minobe M. Trabeculectomy with mitomycin: a comparative study with fluorouracil. Arch Ophthalmol. 1991;109:1693–8.
2. Skuta GL, Beeson CC, Higginbotham EJ, Lichter PR, Musch DC, Bergstrom TJ, Klein TB, Falck FY Jr. Intraoperative mitomycin vs postoperative 5-fluorouracil in high-risk glaucoma filtering surgery. Ophthalmology. 1992;99:438–44.

3. Palmer SS. Mitomycin as adjunct chemotherapy with trabeculectomy. Ophthalmology. 1991;98:317–21.

4. Jampel HD, Friedman DS, Lubomski LH, Kempen JH, Quigley H, Congdon N, Levkovitch-Verbin H, Robinson KA, Bass EB. Effect of technique on intraocular pressure after combined cataract and glaucoma surgery. An evidence-based review. Ophthalmology. 2002;109:2215–24.

5. Wilkins M, Indar A, Wormald R. Intra-operative mitomycin C for glaucoma surgery. Cochrane Database Syst Rev. 2005;4, CD002897.

6. Cheng JW, Xi GL, Wei RL, Cai JP, Li Y. Efficacy and tolerability of nonpenetrating glaucoma surgery augmented with mitomycin C in treatment of open-angle glaucoma: a meta-analysis. Can J Ophthalmol. 2009;44:76–82.

7. Palanca-Capistrano AM, Hall J, Cantor LB, Morgan L, Hoop J, WuDunn D. Long-term outcomes of intraoperative 5-fluorouracil vs intraoperative mitomycin C in primary trabeculectomy surgery. Ophthalmology. 2009;116:185–90.

8. Anand N, Atherley C. Deep sclerectomy augmented with mitomycin C. Eye. 2005;19:442–50.

9. Anand N, Arora S, Clowes M. Mitomycin C augmented glaucoma surgery: evolution of filtering bleb avascularity, transconjunctival oozing, and leaks. Br J Ophthalmol. 2006;90:175–80.

10. Papaconstantinou D, Georgalas I, Karmiris E, Diagourtas A, Koutsandrea C, Ladas I, Apostolopoulos M, Georgopoulos G. Trabeculectomy with OloGen vs trabeculectomy for the treatment of glaucoma: a pilot study. Acta Ophthalmol. 2010;88:80–5.

11. Rosentreter A, Schild AM, Jordan JF, Krieglstein GK, Dietlein TS. A prospective randomised trial of trabeculectomy using mitomycin C vs an ologen implant in open angle glaucoma. Eye (Lond). 2010;24:1449–57.

12. Cillino S, Di Pace F, Cillino G, Casuccio A. Biodegradable collagen matrix implant vs mitomycin-C as an adjuvant in trabeculectomy: a 24-month, randomized clinical trial. Eye (Lond). 2011;25:1598–606.

13. He M, Wang W, Zhang X, Huang W. Ologen implant versus mitomycin C for trabeculectomy: a systematic review and meta-analysis. PLoS One. 2014;9(1):e85782.

14. Nilforushan N, Yadegari M, Hodjat P. Comparison of the success rate of trabeculectomy with OculusGen versus trabeculectomy with mitomycin C. Iranian Journal of Ophthalmology. 2011;23:3–12.

15. Senthil S, Rao HL, Babu JG, Mandal AK, Garudadri CS. Comparison of outcomes of trabeculectomy with mitomycin C vs. ologen implant in primary glaucoma. Indian J Ophthalmol. 2013;61:338–42.

16. Marey HM, Mandour SS, Ellakwa AF. Subscleral trabeculectomy with mitomycin-C versus ologen for treatment of glaucoma. J Ocul Pharmacol Ther. 2013;29:330–34.

17. Johnson MS, Sarkisian Jr SR. Using a Collagen Matrix Implant (Ologen) Versus Mitomycin-C as a Wound Healing Modulator in Trabeculectomy With the Ex-PRESS Mini Glaucoma Device: A 12-Month Retrospective Review. J Glaucoma. 2014;23:649–52.

18. Dada T, Kusumesh R, Bali SJ, Sharma S, Sobti A, Arora V, et al. Trabeculectomy with combined use of subconjunctival collagen implant and low-dose mitomycin C. J Glaucoma. 2013;22:659–62.

19. Narayanaswamy A, Perera SA, Htoon HM, Hoh ST, Seah SK, Wong TT, Aung T. Efficacy and safety of collagen matrix implants in phacotrabeculectomy and comparison with mitomycin C augmented phacotrabeculectomy at 1 year. Clin Experiment Ophthalmol. 2013;41:552–60.

20. Min JK, Kee CW, Sohn SW, Lee HJ, Woo JM, Yim JH. Surgical outcome of mitomycinC-soaked collagen matrix implant in trabeculectomy. J Glaucoma. 2013;22:456–62.

21. Musch DC, Gillespie BW, Lichter PR, Niziol LM, Janz NK, CIGTS Study Investigators. Visual field progression in the Collaborative Initial Glaucoma Treatment Study the impact of treatment and other baseline factors. Ophthalmology. 2009;116(2):200–7.

22. Stalmans I, Gillis A, Lafaut AS, Zeyen T. Safe trabeculectomy technique: long-term outcome. Br J Ophthalmol. 2006;90:44–7.

23. Dhingra S, Khaw PT. The Moorfields safer surgery system. Middle East Afr J Ophthalmol. 2009;16:112–5.

24. Cillino S, Di Pace F, Casuccio A, Lodato G. Deep sclerectomy vs punch trabeculectomy: effect of low-dosage mitomycin C. Ophthalmologica. 2005; 219:281–6.

25. Marquardt D, Lieb WE, Grehn F. Intensified postoperative care vs conventional follow-up: a retrospective long-term analysis of 177 trabeculectomies. Graefes Arch Clin Exp Ophthalmol. 2004;242:106–13.

26. Traverso CE, Greenidge KC, Spaeth GL, Wilson RP. Focal pressure: a new method to encourage filtration after trabeculectomy. Ophthalmic Surg. 1984;15:62–5.

27. Wells AP, Ashraff NN, Hall RC, Purdie G. Comparison of two clinical Bleb grading systems. Ophthalmology. 2006;113:77–83.

28. Kawana K, Kiuchi T, Yasuno Y, Oshika T. Evaluation of trabeculectomy blebs using 3-dimensional cornea and anterior segment optical coherence tomography. Ophthalmology. 2009;116:848–55.

29. Singh M, See JL, Aquino MC, Thean LS, Chew PT. High-definition imaging of trabeculectomy blebs using spectral domain optical coherence tomography adapted for the anterior segment. Clin Exp Ophthalmol. 2009;37:345–51.

30. Jung KI, Lim SA, Park HY, Park CK. Visualization of blebs using anterior-segment optical coherence tomography after glaucoma drainage implant surgery. Ophthalmology. 2013;120:978–83.

31. Brennan P, Silman A. Statistical methods for assessing observer variability in clinical measures. BMJ. 1992;304:1491–4.

32. Lockwood A, Brocchini S, Khaw PT. New developments in the pharmacological modulation of wound healing after glaucoma filtration surgery. Curr Opin Pharmacol. 2013;13:65–71.

33. Patel HY, Danesh-Meyer HV. Incidence and management of cataract after glaucoma surgery. Curr Opin Ophthalmol. 2013;24(1):15–20.

34. Picht G, Grehn F. Classification of filtering blebs in trabeculectomy: biomicroscopy and functionality. Curr Opin Ophthalmol. 1998;9:2–8.

35. Cantor LB, Mantravadi A, WuDunn D, Swamynathan K, Cortes A. Morphologic classification of filtering blebs after glaucoma filtration surgery: the Indiana Bleb Appearance Grading Scale. J Glaucoma. 2003;12:266–71.

36. Lopes JF, Moster MR, Wilson RP, Altangerel U, Alvim HS, Tong MG, Fontanarosa J, Steinmann WC. Subconjunctival sodium hyaluronate 2.3% in trabeculectomy: a prospective randomized clinical trial. Ophthalmology. 2006;113:756–60.

37. Cillino S, Di Pace F, Casuccio A, Calvaruso L, Morreale D, Vadalà M, Lodato G. Deep sclerectomy vs punch trabeculectomy with or without phacoemulsification: a randomized clinical trial. J Glaucoma. 2004;13:500–6.

38. Cillino S, Di Pace F, Casuccio A, Cillino G, Lodato G. Deep sclerectomy vs trabeculectomy with low-dosage mitomycin C: four-year follow-up. Ophthalmologica. 2008;222:81–7.

39. Cillino S, Zeppa L, Di Pace F, Casuccio A, Morreale D, Bocchetta F, Lodato G. E-PTFE (Gore-Tex) implant with or without low-dosage mitomycin-C as an adjuvant in penetrating glaucoma surgery: 2 year randomized clinical trial. Acta Ophthalmol. 2008;86:314–21.

40. Crowston JG, Akbar AN, Constable PH, Occleston NL, Daniels JT, Khaw PT. Antimetabolite-induced apoptosis in Tenon's capsule fibroblasts. Invest Ophthalmol Vis Sci. 1998;39(2):449–54.

41. Boey PY, Narayanaswamy A, Zheng C, Perera SA, Htoon HM, Tun TA, Seah SK, Wong TT, Aung T. Imaging of blebs after phacotrabeculectomy with Ologen collagen matrix implants. Br J Ophthalmol. 2011;95:340–4.

42. Broadway D, Grierson I, Hitchings R. Racial differences in the results of glaucoma filtration surgery: are racial differences in the conjunctival cell profile important? Br J Ophthalmol. 1994;78:466–75.

43. Husain R, Clarke JCK, Seah SKL, Khaw PT. A review of trabeculectomy in East Asian People the influence of race. Eye. 2005;19:243–52.

18

A cross-sectional study of submacular thickening in intermediate uveitis and determination of treatment threshold

Bruno Simonazzi[1], Konstantinos Balaskas[1,2] and Yan Guex-Crosier[1*]

Abstract

Background: The aim of this work is to refine understanding of anatomical and functional alterations in eyes with Intermediate Uveitis (IU), their natural history in mild cases not necessitating treatment and their response to treatment in severely affected eyes with macular edema.

Methods: 61 consecutive patients with IU presenting over a 6-year period were prospectively recruited into the study. Two subgroups of patients with IU were identified on the basis of the need or not for systemic cortico-steroid treatment. A group of healthy volunteers was identified for determining normal average central foveal thickness (CFT) values. Statistical comparisons were sought between patient sub-groups and with the group of normal volunteers for CFT and Best Corrected Visual Acuity (BCVA) at baseline and after 6 months. In a post hoc analysis, a cut-off value of CFT for systemic treatment initiation in IU was statistically identified and its sensitivity and specificity determined.

Results: A statistically significant difference in mean CFT at baseline was observed between patients under systemic treatment and untreated patients ($p = 0.0005$) as well as between untreated patients and healthy volunteers. ($p < 0.001$) After six months difference in CFT between the two patients subgroups was no longer significant ($p = 0.699$). BCVA was worse for patients under systemic treatment. No statistically significant difference could be identified between the subgroup of untreated patients and the group of healthy volunteers either at baseline or after 6 months. Correlation between LogMAR visual acuity and central retinal thickness at baseline was strong ($r = 0.7436$, $p < 0.0001$, Pearson's correlation coefficient). The cut-off value of CFT for initiating systemic treatment was determined at 215.5 μm in a post hoc analysis (sensitivity 62.5 %, specificity 96.4 %).

Conclusions: Subclinical retinal thickening of mildly inflamed eyes with IU can occur though bearing no functional clinical significance and spontaneously resolving within 6 months. A cut-off CFT value for treatment of macular edema in IU, in the presence of other relevant morphological features on Optical Coherence Tomography, seems to emerge from post hoc analysis of collected data demonstrating strong specificity and moderate sensitivity.

Keywords: Optical coherence tomography (OCT), Intermediate uveitis, Pars planitis, Cystoid macular edema, Fluorescein angiography

* Correspondence: yan.guex@fa2.ch
[1]Jules-Gonin Eye Hospital, University of Lausanne, FAA, Av. de France 15, CH-1004 Lausanne, Switzerland
Full list of author information is available at the end of the article

Background

Intermediate uveitis (IU) is a form of chronic ocular inflammation in which the vitreous is the ocular tissue predominantly affected, according to the SUN classification [1]. It usually involves a younger age range and comprises around 10 % of all causes of uveitis. Although unanswered questions persist concerning its etiology, the condition is occasionally associated with certain systemic pathologies, such as sarcoidosis, Lyme disease, Cat-scratch disease and multiple sclerosis [2]. The term pars planitis is used to describe the idiopathic form of IU characterized by the presence of snow-banking and/or snowballs in the vitreous [1]. Common manifestations of IU include retinal vasculitis, mainly involving venous branches and the development of cystoid macular edema (CME). The latter constitutes the principal factor leading to permanent visual loss in the context of IU and its frequency ranges between 30 and 60 % in several studies [2–4]. Despite the high incidence of CME, visual prognosis in IU is favorable with 75 % of patients retaining a visual acuity of 20/40 or better after ten years [3]. Poor visual prognosis is mainly associated with the development of CME, hence the importance of its early detection and treatment. A plethora of reports have underpinned the dominant role of Optical Coherence Tomography (OCT) for the diagnosis of macular edema in the context of ocular inflammation, including IU, and have identified quantitative and qualitative predictors for visual outcome [5–9] and response to treatment [10–12]. In the present prospective study we attempt to refine understanding of the natural history of CME in mild cases of IU not requiring systemic treatment as well as the response to treatment of more severe vision-threatening cases. We emphasize particularly the natural history and clinical significance of subclinical macular thickening not previously described in the context of this condition and we attempt to identify a threshold as regards CFT on OCT for initiating systemic cortico-steroid treatment.

Methods

We conducted a prospective study on patients presenting to the Jules - Gonin Eye Hospital with IU, diagnosed on the basis of clinical criteria proposed by the SUN classification [1]. Inclusion criteria also involved willingness of the patient to offer informed consent and age range between 9 and 77 years. Exclusion criteria were media opacities interfering with reliable OCT measurements and the presence of any other ocular condition associated with CME. All research work adhered to the tenets of the declaration of Helsinki. All patients underwent a full clinical examination, including best-corrected visual acuity (BCVA), tonometry and dilated fundus examination by indirect ophthalmoscopy with pars plana indentation. The following laboratory tests were performed on all patients: complete blood count, erythrocyte sedimentation rate, serum lysozyme, angiotensin converting enzyme, calcium and serologies for syphilis, Lyme disease, Cat-scratch disease. A quantiferon test or a tuberculin skin test to rule out tuberculosis and a chest X-ray were also performed. Fluorescein angiography was performed in all patients presenting with a visual acuity of 0.8 or worse or manifesting clinical signs of vasculitis, severe vitritis or macular edema. The decision to introduce a systemic treatment was based on clinical, OCT and/or angiographic criteria. More precisely, systemic cortico-steroid therapy was introduced in the presence of a loss of visual acuity of one or more lines (each line on the standardized visual acuity chart increasing by 0.1 log units), macular edema detected clinically or on OCT (including any presence of intraretinal cysts, irrespective or central retinal thickness), signs of moderate to severe vasculitis on clinical examination or angiography, more than 2+ of vitreous cells or more than 1 + of vitreous haze (assessed clinically on the basis of the SUN) classification, peripheral serous retinal detachment or papillitis. Systemic corticosteroids were used as first line therapy. Posterior subtenon's steroid injections were used as second line therapy in view of the commonly bilateral nature of IU and the potential steroid responsiveness to subtenon's injections. Steroid sparing agents were introduced in a second line therapy, when corticosteroids could not be tapered off after more than 3 months according to international guidelines. None of the patients were on immunosuppressive therapy during their inclusion in the study. A Stratus OCT was used (*Zeiss Humphrey Systems, San Leandro, CA*) with a cross-sectional scan performed at the macula to measure CFT (Fig. 1). In the presence of bilateral ocular inflammation, only the more severely inflamed eye was considered as the study eye, so as to account for inter-eye correlation in cases of bilateral involvement. The same evaluations as the ones performed at baseline were repeated 5 ± 1.6 months after initial evaluation. A group of 27 age-matched healthy volunteers without any ocular disease was included in the study. 6–10 OCT measurements per eye of the healthy volunteers were performed and averaged to determine normal values of central foveal thickness. For the purposes of refining understanding of disease behaviour, two sub-groups of patients were considered on the basis of the need or not of systemic treatment for IU. The first sub-group consisted of patients to whom systemic corticosteroids were administered and the second of patients without treatment, other than a short course of topical corticosteroids. This consisted of a course of prednisolone 1 % drops QDS on a tapering regimen over a period of 4–6 weeks. The amount of topical steroids did not vary between the two patient groups. Statistical significance of difference in mean CFT between the two patient sub-groups, as well as between each patient sub-group and the group of healthy volunteers was assessed at baseline and at the end of follow-up. The same statistical analysis was performed for difference in mean

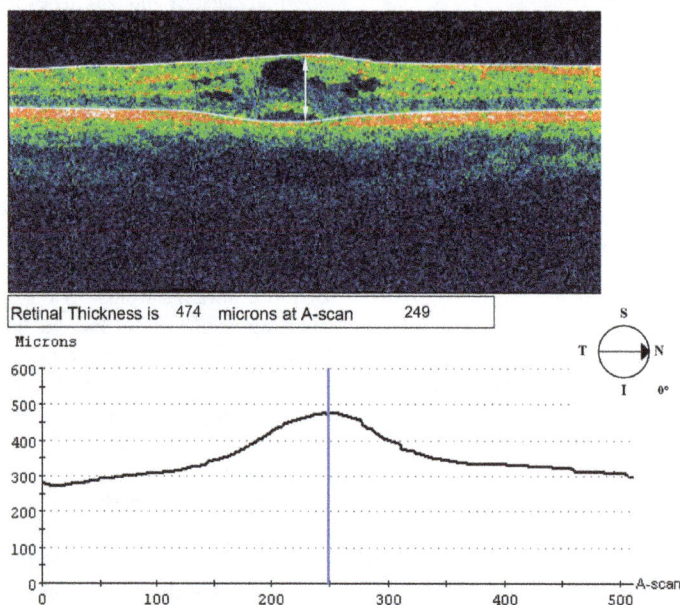

Fig. 1 OCT Measurement of central foveal thickness. A cross sectional scan was performed at the macula (white double arrow). Central foveal thickness was determined by automated segmentation of retinal layers and positioning of the marker at the apex of the curve in the thickness chart. Central foveal thickness of 249 microns was measured in this case

BCVA between the various groups at baseline and at the end of follow-up. The correlation between visual acuity and central foveal thickness at baseline was also evaluated. For purposes of statistical analysis Snellen visual acuity values were converted to the LogMAR scale. A post hoc analysis was performed in order to identify a cut-off value of CFT for initiating systemic cortico-steroid treatment. The sensitivity and specificity of this cut-off value were evaluated against the actual presence or absence of severe disease warranting systemic treatment in this patient cohort. Mann-Whitney-Wilcoxon test for independent samples (MWW), Wilcoxon matched pairs test and Pearson's correlation coefficient were appropriately applied. Level of statistical significance was set to 5 %. Statistical analysis was performed with the use of the JMP software (JMP 8.0.1 copyright 2009 SAS institutes (www.jmp.com)).

Results

The study sample consisted of 61 consecutive patients, of which 31 males and 30 females with a mean age of 30 ± 17 years, prospectively followed for a period of 6 months. There were 57 patients with pars planitis, 2 were diagnosed with sarcoidosis and 2 with Lyme disease. 29 patients did not receive systemic treatment, while 32 patients received systemic cortico-steroid treatment with an initial dosage of 1 mg/kg/day. A progressive tapering regimen was used with a decrease of 5 mg every three to four weeks. The control group of 27 healthy subjects consisted of 12 men and 15 women with a mean age of 36 ± 16 years (($p = 0.139$)

for mean age difference between patient and control group, t-test). All patients were phakic. CFT was 176 ± 16 μm for the normal volunteers ($n = 27$), while it was 310 ± 182 μm for the group of patients under systemic treatment ($n = 32$) and 183 ± 24 μm for the group of untreated patients ($n = 29$). Difference in CFT at baseline was statistically significant between normal subjects and untreated patients ($p < 0.0001$, MWW), normal subjects and patients under systemic treatment ($p < 0.0001$, MWW) and between treated and untreated patients ($p = 0.0005$, MWW) [Table 1].

15 patients did not complete the full 6 months follow-up period (8 patients in the group of untreated patients and 7 patients in the group of systemically treated patients). For patients available for the 6-months follow-up visit (mean CFT of 325 ± 122 at baseline) mean CFT decreased in a statistically significant manner to 209 ± 86 μm for the group of treated patients ($n = 25$, $p = 0.0004$, Wilcoxon matched

Table 1 Statistical significance of difference in central retinal thickness between the various groups

	Untreated patients	Treated patients		Control group
Untreated patients		Baseline $p = 0.0005$	6 months $p = 0.699$	Baseline $p < 0.0001$
Treated patients				Baseline $p < 0.0001$
Control group				

p-values derived from Mann-Whitney-Wilcoxon test

pairs), while it remained practically unchanged in the group of untreated patients (181 ± 29 μm from 179 ± 18 at baseline) ($n = 21$, $p = 0.561$, Wilcoxon matched pairs). Difference in CFT was no longer statistically significant between the two patient subgroups ($p = 0.699$, MMW).

Mean initial BCVA differed in a statistically significant manner between the two patient sub-groups ($p < 0.0001$, MWW), but not between untreated patients and the group of normal volunteers ($p = 0.085$, MWW) [Table 2]. Mean BCVA slightly, though statistically significantly, improved in the group of treated patients, passing from 0.222 ± 0.249 to 0.087 ± 0.125 ($p = 0.0075$, Wilcoxon matched pairs), while it remained practically unchanged in the group of untreated patients, passing from 0.024 ± 0.085 to 0.015 ± 0.060 ($p = 0.644$, Wilcoxon matched pairs). Changes in CFT and BCVA for the two patient subgroups over the follow-up period are summarized in Table 3. Difference in BCVA between the two patient subgroups remained statistically significant at the end of follow-up ($p = 0.032$, MMW). There was a strong correlation between baseline BCVA and CFT on OCT ($r = 0.743$, $p < 0.0001$ Pearson's correlation coefficient). Comparisons bear on patients that completed the 6 months of follow up only. In the post hoc analysis a CFT cut-off for initiating treatment with systemic cortico-steroids was determined at 215.5 μm in the present cohort. The sensitivity of this value was moderate at 62.5 %, yet its specificity was strong at 96.4 %.

Discussion

The present study accrues useful additional clues in our understanding of the anatomical and functional repercussions of IU and its response to cortico-steroid treatment. Segregating patients with respect to the need for systemic treatment for CME and comparing anatomical and functional outcomes between patient sub-groups and with a group of healthy volunteers in a prospective study design allowed identifying the presence of subclinical retinal thickening in milder, not systemically treated cases as well as the clinical significance of this phenomenon. Re-affirming the established favorable prognosis to systemic treatment of CME secondary to IU, there was a statistically significant decrease in CFT after a period of 6 months in the sub-

Table 2 Statistical significance of difference in LogMAR BCVA between the various groups

	Untreated patients	Treated patients		Control group
Untreated patients		Baseline $p < 0.0001$	6 months $p = 0.032$	Baseline $p = 0.085$
Treated patients				Baseline $p < 0.0001$
Control group				

p-values derived from Mann-Whitney-Wilcoxon test

Table 3 Statistical significance of change in central retinal thickness and BCVA between baseline/end of follow-up. (Patients who completed 6 months of follow-up)

	Baseline	6-months	p
Untreated patients			
Central foveal thickness (μm)	179 ± 18	181 ± 29	0.561
BCVA (LogMAR)	0.024 ± 0.085	0.015 ± 0.060	0.644
Treated patients			
Central foveal thickness (μm)	325 ± 122	209 ± 86	0.0004
BCVA (LogMAR)	0.222 ± 0.249	0.087 ± 0.125	0.0075

p-values derived from Wilcoxon matched pairs test

group of more severely affected patients, which translated into a significant, though slight, improvement in BCVA. Although in the group of patients that did not receive systemic treatment mean CFT was significantly inferior to that of the treated group, it was, nevertheless, significantly superior to that of the group of healthy volunteers. Despite this marginal retinal thickening in the group of untreated patients, retinal thickness did not increase further in the course of follow-up, nor was there a significant drop in visual acuity suggesting no clinical significance of subclinical retinal thickening in milder cases of IU. This slight, though statistically significant, macular thickening in the group of patients with mild disease, not necessitating systemic treatment, is a striking finding not previously identified in the context of IU. This patient sub-group presented subclinical macular thickening, as evidenced by the absence of visual acuity loss in these patients, compared to the group of normal volunteers. Few studies have tackled the issue of subclinical retinal thickening in other forms of intraocular inflammation, such as acute anterior uveitis (AAU) [13, 14]. These include a retrospective study by Castellano [13], demonstrating a statistically significant difference in retinal thickness between the study and fellow eye for all OCT subfields in patients with acute anterior uveitis and the prospective study by Balaskas et al. [15] that offered a model of quantification of retinal thickness asymmetry between fellow eyes in the course of an episode of AAU. The identification of a critical value of retinal thickness beyond which systemic treatment is clearly indicated in patients with IU has yet to be determined, though it would constitute a powerful clinical tool. Although a precise CFT threshold for treatment cannot be envisaged in isolation, our post hoc analysis determined a cut-off value of 215.5 μm for commencing treatment in the present cohort. Clinical management decisions cannot be based on CFT values alone, however CFT should be taken into consideration when reaching management decisions alongside other qualitative morphological features on OCT, most importantly the presence of cystoid spaces. In the presence of cystic changes on OCT, however, determining a cut-off CFT value beyond which the risk-benefit ratio is tipped in favour of systemic treatment is of particular clinical relevance. When analysed against the actual presence or absence of severe disease requiring systemic treatment in our series, this cut-off value for CFT exhibited strong specificity, yet moderate sensitivity. This may indicate that cases requiring systemic treatment may occasionally be missed on the basis of this cut-off value if considered in isolation, while, on the other hand, this value is an accurate indicator of severe disease warranting systemic treatment in the vast majority of such cases. Taking into account that in a real-life scenario, clinical management decisions will be based on a multitude of factors rather than on CFT alone, the strong specificity of this cut-off value may offer a useful tool to clinicians as an additional argument in favour of systemic treatment in relevant cases that are more likely to benefit from it. Strong correlation between CFT thickness and mean logMAR visual acuity at baseline was observed in the present study. The issue of correlation between retinal thickness and visual acuity remains controversial with some studies reporting a high [16] negative correlation and others failing to verify this finding [17]. Several factors may play a role in the observed discrepancy, such as structural characteristics of macular edema, chronicity and underlying pathology. The high specificity of the identified CFT cut-off value for initiating systemic treatment in this study suggests that almost all cases deemed of sufficient severity to warrant systemic treatment in our practice, on the basis of various clinical indicators and not just OCT findings, had a CFT that exceeded the determined cut-off value. Although clinical application of this cut-off CFT value needs to be in conjunction with other clinical and imaging features rather than in isolation, its high specificity renders it a useful adjunct in the decision making process for commencing systemic treatment in IU. From a practical point of view, CFT values can be obtained on newer generation OCT technology as well and can be evaluated against the cut-off value suggested in this work employing conversion algorithms already reported in the literature, hence retaining their clinical relevance and usefulness [18, 19]. The present study has certain limitations. Patients with advanced media opacities preventing clear visualization of the fundus and interfering with OCT measurements were excluded. The use of CFT as a marker of retinal thickness, although not uncommon in the literature, is a rather less frequently used clinical endpoint for research when compared to the more familiar central macular thickness (CMT) value. The choice of CFT in this work as clinical endpoint resides in the researcher's reliance on this marker for clinical decision making in the era of the Stratus OCT. The age-matched group of healthy volunteers randomly selected may not be representative of the general population for determining normal CFT range, although very similar values for CFT in healthy eyes have been previously reported [20].

Conclusions

Present study contributes two novel concepts in our understanding of macular thickening in the context of IU:

1. Subclinical retinal thickening of mildly inflamed eyes with IU is a previously unreported phenomenon, with however no functional clinical significance and spontaneous resolution by 6 months.
2. A cut-off value of CFT for initiating systemic treatment of 215.5 μm was identified in the present cohort exhibiting strong specificity and moderate sensitivity. This may serve as a useful additional clinical tool aiding clinicians in reaching therapeutic decisions in patients with IU.

Ethics approval and consent to participate

Ethics approval was obtained by the Ethics Committee of the University of Lausanne, Switzerland (reference number VD 33/09). Informed consent has been obtained for all participants. For patients under 16 years of age, consent has been obtained from their parents/guardians.

Consent for publication

Not applicable (no identifying patient data).

Abbreviations

AAU: acute anterior uveitis; BCVA: best-corrected visual acuity; CME: cystoid macula edema; CFT: central foveal thickness, mean thickness at the intersection of radial scans; CMT: central macular thickness; IU: intermediate uveitis; LogMAR: log (decimal acuity) = −log of the minimal angle resolution; MWW: Mann-Whitney-Wilcoxon test; OCT: optical coherence tomography; SUN: standardization of uveitis nomenclature (SUN).

Competing interests

No financial support or funding was received in support of this study. None of the authors have any financial or property interest on any product, method or material presented in this paper. No conflicting relationship exists for any author. The authors have no conflict of interest to declare.

Authors' contributions

BS, YGC conceived the study, proposed its design, made OCT measurement, and participated in drafting the manuscript. BS, KB collected the clinical data, participated in study design and drafted the manuscript. All authors read and approved the final manuscript.

Acknowledgements

We thank Ciara Bergin who provided expert statistical input.

Funding

No funding was obtained for this study.

Author details

[1]Jules-Gonin Eye Hospital, University of Lausanne, FAA, Av. de France 15, CH-1004 Lausanne, Switzerland. [2]Manchester Royal Eye Hospital, Manchester, UK.

References

1. Jabs DA, Nussenblatt RB, Rosenbaum JT. Standardization of uveitis nomenclature for reporting clinical data. Results of the First International Workshop. Am J Ophthalmol. 2005;140:509–16.

2. Vidovic-Valentincic N, Kraut A, Hawlina M, et al. Intermediate uveitis: long-term course and visual outcome. Br J Ophthalmol. 2009;93:477–80.

3. Donaldson MJ, Pulido JS, Herman DC, Diehl N, Hodge D. Pars planitis: a 20-year study of incidence, clinical features, and outcomes. Am J Ophthalmol. 2007;144:812–7.

4. Rothova A, Suttorp-van Schulten MS, Frits TW, Kijlstra A. Causes and frequency of blindness in patients with intraocular inflammatory disease. Br J Ophthalmol. 1996;80:332–6.

5. Puliafito CA, Hee MR, Lin CP, Reichel E, Schuman JS, Duker JS, Izatt JA, Swanson EA, Fujimoto JG. Imaging of macular diseases with optical coherence tomography. Ophthalmology. 1995;102:217–29.

6. Schneeberg AE, Gobel W. Diagnosis and follow-up of non-diabetic macular edema with optical coherence tomography (OCT). Ophthalmologe. 2003;100:960–6.

7. Hee MR, Puliafito CA, Wong C, Duker JS, Reichel E, Rutledge B, Schuman JS, Swanson EA, Fujimoto JG. Quantitative assessment of macular edema with optical coherence tomography. Arch Ophthalmol. 1995;113:1019–29.

8. Reinthal EK, Volker M, Freudenthaler N, Grüb M, Zierhut M, Schlote T. Optical coherence tomography in the diagnosis and follow-up of patients with uveitic macular edema. Ophthalmologe. 2004;101:1181–8.

9. Markomichelakis NN, Halkiadakis I, Pantelia E, Peponis V, Patelis A, Theodossiadis P, Theodossiadis G. Patterns of macular edema in patients with uveitis: qualitative and quantitative assessment using optical coherence tomography. Ophthalmology. 2004;111:946–53.

10. Venkatesh P, Abhas Z, Garg S, Vohra R. Prospective optical coherence tomographic evaluation of the efficacy of oral and posterior subtenon corticosteroids in patients with intermediate uveitis. Graefes Arch Clin Exp Ophthalmol. 2007;245:59–67.

11. Antcliff RJ, Spalton DJ, Stanford MR, Graham EM, ffytche TJ, Marshall J. Intravitreal triamcinolone for uveitic cystoid macular edema: an optical coherence tomography study. Ophthalmology. 2001;108:765–72.

12. Sivaprasad S, Ikeji F, Xing W, Lightman S. Tomographic assessment of therapeutic response to uveitic macular oedema. Clin Experiment Ophthalmol. 2007;35:719–23.

13. Castellano CG, Stinnett SS, Mettu PS, McCallum RM, Jaffe GJ. Retinal thickening in iridocyclitis. Am J Ophthalmol. 2009;148:341–9.

14. Traill A, Stawell R, Hall A, Zamir E. Macular thickening in acute anterior uveitis. Ophthalmology. 2007;114:402.

15. Balaskas K, Ballabeni P, Guex-Crosier Y. Retinal thickening in HLA-B27-associated acute anterior uveitis: evolution with time and association with severity of inflammatory activity. Invest Ophthalmol Vis Sci. 2012; 53(10):6171–7.

16. Tran TH, de Smet MD, Bodaghi B, Fardeau C, Cassoux N, Lehoang P. Uveitic macular oedema: correlation between optical coherence tomography patterns with visual acuity and fluorescein angiography. Br J Ophthalmol. 2008;92:922–7.

17. Nussenblatt RB, Kaufman SC, Palestine AG, Davis MD, Ferris 3rd FL. Macular thickening and visual acuity. Measurement in patients with cystoid macular edema. Ophthalmology. 1987;94:1134–9.

18. Roh YR, Park KH, Woo SJ. Foveal thickness between stratus and spectralis optical coherence tomography in retinal diseases. Korean J Ophthalmol. 2013;27(4):268–27.

19. Sull A, Vuong L, Price LL. Comparison of Spectral/Fourier domain optical coherence tomography instruments for assessment of normal macular thickness. Retina. 2010;30(2):235.

20. Chan A, Duker J, Ko TH, Fujimoto JG, Schuman JS. Normal Macular Thickness Measurements in Healthy Eyes Using Stratus Optical Coherence Tomography. Arch Ophthalmol. 2006;124(2):193–8.

19

Induced Higher-order aberrations after Laser In Situ Keratomileusis (LASIK) Performed with Wavefront-Guided IntraLase Femtosecond Laser in moderate to high Astigmatism

Ferial M. Al-Zeraid[1] and Uchechukwu L. Osuagwu[2]* (iD)

Abstract

Background: Wavefront-guided Laser-assisted in situ keratomileusis (LASIK) is a widespread and effective surgical treatment for myopia and astigmatic correction but whether it induces higher-order aberrations remains controversial. The study was designed to evaluate the changes in higher-order aberrations after wavefront-guided ablation with IntraLase femtosecond laser in moderate to high astigmatism.

Methods: Twenty-three eyes of 15 patients with moderate to high astigmatism (mean cylinder, -3.22 ± 0.59 dioptres) aged between 19 and 35 years (mean age, 25.6 ± 4.9 years) were included in this prospective study. Subjects with cylinder ≥ 1.5 and ≤ 2.75 D were classified as moderate astigmatism while high astigmatism was ≥ 3.00 D. All patients underwent a femtosecond laser–enabled (150-kHz IntraLase iFS; Abbott Medical Optics Inc) wavefront-guided ablation. Uncorrected (UDVA), corrected (CDVA) distance visual acuity in logMAR, keratometry, central corneal thickness (CCT) and higher-order aberrations (HOAs) over a 6 mm pupil, were assessed before and 6 months, postoperatively. The relationship between postoperative change in HOA and preoperative mean spherical equivalent refraction, mean astigmatism, and postoperative CCT were tested.

Results: At the last follow-up, the mean UDVA was increased ($P < 0.0001$) but CDVA remained unchanged ($P = 0.48$) and no eyes lost ≥ 2 lines of CDVA. Mean spherical equivalent refraction was reduced ($P < 0.0001$) and was within ± 0.50 D range in 61 % of eyes. The average corneal curvature was flatter by 4 D and CCT was reduced by 83 μm ($P < 0.0001$, for all), postoperatively. Coma aberrations remained unchanged ($P = 0.07$) while the change in trefoil ($P = 0.047$) postoperatively, was not clinically significant. The 4th order HOAs (spherical aberration and secondary astigmatism) and the HOA root mean square (RMS) increased from -0.18 ± 0.07 μm, 0.04 ± 0.03 μm and 0.47 ± 0.11 μm, preoperatively, to 0.33 ± 0.19 μm ($P = 0.004$), 0.21 ± 0.09 μm ($P < 0.0001$) and 0.77 ± 0.27 μm ($P < 0.0001$), six months postoperatively. The change in spherical aberration after the procedure increased with an increase in the degree of preoperative myopia. (Continued on next page)

* Correspondence: osuagoul@aston.ac.uk
[2]Department of Optometry & Vision Sciences, Faculty of Health, Ophthalmic and Visual Optics Laboratory Group (Chronic Disease & Ageing), Institute of Health and Biomedical Innovation, Q Block, Room 5WS36 60 Musk Avenue Kelvin Grove, Brisbane, QLD 4059, Australia
Full list of author information is available at the end of the article

(Continued from previous page)

Conclusions: Wavefront-guided IntraLASIK offers a safe and effective option for vision and visual function improvement in astigmatism. Although, reduction of HOA is possible in a few eyes, spherical-like aberrations are increased in majority of the treated eyes.

Keywords: Laser-assisted in situ keratomileusis, Wavefront-guided, Myopia, Astigmatism, Intralase, Femtosecond laser, Distance visual acuity, Coma, Spherical aberration, Higher-order aberration

Background

Laser-assisted in situ keratomileusis (LASIK) has become a widespread and effective surgical treatment to correct myopia and astigmatism [1–6]. Like other corneal refractive surgeries (such as radial keratotomy, photorefractive keratectomy), it is designed to modify the central corneal curvature, making it flatter to correct myopia and steeper to correct hyperopia [7]. This surgical modification might influence the optical quality of the cornea, creating aberrations that will lead to distorted images [8].

Conventional LASIK involved mainly the creation of a stromal flap with the aid of a mechanical microkeratome. Like most standard laser refractive surgery, it eliminates conventional refractive errors (lower order aberration like myopia, hyperopia and astigmatism) leaving higher-order aberrations uncorrected or inducing some higher order aberrations (HOAs) particularly spherical aberrations [3, 9–11] which are thought to be responsible for the patients' complaints of poor quality of vision, even with visual acuity of 20/25 or 20/20, postoperatively.

Femtosecond laser and wavefront-guided ablations are two new technologies for flap creation [3, 4, 6, 12–14] designed to improve the patients' quality of vision. Femtosecond laser is a solid-state laser [6, 15, 16] used for flap creation in LASIK procedures. Compared with the conventional LASIK (mechanical microkeratome technology), femtosecond laser create flaps with good predictability of thickness and has rare incidence of flap-related complications [3, 4, 11]. In the wavefront-guided ablation technique, the source of the input data is the objective data from an aberrometer [7] in contrast to the subjective refraction data in the standard excimer treatment. The wavefront-guided ablation technique is targeted at correcting optical aberrations of the eye in order to increase retinal image resolution while offering a more accurate refractive correction with fewer optical side effects than with non-wavefront guided femtosecond laser [1, 7, 17].

High astigmatism is one of the most significant obstacles for achieving satisfactory visual function following refractive surgery [18]. It is associated with high amounts of coma aberrations [19] and affects about 62 % of cases seen in optometry practices [20]. Keratoconus has a high incidence and severity in Saudi Arabia, with an early onset. The disease progresses very rapidly to its severe form at a young age [21] and astigmatism is

the hallmark sign of this disease [22]. Wavefront-guided ablations for intraLase treatment has been shown to be effective and predictable in reducing the astigmatism and higher order aberrations [4, 6, 13, 14, 23] in the eye. Assessing the effects of intraLase treatment for treatment of moderate to high astigmatism and higher-order aberrations in our population is important. The aim of this study was to: a), assess the changes in vision and visual outcomes after wavefront-guided IntraLase for high astigmatism; b), evaluate the higher-order aberrational changes using the SCHWIND CAM (Eye-tech-Solutions, GmbH & Co. Kleinostheim, Germany); and c), evaluate the relationship between any observed aberrational changes and the changes in other clinical outcomes, postoperatively. The result could provide a better platform than using sphere and cylinder to evaluate the effectivity of this technique and comparison can be made between this technique and other laser techniques.

Methods
Study population
Twenty-three eyes of 15 patients [six males (40 %) and nine females (60 %)] mean age of 25.6 ± 4.9 years (ranging from 19 to 35 years) were randomly recruited from patients already scheduled to undergo the surgery technique in the University hospital. The study was conducted between June 2014 and February 2015. The protocol conformed to the tenets of the Declaration of Helsinki 1975 as revised in Fortaleza 2013 and was approved by the Research Ethics Review Board of the College of Applied Medical Sciences, King Saud University. Before participating in this study, the nature of the study was explained and each patient gave a written informed consent.

Pre-treatment mean refraction spherical equivalent obtained with subjective refraction was −4.12 ± 2.55 D (range from −10.00 to +0.75 D). All patients underwent laser treatment using IntraLase FS60 laser (a 60-kHz platform). Patients were included in this study if they: are aged between 18 and 40 years, had astigmatism above 1.50 D, had no current eye disease or injury, are not on any ocular or systemic medication, and agreed to participate in the study, Soft contact lens wearer had to discontinue contact lens wear 2 weeks prior to surgery and patients were required to come for follow-up examinations up to 6 months after surgery. Astigmatism was defined as moderate for

Table 1 Summary statistics (mean ± standard deviation) preoperatively ($n = 23$), six months postoperatively and results of comparative analysis

Measured outcome	Sphere	Cylinder	MRSE	J_{180}	J_{45}	UDVA	CDVA	K_{steep}	K_{flat}	$K_{average}$	CCT
Preop	−2.5 ± 2.5	−3.22 ± 0.59	−4.12 ± 2.55	−0.16 ± 0.92	−0.26 ± 1.36	−0.94 ± 0.35	+0.01 ± 0.09	44.80 ± 1.56	42.16 ± 1.49	43.48 ± 1.47	547.00 ± 21.65
Postop	+0.04 ± 0.48	−0.72 ± 0.46	−0.31 ± 0.56	−0.03 ± 0.25	−0.02 ± 0.07	−0.04 ± 0.07	−0.00 ± 0.02	39.97 ± 2.18	39.06 ± 2.01	39.51 ± 2.08	464.20 ± 48.07
Post-Pre	+2.55 ± 2.65	+2.52 ± 0.69	+3.82 ± 2.82	+0.13 ± 0.94	+0.27 ± 1.39	+0.90 ± 0.35	−0.01 ± 0.09	−4.83 ± 2.36	−3.11 ± 1.93	−3.97 ± 2.12	−82.74 ± 41.45
P value	<0.0001	<0.0001	<0.0001	0.51	0.35	<0.0001	0.48	<0.0001	<0.0001	<0.0001	<0.0001

MRSE mean refraction spherical equivalent, J_{180} and J_{45} Jackson cross cylinder vector components at 180° and 45° respectively, CDVA unaided distance visual acuity, CDVA corrected distance visual acuity, K keratometry, CCT central corneal thickness, Pre preoperative and postop = postoperative eyes with a cylinder ≥ 1.5 and ≤2.75 D, while high astigmatism was ≥3.00 D [24]. The range of cylinders was from 2.5 D to 4.5 D. Patients were excluded in the presence of any of the following conditions: a systemic or ocular disease likely to influence corneal healing; glaucoma; retinal disorders that might reduce visual acuity (such as myopic maculopathy) or complicate LASIK (eg, equatorial degenerations); history of ocular surgery, or history of dry eyes confirmed by an abnormal Schirmer test.

All surgeries were performed at King Saud University Ophthalmology Department by a single surgeon (ALS). LASIK flaps were created using the 150-kHz IntraLase iFS (Abbott Medical Optics Inc. Santa Ana, CA, USA). A 9.0 mm diameter superior hinge, programmed flap thickness of 105 μm, and an inverted side-cut angle of 130° were created. The bed laser pulse energy was 0.75 μJ with bed separation, spot, and line separations of 7 μm. The side-cut spot and line separation were both set at 5 μm with the same bed laser pulse energy. Postoperatively, patients were evaluated at one day, 1 week, 1 month, 3 months and 6 months. Preoperative and six months postoperative data were used in this study. Postoperative medications included 4 times daily dosage of topical moxifloxacin for 4 days and prednisolone acetate 1.0 % (Predforte) for 7 days.

Data collection

Clinical evaluation of general and ocular health was performed pre-operatively. For all patients, the same optometrists assessed the following visual parameters, at baseline, after the procedure and at last follow-up (range of 6 – 8 months): uncorrected [UDVA(logMAR)], corrected distance visual acuity [CDVA(logMAR)] obtained by the Snellen projected eye chart; cylinder and sphere by subjective refraction with best sphere maximum visual acuity technique; topographical keratometry values (D), higher-order aberrations [only third to fourth order individual aberrations were considered since they are the most important of the HOAs and are present in higher amounts than other HOAs [25]], and higher-order aberrations RMS were once obtained by SCHWIND Ocular analyzer (Eye-tech-Solutions, GmbH & Co. Kleinostheim, Germany); and applanation tonometry. The wavefront aberration data captured when the entrance pupils were at least 6.0 mm were analysed with a 6.0 mm pupil diameter.

Statistical analysis

All data were entered into a Microsoft Excel 2007 spreadsheet (Microsoft, Inc, Redmond, Washington, USA) and analysed using the Graphpad Instat software (version 3.00-Graph pad Software Inc., San Diego, CA, USA). A P value <0.05 (α) was considered statistically significant, and with 23 eyes the study had a power of 80 % as calculated using the G power software 3.1.3

version. Kolmogorov-Smirnov Test was applied to evaluate the normality of data distribution. Results were presented descriptively as mean and standard deviation (SD) in a table and figure where applicable. The refraction vector components were analysed according to Fourier analysis [26, 27]. The sphere (s), cylinder (C), and axis (θ) were represented as the mean refraction spherical equivalent MRSE, 180° to 90° astigmatism J_{180}, and 45° to 135° astigmatism J_{45} components, calculated with the following equations [27]:

$$MSER = S + C/2$$

$$J_{180} = -(C/2) \cos(2\theta)$$

$$J_{45} = -(C/2) \sin(2\theta)$$

To assess the changes in tested parameters postoperatively, Student's t-test was used to compare preoperative and postoperative mean values. To determine whether any higher-order aberration changed differently from the others, the change (Δ) in higher-order aberration calculated as difference between postoperative and preoperative mean HOA value were compared using one way ANOVA. The changes were plotted against the preoperative mean values and the regression coefficient obtained equals the slope of the regression line and gives the predictability metrics for the HOA correction. The mean difference between pre and post-operative HOA were also determined and the associations between the changes in HOAs and preoperative MRSE and astigmatism were tested using Pearson correlation coefficient.

Results

Table 1 shows the descriptive statistics and results of comparative analysis of refractive components (MSER, J_{180} and J_{45}), visual acuities, keratometry readings and CCT values before and six months after surgery. All patients achieved successful correction (postoperative MRSE = −0.30 ± 0.56 D) showing unaided visual acuity

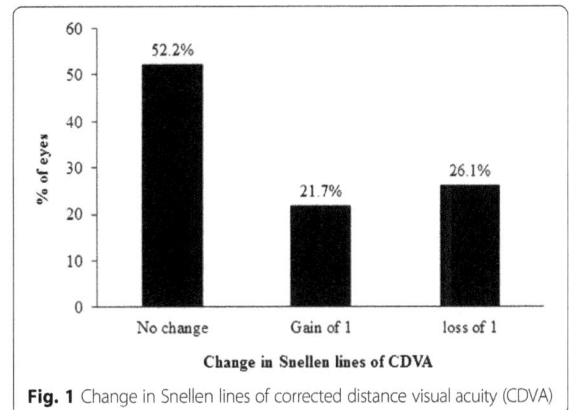

Fig. 1 Change in Snellen lines of corrected distance visual acuity (CDVA)

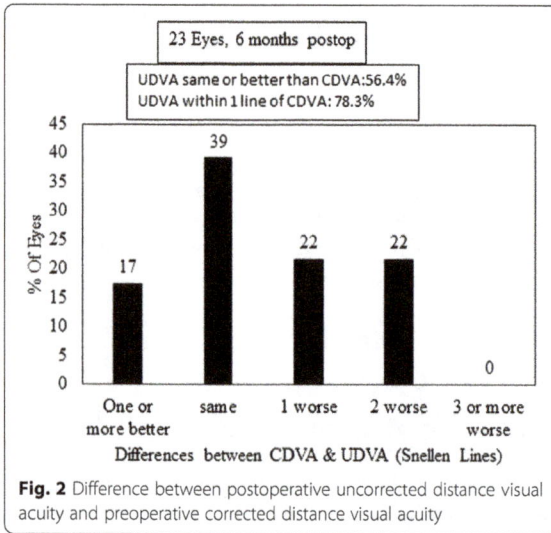

Fig. 2 Difference between postoperative uncorrected distance visual acuity and preoperative corrected distance visual acuity

equal or better than 0.00 log-MAR. Data from two patients were not included in this analysis data after they failed to attend the six months postoperative visit.

Efficacy & safety

Figure 1 shows the percentage change in CDVA following the procedure. Regarding the method safety, CDVA was unchanged postoperatively (p > 0.05) and remained the same in 12 eyes (52.2 %). Twenty two percent (5/23) of eyes gained at least one line of CDVA and no eye lost ≥2 lines of CDVA. No patient reported any complications at final visit. Preoperative CDVA was not different from postoperative UDVA (Table 1) and none of the eyes experienced supranormal VA of 20/12 or higher.

Figure 2 shows the difference between postoperative UDVA and preoperative CDVA. UDVA was the same or better than CDVA in 56 % of eyes and in 78.3 % of eyes, UDVA was within one line of CDVA. Six months postoperatively, 69.6 % of eyes had UDVA of 20/20 and 100 % of eyes had 20/32 or better (Fig. 3). As expected, UDVA increased by about 0.90 logMAR (p < 0.0001). The efficacy index was 5.6.

Predictability

The MSER was within ±1.00 in 91 % of eyes, within ±0.50 D in 61 % of eyes and 39 % of eyes achieved absolute emmetropia (+0.50 to −0.25 D), six months postoperatively (Fig. 4). All refractive outcomes were significantly improved (p < 0.0001) except for the J_{180} and J_{45} which remained unchanged (p > 0.05, for both), postoperatively (Table 1). The mean difference (±SD) between preoperative and postoperative MSER was 3.82 ± 2.82 D (95 % confidence interval of −1.70 to 9.31 D). For sphere refraction, it was 2.55 ± 2.65 D (95 % confidence interval of −2.64 to 7.75D) and for cylinder it was, 2.50 ± 0.69 (95 % confidence interval of 1.14 to 3.86 D). Following the procedure, the postoperative refractive astigmatism was ≤1.00D in 83 % of eyes (Fig. 5).

Keratometry and central corneal thickness changes

All keratometry readings (K steep, K flat, K average) were significantly decreased (p < 0.0001), six months after the procedure with the corneal curvature becoming flatter by about 4.00 D. Also, the mean CCT was significantly decreased by about 82 μm (p < 0.0001), six months postoperatively (Table 1).

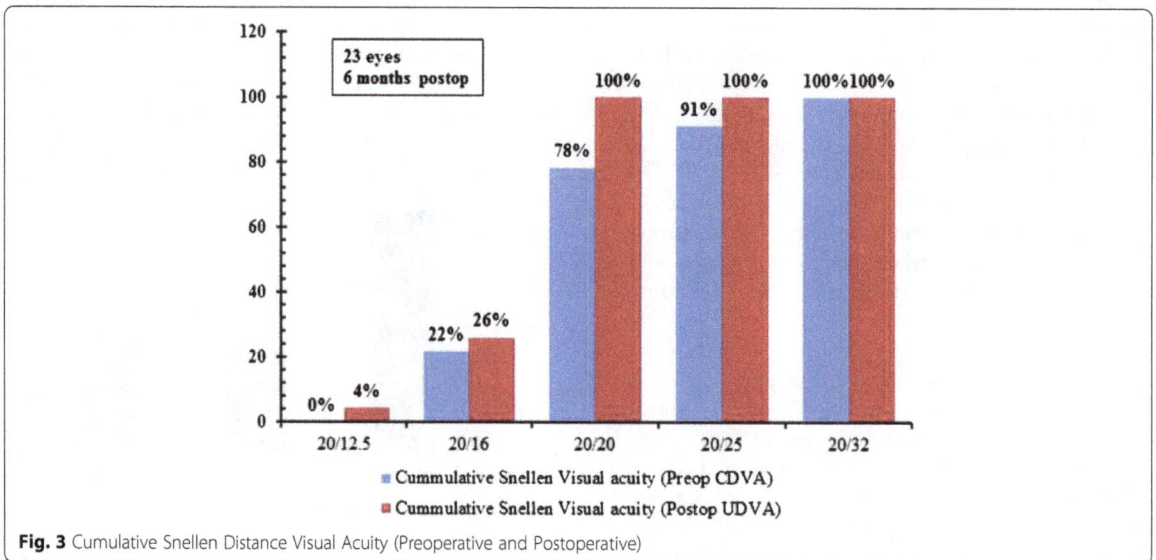

Fig. 3 Cumulative Snellen Distance Visual Acuity (Preoperative and Postoperative)

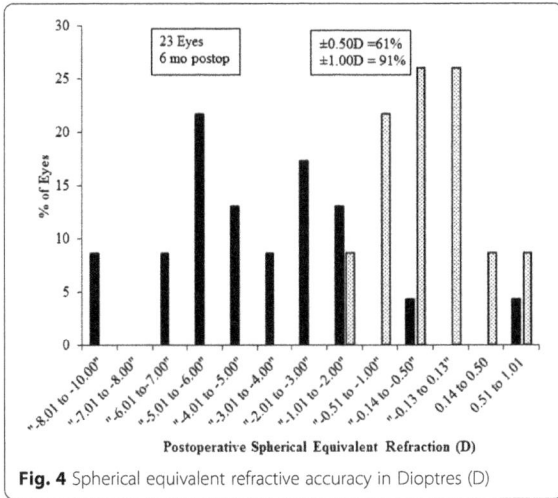

Fig. 4 Spherical equivalent refractive accuracy in Dioptres (D)

0.31 μm to 0.76 μm but following the procedure it ranged from 0.40 μm to 1.39 μm. The mean change in HOA was highest for total higher-order RMS (0.3 μm) which was reduced in 13 % of eyes. This was followed by secondary astigmatism and spherical aberration with 0.2 μm mean change for both coefficients. Secondary astigmatism was increased in all eyes postoperatively and spherical aberration was also increased in majority of eyes (69.6 %). Trefoil and coma aberrations were considerably reduced in 39.1 and 34.8 % of eyes. The change in HOAs varied significantly ($p = 0.0007$) but post-hoc analysis using Tukey's multiple comparison tests (Table 3) found statistically significant differences only in the comparison between changes in higher-order aberration RMS and either coma ($p < 0.05$) or trefoil ($p < 0.05$).

The preoperative third-order HOAs and the higher-order aberration RMS were moderately related with the change in HOA, following the procedure. For the fourth-order aberrations, a strong relationship was also observed between the preoperative mean spherical aberration and the change in aberration but the relationship between preoperative mean secondary astigmatism and its corresponding change postoperatively, was weak (Fig. 7a-c). Regarding the preoperative MSER (Fig. 7d), it was negatively associated with the change in measured HOAs but this association was significant only with the change in spherical aberration ($r = -0.57$, $p = 0.004$), and higher-order aberration RMS ($r = -0.43$, $p = 0.041$) (Table 4). In contrast, the association between preoperative astigmatism and the changes in measured HOAs were not significant ($p > 0.05$, for all).

The preoperative CCT was not significantly related with any of the measured HOAs ($p > 0.05$, for all), but the postoperative change in CCT (reduction) was significantly associated with the postoperative increases in trefoil ($r = -0.42$, $p = 0.046$), spherical aberration ($r = -0.59$, $p = 0.003$), secondary astigmatism ($r = -0.45$,

Changes in higher-order aberrations

Table 2 shows the preoperative and postoperative mean HOA measurements (over a 6 mm pupil) together with the results of paired *t*-test. There were individual variations in measured higher-order aberration RMS preoperatively (as indicated by the standard deviation of 0.11 μm) which was further widened postoperatively (standard deviation of 0.27 μm). Compared with the preoperative values, the third-order HOAs (coma-like aberrations) were not significantly affected postoperatively although the trefoil aberration just approached a borderline of significance which was considered non-clinically significant. In contrast, the fourth-order aberrations were significantly increased ($p < 0.0001$), postoperatively. The individual variations in higher-order aberrations six months postoperatively are shown in Fig. 6. The mean higher-order aberration RMS changed significantly ($p < 0.0001$) postoperatively. The preoperative higher-order aberration RMS ranged from

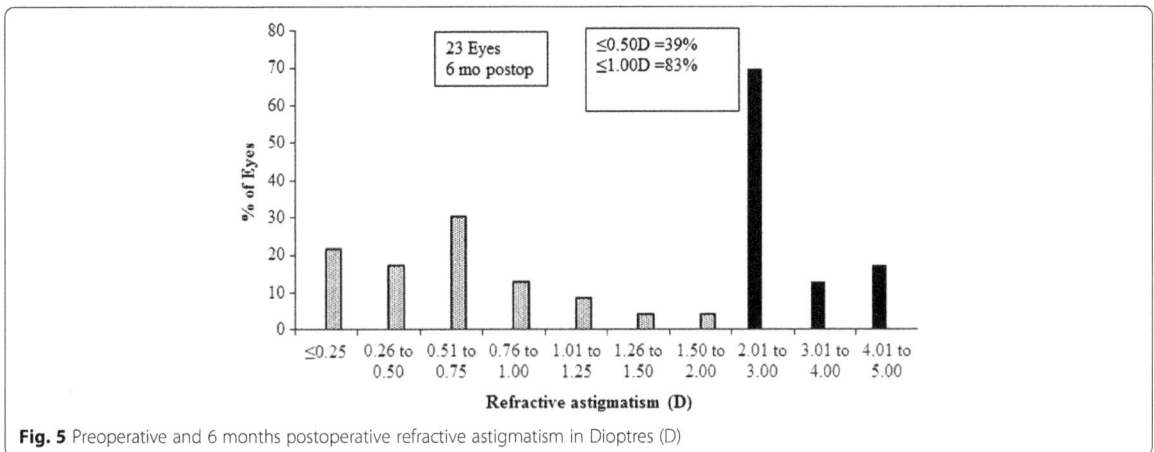

Fig. 5 Preoperative and 6 months postoperative refractive astigmatism in Dioptres (D)

Table 2 Summary statistics (mean ± standard deviation) preoperatively ($n = 23$), six months postoperatively and results of comparative analysis of higher-order aberrations across a 6 mm pupil

Measured outcome	Coma	Trefoil	Spherical Aberration	Secondary Astigmatism	HOA root- mean-square
Preoperative	0.22 ± 0.11	0.11 ± 0.07	0.18 ± 0.07	0.04 ± 0.03	0.47 ± 0.11
Postoperative	0.31 ± 0.18	0.16 ± 0.10	0.33 ± 0.19	0.21 ± 0.09	0.77 ± 0.27
p-value	0.07	0.047	0.004	<0.0001	<0.0001

$p = 0.03$) and higher-order RMS ($r = -0.66$, $p = 0.0007$) but not with coma ($r = -0.27$, $p = 0.21$), Fig. 8.

Discussion

The 150 kHz iFS Advanced femtosecond laser used in this study is a new generation system. It was shown to be comparable in performance with the Wavelight FS200 system [28]. In this prospective study, the procedure improved reduced all refraction components (MRSE, mean sphere, mean cylinder) except for J_{180} and J_{45} astigmatism vector components which were unaffected. The mean corneal curvature became flatter by about 3.97 D, while the CCT was reduced from 547.00 D to 464.20 D, six months, postoperatively. Refractive astigmatism ranged from –2.50 D to –4.50 D preoperatively, but was considerably reduced by up to –1.75 D, postoperatively. Eighty-three and thirty nine percent of eyes had astigmatism of ≤1.00 D and ≤0.50 D, respectively 6 months following the procedure.

Safety of this procedure (defined as the number and percentage of eyes losing 2 or more lines of CDVA) [1, 29] was excellent as no eyes lost ≥2 lines of CDVA, rather, lines of CDVA were unchanged in one-half of the eyes (12 eyes, 52 %) and in 5 eyes (22 %), a gain of at least one line of CDVA was observed. The safety calculated in this study was slightly better than previous reports six months after LASIK procedure (a loss of two lines of CDVA in 0.6 % of myopic and 0.9 % of

astigmatic eyes) in eyes with preoperative sphere and cylinder of up to –11.00 D and –5.00 D, preoperatively [30]. Safety ranges for low to moderate myopia treated with LASIK are between 0 and 7 % and for efficacy, the reported values range from 45 to 79 % for a CDVA of 20/20 [29]. In this study, the safety was calculated to be 5.6 % and the efficacy (defined as the percentage of eyes with an UDVA of 20/20 or better) was 69.6 %. These values are in the upper limits of the reported ranges suggesting that wavefront-guided ablation with IntraLase femtosecond laser is safe and effective for use in the management of eyes with moderate to high astigmatism.

Continuing this, predictability was good in this study, as 61 % of eyes achieved MRSE that was within ±0.50 D while 39 % of eyes achieved absolute emmetropia, postoperatively. A significant hyperopic shift in refraction was observed. The changes observed in this study are comparable with previous reports [1, 30, 31] and are not expected to change significantly after completion of this study. This is because, LASIK eyes were stable from 1 to 3 months after surgery [30, 32].

Higher-order aberration changes

Patients with moderate to high astigmatism were recruited because of the known presence of above average preoperative higher-order aberrations [33] in these eyes. Although several studies have assessed the wavefront aberrations induced by different LASIK techniques

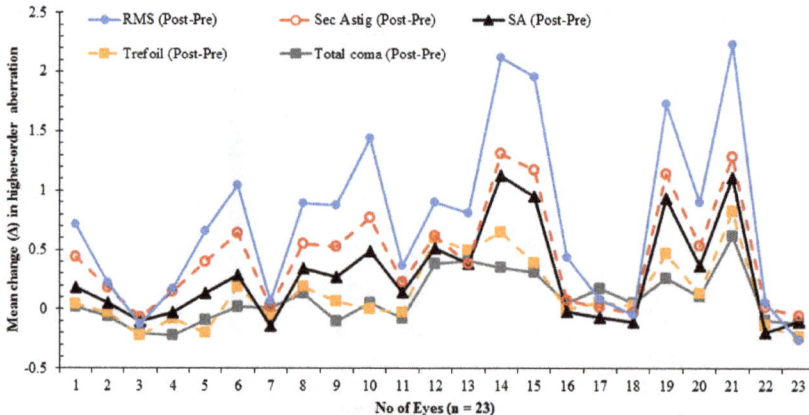

Fig. 6 Changes in higher-order aberrations in micrometres (μm), 6 months postoperative

Table 3 Tukey's multiple comparison between mean changes (postoperative minus preoperative values) in higher order aberrations (HOAs) postoperative

Change (Δ) in higher-order aberrations	Mean Diff.	95 % CI of diff.	Significant?
Δ Coma vs. Δ Trefoil	+0.03	−0.13 to 0.20	No
Δ Coma vs Δ Spherical Aberration	−0.06	−0.23 to 0.11	No
Δ Coma vs Δ Secondary Astigmatism	−0.08	−0.25 to 0.09	No
Δ coma vs. Δ HOA root-mean-square	−0.22	−0.38 to −0.05	Yes
Δ Trefoil vs Δ Spherical Aberration	−0.09	−0.26 to 0.07	No
Δ Trefoil vs. Δ Secondary Astigmatism	−0.12	−0.28 to 0.05	No
Δ Trefoil vs. Δ HOA root-mean-square	−0.25	−0.42 to −0.08	Yes
Δ Spherical Aberration vs. Δ Secondary Astigmatism	−0.02	−0.19 to 0.14	No
Δ Spherical Aberration vs Δ HOA root-mean-square	−0.16	−0.32 to 0.01	No
Δ Secondary Astigmatism vs. Δ HOA root-mean-square	−0.14	−0.30 to 0.03	No

The Mean difference (Mean diff) and 95 % confidence interval (CI) of mean difference are shown

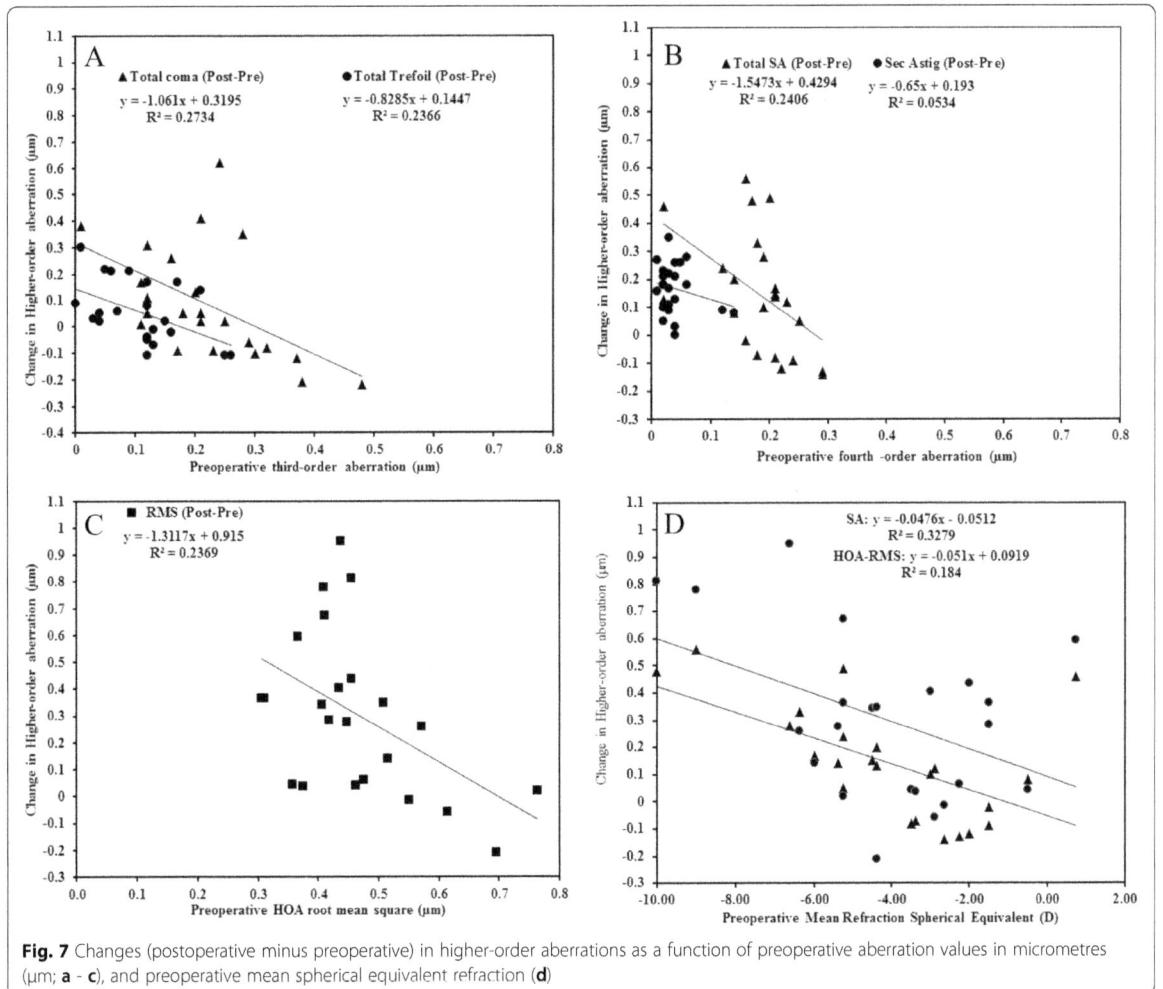

Fig. 7 Changes (postoperative minus preoperative) in higher-order aberrations as a function of preoperative aberration values in micrometres (μm; **a** - **c**), and preoperative mean spherical equivalent refraction (**d**)

Table 4 Association between changes in higher-order aberrations and preoperative mean spherical equivalent refraction, mean astigmatism, six months following the procedure

Pearson r	Coma (Post-Pre)	Trefoil (Post-Pre)	SA (Post-Pre)	Sec Astig (Post-Pre)	RMS (Post-Pre)
MSER	−0.13 (−0.52 to +0.30)	−0.16 (−0.54 to +0.27)	−0.57 (−0.80 to −0.21)	−0.32 (−0.65 to 0.11)	−0.43 (−0.72 to −0.02)
p-value	0.55	0.46	0.004	0.14	0.04
Astigmatism	−0.18 (−0.55 to 0.25)	−0.36 (−0.67 to 0.06)	−0.08 (−0.48 to 0.34)	−0.38 (−0.69 to 0.03)	−0.31 (−0.64 to 0.12)
p-value	0.41	0.09	0.72	0.07	0.15

Correlation coefficients r (95 % confidence intervals) are shown

including IntraLase femtosecond laser flap creation, there are no consensus results regarding the changes in individual aberration terms [34]. The difference in the previous reports may be related to the different levels of preoperative aberrations and the pupil analysis diameter used. In agreement with previous reports [1, 32, 35, 36], the preoperative wavefront aberrations in our patients (for a 6 mm pupil) varied widely between patients (SD of 0.11 μm for the higher-order aberration RMS). This inter-individual variation was more pronounced following the procedure (SD of 0.27 μm). The changes in third-order aberrations ranged between −0.34 and 0.51 μm (95 % confidence intervals of mean difference) for coma, and between −0.18 to 0.29 μm for trefoil, but fourth-order aberrations (particularly spherical aberration) were dominant in the eye, postoperatively. Spherical aberration was slightly reduced in few eyes but it increased in majority of eyes by as much as 0.56 μm. Secondary astigmatism was increased in all eyes but the increase was much smaller than previous reports (mean change was 0.4 μm vs 0.2 μm) on wavefront-guided LASIK performed on fewer eyes (n = 6) with moderate to high astigmatism [37]. In 87 % of eyes enrolled in this study, higher-order aberration RMS was induced and in

few eyes, the increase reached 0.90 μm, postoperatively. These changes in higher-order aberration RMS is consistent with previous reports [1, 8, 11, 32, 38] but it was markedly lower than results from conventional LASIK [3, 8, 11]. Although third and fourth-order aberrations increased only moderately or could be reduced in about one third of the eyes, the increase in spherical-like aberrations was statistically significant. Postoperative spherical aberration increased in eyes with high preoperative higher-order aberration. On the average, all individual higher-order aberrations changed by similar amounts at final visit (Table 3) and the increase in spherical-like aberrations corresponds to the thin central cornea observed in this study, postoperatively [32] (Fig. 8).

Induced HOAs after LASIK procedures have been attributed to various factors including: variations in measurement of HOAs due to fluctuations in accommodation and tear film changes [39]; discrepancy of measurement and treatment position of the eye due to laser misalignment or cyclotorsion [40]; and the ablation rate per excimer pulse since single excimer laser pulse delivered to the cornea which might have different effects at different corneal areas [1]. In the present study, only the spherical-like aberrations were significantly altered, postoperatively and the induced amount was increased as the degree of myopia increased (Fig. 7). This is because, following LASIK, the cornea becomes more prolate as compared to normal corneas [41] and this exposes it to higher amounts of induced spherical aberration [8].

Despite the induced HOAs, the femtosecond laser technique used in this study provided a relatively effective wavefront-guided correction with final outcomes that were not affected by HOA changes. [1, 3, 11, 34, 42]. This technique was shown to yield better postoperative aberration profile than wavefront-optimized LASIK in eyes with higher-order aberration RMS errors >0.3 μm [34]. In this study, the mean preoperative higher-order aberration RMS error was 0.47 μm.

Conclusions

Wavefront-guided ablation with IntraLase femtosecond laser is a safe and effective option with predictable improvements in visual outcomes in cases with moderate to high astigmatism. Although reduction of higher-order

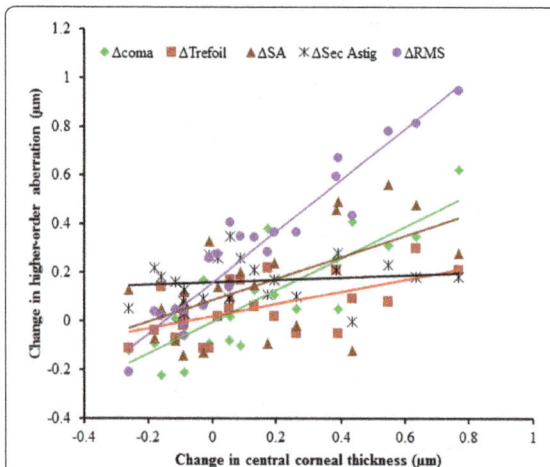

Fig. 8 Changes (postoperative minus preoperative) in higher-order aberrations as a function of change in central corneal thickness CCT in micrometres (μm)

aberration is possible in a few eyes, the technique induced spherical-like aberrations in majority of the treated eyes and increased the higher-order aberration RMS. This increase in higher-order aberrations RMS was linearly related with the degree of preoperative myopia and the postoperative change in central corneal thickness. There is need for further improvement in the predictability of the treatment algorithm used in this procedure.

Ethics approval and consent to participate
This study was approved by the Research Ethics Review Board of the College of Applied Medical Sciences, King Saud University and all participants gave written informed consent after the study protocol had been explained.

Abbreviations
logMAR: logarithm of minimum angle resolution; CCT: central corneal thickness; CDVA: corrected distance visual acuity; HOA: higher-order aberration; LASIK: laser in situ Keratomileusis; MSER: Mmean spherical equivalent refraction; RMS: root mean square; SA: spherical aberration; UDVA: uncorrected distance visual acuity.

Competing interests
The authors declare that they have no competing interest.

Authors' contributions
FA conceived of the study and carried out the data collection. FA carried out the entry of data into excel for analysis and helped to draft the manuscript. OU participated in the study design and coordination during data collection. OU performed the statistical analysis and drafted the manuscript. All authors read and approved the final manuscript.

Acknowledgment
The authors appreciate Lama Alsubaei for help during data collection.

Funding
The authors extend their appreciation to the Research Centre at Sciences Divisions & Medical Studies Center (Female Center) King Saud University, for funding this research.

Author details
[1]Department of Optometry & Vision Sciences, College of Applied Medical Sciences, King Saud University, Riyadh, P.O Box 10219, Riyadh 11433, Saudi Arabia. [2]Department of Optometry & Vision Sciences, Faculty of Health, Ophthalmic and Visual Optics Laboratory Group (Chronic Disease & Ageing), Institute of Health and Biomedical Innovation, Q Block, Room 5WS36 60 Musk Avenue Kelvin Grove, Brisbane, QLD 4059, Australia.

References
1. Kohnen T, Bühren J, Kühne C, Mirshahi A. Wavefront-guided LASIK with the Zyoptix 3.1 system for the correction of myopia and compound myopic astigmatism with 1-year follow-up: clinical outcome and change in higher order aberrations. Ophthalmology. 2004;111(12):2175–85.
2. Kohnen T, Mahmoud K, Bühren J. Comparison of corneal higher-order aberrations induced by myopic and hyperopic LASIK. Ophthalmology. 2005; 112(10):1692. e1691-1692. e1611.
3. Tran DB, Sarayba MA, Bor Z, Garufis C, Duh Y-J, Soltes CR, Juhasz T, Kurtz RM. Randomized prospective clinical study comparing induced aberrations with IntraLase and Hansatome flap creation in fellow eyes: potential impact on wavefront-guided laser in situ keratomileusis. J Cataract Refract Surg. 2005;31(1):97–105.
4. Stonecipher K, Ignacio TS, Stonecipher M. Advances in refractive surgery: microkeratome and femtosecond laser flap creation in relation to safety, efficacy, predictability, and biomechanical stability. Curr Opin Ophthalmol. 2006;17(4):368–72.
5. Sugar A, Rapuano CJ, Culbertson WW, Huang D, Varley GA, Agapitos PJ, de Luise VP, Koch DD. Laser in situ keratomileusis for myopia and astigmatism: safety and efficacy: a report by the American Academy of Ophthalmology. Ophthalmology. 2002;109(1):175–87.
6. Farjo AA, Sugar A, Schallhorn SC, Majmudar PA, Tanzer DJ, Trattler WB, Cason JB, Donaldson KE, Kymionis GD. Femtosecond lasers for LASIK flap creation: a report by the American Academy of Ophthalmology. Ophthalmology. 2013;120(3):e5–20.
7. Chalita MR, Chavala S, Xu M, Krueger RR. Wavefront analysis in post-LASIK eyes and its correlation with visual symptoms, refraction, and topography. Ophthalmology. 2004;111(3):447–53.
8. Oshika T, Miyata K, Tokunaga T, Samejima T, Amano S, Tanaka S, Hirohara Y, Mihashi T, Maeda N, Fujikado T. Higher order wavefront aberrations of cornea and magnitude of refractive correction in laser in situ keratomileusis. Ophthalmology. 2002;109(6):1154–8.
9. Moreno-Barriuso E, Lloves JM, Marcos S, Navarro R, Llorente L, Barbero S. Ocular aberrations before and after myopic corneal refractive surgery: LASIK-induced changes measured with laser ray tracing. Invest Ophthalmol Vis Sci. 2001;42(6):1396–403.
10. Ma L, Atchison DA, Albietz JM, Lenton LM, McLennan SG. Wavefront aberrations following laser in situ keratomileusis and refractive lens exchange for hypermetropia. J Refract Surg. 2003;20(4):307–16.
11. Buzzonetti L, Petrocelli G, Valente P, Tamburrelli C, Mosca L, Laborante A, Balestrazzi E. Comparison of corneal aberration changes after laser in situ keratomileusis performed with mechanical microkeratome and IntraLase femtosecond laser: 1-year follow-up. Cornea. 2008;27(2):174–9.
12. Kezirian GM, Stonecipher KG. Comparison of the IntraLase femtosecond laser and mechanical keratomes for laser in situ keratomileusis. J Cataract Refract Surg. 2004; 30(4): 804-11.
13. Sáles CS, Manche EE. One-year eye-to-eye comparison of wavefront-guided versus wavefront-optimized laser in situ keratomileusis in hyperopes. Clin Ophthalmol. 2014;8:2229.
14. Padmanabhan P, Mrochen M, Basuthkar S, Viswanathan D, Joseph R. Wavefront-guided versus wavefront-optimized laser in situ keratomileusis: contralateral comparative study. J Cataract Refract Surg. 2008;34(3):389–97.
15. Binder PS. One thousand consecutive IntraLase laser in situ keratomileusis flaps. J Cataract Refract Surg. 2006;32(6):962–9.
16. Ratkay-Traub I, Ferincz IE, Juhasz T, Kurtz RM, Krueger RR. First clinical results with the femtosecond neodynium-glass laser in refractive surgery. J Refract Surg. 2002;19(2):94–103.
17. Pesudovs K. Wavefront aberration outcomes of LASIK for high myopia and high hyperopia. Pergamon: Elsevier; 2005.
18. Zheng G, Du J, Zhang J, Liu S, Nie X, Zhu X, Tang X, Xin B, Mai Z, Zhang W. Contrast sensitivity and higher-order aberrations in patients with astigmatism. Chin Med J. 2007;120(10):882–5.
19. Hu J, Yan Z, Liu C, Huang L. Higher-order aberrations in myopic and astigmatism eyes. Zhonghua Yan Ke Za Zhi. 2004;40(1):13–6.
20. Dobson V, Tyszko R, Miller J, Harvey E. Astigmatism, amblyopia, and visual disability among a Native American population. Vision Sci Appli. 1996;1:139–42.
21. Assiri AA, Yousuf BI, Quantock AJ, Murphy PJ. Incidence and severity of keratoconus in Asir province, Saudi Arabia. Br J Ophthalmol. 2005;89(11):1403–6.
22. Rabinowitz YS. Keratoconus. Surv Ophthalmol. 1998;42(4):297–319.
23. Tran DB, Shah V. Higher order aberrations comparison in fellow eyes following intraLase LASIK with wavelight allegretto and customcornea LADArvision4000 systems. J Refract Surg. 2006;22:S961.
24. Mendoza G, Lozano JF, Tamez A, Lozano J, Zavala J, Valdez JE. Comparative study of the outcome of LASIK in Moderate versus High Astigmatism. Invest Ophthalmol Vis Sci. 2014;55(13):1557–7.
25. Thibos LN, Applegate RA, Schwiegerling JT, Webb R. Standards for reporting the optical aberrations of eyes. J Refract Surg. 2002;18(5):652–60.
26. Thibos LN, Wheeler W, Horner D. Power vectors: an application of Fourier analysis to the description and statistical analysis of refractive error. Optom Vis Sci. 1997;74(6):367–75.
27. Thibos LN, Horner D. Power vector analysis of the optical outcome of refractive surgery. J Cataract Refract Surg. 2001;27(1):80–5.

28. Kymionis GD, Kontadakis GA, Naoumidi I, Kankariya VP, Panagopoulou S, Manousaki A, Grentzelos MA, Pallikaris IG. Comparative study of stromal bed of LASIK flaps created with femtosecond lasers (IntraLase FS150, WaveLight FS200) and mechanical microkeratome. Br J Ophthalmol. 2013;98(1):133–7. bjophthalmol-2013-304023.

29. Huang SC, Chen HC. Overview of laser refractive surgery. Chang Gung Med J. 2008;31(3):237–52.

30. McDonald MB, Carr JD, Frantz JM, Kozarsky AM, Maguen E, Nesburn AB, Rabinowitz YS, Salz JJ, Stulting RD, Thompson KP. Laser in situ keratomileusis for myopia up to −11 diopters with up to −5 diopters of astigmatism with the summit autonomous LADARVision excimer laser system. Ophthalmology. 2001;108(2):309–16.

31. Kohnen T, Steinkamp G, Schnitzler E-M, Baumeister M, Wellermann G, Bühren J, Brieden M, Herting S, Mirshahi A, Ohrloff C. LASIK mit superiorem Hinge und Scanning-Spot-Excimerlaserablation zur Korrektur von Myopie und myopem Astigmatismus Einjahresergebnisse einer prospektiven klinischen Studie an 100 Augen. Ophthalmologe. 2001;98(11):1044–54.

32. Hjortdal JØ, Møller-Pedersen T, Ivarsen A, Ehlers N. Corneal power, thickness, and stiffness: Results of a prospective randomized controlled trial of PRK and LASIK for myopia. J Cataract Refract Surg. 2005;31(1):21–9.

33. Myrowitz EH, Chuck RS. A comparison of wavefront-optimized and wavefront-guided ablations. Curr Opin Ophthalmol. 2009;20(4):247–50.

34. Feng Y, Yu J, Wang Q. Meta-analysis of wavefront-guided vs. wavefront-optimized LASIK for myopia. Optom Vis Sci. 2011;88(12):1463–9.

35. Hashemian SJ, Soleimani M, Foroutan A, Joshaghani M, Ghaempanah MJ, Jafari ME, Yaseri M. Ocular higher-order aberrations and mesopic pupil size in individuals screened for refractive surgery. Ophthalmologica. 2012;5(2):222.

36. Castejon-Mochon JF, Lopez-Gil N, Benito A, Artal P. Ocular wave-front aberration statistics in a normal young population. Vision Res. 2002;42(13): 1611–7.

37. Mohammadi S-F, Tahvildari M, Abdolahinia T. Induced Secondary Astigmatism and Horizontal Coma after LASIK for Mixed Astigmatism. Iran J Ophthalmol. 2012;24(3):52–6.

38. Yamane N, Miyata K, Samejima T, Hiraoka T, Kiuchi T, Okamoto F, Hirohara Y, Mihashi T, Oshika T. Ocular higher-order aberrations and contrast sensitivity after conventional laser in situ keratomileusis. Invest Ophthalmol Vis Sci. 2004;45(11):3986–90.

39. Artal P, Chen L, Fernandez EJ, Singer B, Manzanera S, Williams DR. Adaptive optics for vision: the eye's adaptation to point spread function. J Refract Surg. 2003;19(5):S585–7.

40. Pansell T, Schworm HD, Ygge J. Torsional and vertical eye movements during head tilt dynamic characteristics. Invest Ophthalmol Vis Sci. 2003; 44(7):2986–90.

41. Mathur A, Atchison DA. Effect of orthokeratology on peripheral aberrations of the eye. Optom Vis Sci. 2009;86(5):E476–84.

42. Porter J, MacRae S, Yoon G, Roberts C, Cox IG, Williams DR. Separate effects of the microkeratome incision and laser ablation on the eye's wave aberration. Am J Ophthalmol. 2003;136(2):327–37.

20

Comparison of the Orbscan II topographer and the iTrace aberrometer for the measurements of keratometry and corneal diameter in myopic patients

Yao Chen and Xiaobo Xia[*]

Abstract

Background: The purpose of this study was to compare corneal power and horizontal corneal diameter (white-to-white [WTW] distance) readings obtained by the Orbscan II topographer and the iTrace aberrometer.

Methods: Keratometry readings in the flat (Kf) and steep (Ks) meridians and WTW distance were measured with the Orbscan II and iTrace systems in 100 myopic patients. Statistical evaluation was performed using the paired t test, Pearson correlation, and Bland-Altman analysis for comparison of measurement techniques.

Results: The mean keratometry values with the Orbscan II and iTrace were 43.16 ± 1.44 and 42.64 ± 1.43 diopter (D), respectively ($P < 0.0001$). The mean WTW distance measurements with the Orbscan II and iTrace were 11.57 ± 0.34 and 11.33 ± 0.36 mm, respectively ($P < 0.0001$). For the measurement of corneal power, the 95 % limits of agreement (LoA) between the Orbscan II and iTrace were -0.21 to 1.21 D for the flat meridian and -0.15 to 1.25 D for the steep meridian. For the measurement of WTW distance, the range of the 95 % LoA between the two devices was 0.47 mm.

Conclusions: For some clinical applications, the keratometry and WTW distance measurements obtained by the Orbscan II topographer and the iTrace aberrometer differed greatly and therefore were not interchangeable.

Trial registration: Clinical trials number: ChiCTR-OCS-14005077 (August 2nd, 2014).

Keywords: Keratometry, White-to-white distance, Orbscan II, iTrace

Background

Measurements of corneal power and WTW distance are important prior to either cataract or refractive surgery. Accurate intraocular lens (IOL) power calculations, contact lens fitting, and monitoring postoperative cornea are major clinical applications of these parameters [1, 2]. The IOL power is usually calculated using standard IOL calculation formulas, which are based on the value of corneal power [3]. Precise keratometry measurements are particularly crucial in determining the correct IOL power for patients who had previously undergone corneal refractive surgery [4, 5]. With the wider use of phakic IOLs, accurate determination of the WTW

distance has gained increased attention in sizing posterior chamber phakic IOLs [6, 7] and estimating the postoperative vault height in eyes with implantable collamer lenses (ICL; STAAR Surgical AG, Nidau, Switzerland) [8, 9].

Until recently, the Orbscan II topography system (Bausch & Lomb, Orbtek Inc., UT, USA) has been widely applied for measuring the corneal power and WTW distance and is considered accurate and reproducible [10–14]. Currently, corneal wavefront analysis has gained increased importance in-line with the development of wavefront sensing technology [15, 16]. Clinical wavefront aberrometers allow an objective measurement of optical aberrations other than sphere and cylinder, such as spherical aberration, coma, trefoil, and other higher-order optical aberrations (HOAs), which present diagnostic and therapeutic applications [17].

* Correspondence: xbxia21@163.com
Department of Ophthalmology, Xiangya Hospital, Central South University, Changsha, Hunan, China

The commercially available iTrace system (Tracey Technologies Corp. TX, USA) integrates corneal topography with a ray-tracing aberrometer, yielding information about refractive, wavefront and corneal topographic data of the human optical system [18, 19]. Visser et al. [20] showed that the iTrace device exhibits a high level of repeatability for measuring corneal aberrations. However, the measurements of corneal power and WTW distance is seldom reported. Moreover, it remains unclear whether or not the iTrace aberrometer could be considered as an alternative instrument for IOL power calculations in clinical practice. Therefore, the purpose of this study was to compare the corneal power and WTW distance measurements using the Orbscan II topographer and the iTrace aberrometer.

Methods

Subjects

One hundred right eyes of 100 myopic patients (51 male, 49 female, age 20.18 ± 5.12 years, age range, 8 to 39 years old) were included in this study. Each subject underwent full ophthalmic examinations, including vision, subjective refraction, slit-lamp and fundus examinations, and corneal topography by the Orbscan II topographer and the iTrace aberrometer. All subjects had good best corrected distance visual acuity (BCVA) equal to or better than 20/20 to allow for adequate fixation. Exclusion criteria included coexisting ocular diseases or a dry eye, corneal anomalies, contact lens wear within the preceding 2 weeks, any history of ocular surgery or trauma. The ethics committee of Xiangya Hospital approved this study. Adults and parents of juveniles provided the written informed consent in accordance with the Declaration of Helsinki before the measurements were carried out.

Instruments

The Orbscan II topographer, combined slit-scanning with a Placido disk, has the capacity to directly acquire elevation and curvature data of both anterior and posterior corneal surfaces [11]. The Placido disk and 40 slits are sequentially projected on the cornea, then the anterior and posterior edges of the slits are captured and analyzed, and eventually, elevation and curvature topographic maps are generated. The corneal limbus (the border of the cornea and the sclera) is automatically detected to calculate the WTW distance.

The iTrace aberrometer utilizes a Placido disk format named Vista developed by EyeSys Vision Inc. (Houston, TX, USA) with a laser diode at the wavelength of 655 nm for corneal topography assessment. The iTrace software then defines the ring edges and calculates corneal curvature, corneal wavefront data and detects the WTW distance.

Measurements

The refraction of each eye was determined with subjective manifest refraction. Three repeated consecutive measurements were performed independently by two experienced operators for both eyes of all subjects using the Orbscan II topographer and the iTrace aberrometer. The sequence of the measurements with the two devices was randomly chosen. In this study, the following parameters were recorded, the keratometry readings in the flat (Kf) and steep (Ks) meridians, and the WTW distance. The mean keratometry value was calculated using the following formula: (Kf + Ks)/2. Only the right eye of each subject was calculated and analyzed. All participants underwent measurements approximately 5 min apart between 8 AM and 12 AM.

For the Orbscan II topographer measurements, the operator adjusted the distance between the corneal apex and the center of the moving slit for correct alignment. Then the subjects were asked to keep their eyes open and not move their eyes once the scan had started. The device detected excessive eye movement and discarded low-quality or incomplete images.

For the iTrace aberrometer measurements, the internal optometer incorporated in the device was used for alignment of the patient's line of sight with the laser axis. Then the iTrace aberrometer automatically centered onto the pupil and verified focus and alignment, and captured the data. The best scan, defined as all of the reflected Placido rings devoid of missing ring edges, was chosen for the final analysis.

Statistical analysis

Statistical analysis was performed using SPSS software (version 19.0, SPSS, Inc.) and MedCalc (version 13.0, MedCalc software bvba, Inc.). The Kolmogorov-Smirnov test was used to confirm the normality of all data distribution. Differences between the devices were assessed using the paired t test. All tests were two tailed, P values less than 0.05 were considered statistically significant. The Pearson correlation coefficient was determined to show the correlation between the two measurements for each subject. The Bland-Altman plots with 95 % limits of agreement (LoA; mean difference of two methods ± 1.96 standard deviation) [21] were calculated to evaluate interdevice agreement and interchangeability.

Results

For 100 right eyes of 100 myopic patients, the mean spherical equivalent refraction was -5.33 ± 2.42 diopter (D) (range,-12.50 to -0.75 D). The mean examination time was 10 min, and the iTrace aberrometer was quicker than the Orbscan II topographer for all measurements. No significant deviation from a normal distribution pattern was observed in the corneal power and WTW distance (Kolmogorov-Smirnov tests, $P > 0.1$).

The corneal power and WTW distance readings assessed with the Orbscan II topographer and the iTrace aberrometer are summarized in Table 1. The Kf, Ks, and WTW distance measurements taken with the Orbscan II topographer were greater in magnitude than those measured by the iTrace aberrometer ($P < 0.0001$ for all pairwise comparisons; paired t test). The mean keratometry values obtained with the Orbscan II topographer and the iTrace aberrometer were 43.16 ± 1.44 and 42.64 ± 1.43 D, respectively. A statistically significant difference between the two instruments was noted ($P < 0.0001$, paired t test). The mean difference (with 95 % LoA) in the mean keratometry measurements between the two instruments was 0.52 D (range:−0.16 to 1.21 D).

Pearson correlation coefficients and Bland-Altman plots for the measurements of corneal power and WTW distance are shown in Figs. 1, 2 and 3. Results with the Orbscan II topographer and the iTrace aberrometer correlated closely, with Pearson correlation coefficients ranging from 0.9426 to 0.9743. The Bland-Altman plots revealed a fixed bias towards the Orbscan II topographer for the measurements of Kf, Ks and WTW distance. Mean differences (with 95 % LoA) between the Orbscan II topographer and the iTrace aberrometer were 0.50 D (range:−0.21 to 1.21 D) for Kf and 0.55 D (range:−0.15 to 1.25 D) for Ks measurements. The mean difference (with 95 % LoA) in the WTW distance measurements between the two devices was 0.24 mm (range: 0.00 to 0.47 mm).

Based on the median age (19 years), the subjects were divided into age <19 years old (less than 19 years old; mean age, 15.95 ± 2.92; $n = 40$) and age ≥19 years old groups (19 years or older; mean age, 23.00 ± 4.27; $n = 60$). We evaluated the effects of age on the corneal power and WTW distance measured by the Orbscan II topographer and the iTrace aberrometer. The Orbscan II topographer generated larger values when compared with those of the iTrace aberrometer for both age <19 years old and age ≥19 years old groups ($P < 0.0001$ for all pairwise comparisons; paired t test; Table 2). The 95 % LoA between the Orbscan II and iTrace were almost larger than 1.20 D for Kf and Ks measurements for both age <19 years old and age ≥19 years old groups.

Table 1 Comparison of the corneal power and WTW distance values measured by the 2 devices

Parameters	Orbscan II	iTrace	P value[a]
Kf (D)	42.56 ± 1.34	42.06 ± 1.34	<0.0001
Ks (D)	43.76 ± 1.58	43.21 ± 1.57	<0.0001
WTW (mm)	11.57 ± 0.34	11.33 ± 0.36	<0.0001

Data are expressed as mean ± SD; [a]paired t test <0.05 considered significant; Kf = flat axis power; Ks = steep axis power, D = diopter

The 95 % LoA for the WTW distance mesurements were equal to or larger than 0.45 mm for both groups.

As shown in Table 3, there were statistically significant differences in the Kf, Ks, and WTW distance mesurements between the Orbscan II topographer and the iTrace aberrometer ($P < 0.0001$ for all pairwise comparisons; paired t test) for both male and female subjects. The 95 % LoA for the Kf and Ks mesurements between the Orbscan II and iTrace were equal to or larger than 1.29 D for both male and female subjects. As regards the WTW distance mesurements, the 95 % LoA were equal to or larger than 0.47 mm for both male and female subjects.

Discussion

Refractive considerations are integrated in modern cataract surgery as a result of the increased application of advanced IOLs, progresses in surgical techniques, and use of new preoperative biometry instruments [22, 23]. The final refractive outcome following cataract surgery is affected by various factors such as IOL power calculations, selection of the proper IOL formula, and the quality of the IOL. Of these factors, inaccurate computation of IOL power contributes to the prediction deviations of refractive outcome the most [3]. The accuracy of optical IOL power calculation depends on the preoperative biometric measurements of the eye. Norrby et al. [24] demonstrated that inaccurate corneal power is a major cause of error in IOL power calculations. A 1 D error in the corneal power mesurement will induce approximately a 1 D error in the calculation of the IOL power [25]. Thus, precise postoperative refractive outcomes depend on the improvements in biometry and IOL power calculations.

In this study, measurements of the corneal power and WTW distance obtained by the Orbscan II topographer differed significantly from those of the iTrace aberrometer. Despite a strong positive correlation, almost all plots lied by one side towards the Orbscan II topographer along the equality line (the right-hand side of Figs. 1, 2 and 3). As Bland and Altman [21] pointed out, perfect agreement merely exists if all points lie along the equality line, but perfect correlation will occur if points lie along any straight line. They advocated the use of the 95 % LoA as a more accurate method for assessing agreement. A narrower 95 % LoA indicates better agreement between devices. The acceptable range of agreement between two devices partly depends on clinical practice, that is, if the range of the 95 % LoA is small enough to avoid problems with clinical interpretation, they may be used interchangeably. However, if the range of the 95 % LoA has significant clinical implications, the two methodologies cannot be used interchangeably [26].

Shirayama et al. [27] used the Galilei dual-Scheimpflug Analyzer, the Humphrey Atlas corneal topographer, the

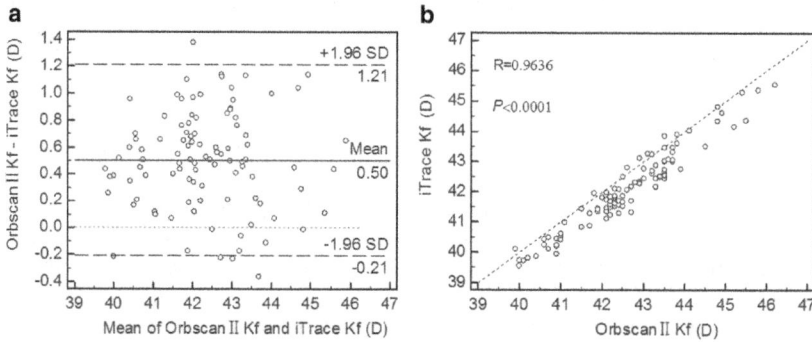

Fig. 1 Kf measurements by the Orbsan II versus the iTrace. **a** Bland-Altman plot showing the mean difference and the limits of agreement. **b** Scatter diagram and Pearson correlation analysis

IOLMaster, and a manual keratometer to assess the repeatability and comparability of anterior corneal power values. For the mean keratometry values, each pair of devices recorded a 95 % LoA range of <0.5 D. The corneal measurements from the four devices were found to be highly reproducible and comparable. Another study by Tajbakhsh et al. [28] found that the 95 % LoA range of the keratometry values between the TMS-4 (a Placido disc-based system) and the Orbscan IIz was 0.8 D which implied that they could not be used interchangeably in clinical practice. In the present study, the 95 % LoA range of the mean keratometry values was approximately 1.37 D with a mean difference of 0.52 D. Classic IOL power calculation formulas usually multiply the keratometry reading by approximately 0.9 [3], so this would translate into a mean difference in lens power prediction of 0.47 D, with 95 % of differences falling within 1.23 D of the spherical equivalent refraction. Because most IOLs are currently available in 0.5 D gradations, these discrepancies might lead to errors in IOL power calculations and cause hyperopia after cataract surgery. According to our data, the mean differences in the corneal

power mesurements between the Orbscan II topographer and the iTrace aberrometer were 0.50 (Kf) to 0.55 D (Ks), and the range of the 95 % LoA was 1.40 (Ks) to 1.42 D (Kf). Also, the differences were consistent in both age groups.and in both gender groups. As a consequence, the wide limits of agreement of corneal power mesurements between the two devices observed in the current study were beyond clinically acceptable levels in the prediction of the IOL power.

For the WTW distance measurements, previous studies have verified the accuracy and repeatability obtained with the Orbscan II topographer [10, 12]. Although our study did not demonstrate which device measured the WTW distance more accurately, it should be noted that the iTrace aberrometer measurements were smaller than those of the Orbscan II topographer. Martin et al. [29] found that the mean difference in the WTW distance measurements between the Orbscan and IOLMaster was 0.50 mm (with 95 % LoA of 0.01 to – 1.01 mm), this difference could have practical relevance and they suggested the two devices were not interchangeable for WTW assessment in clinical practice. Another study by

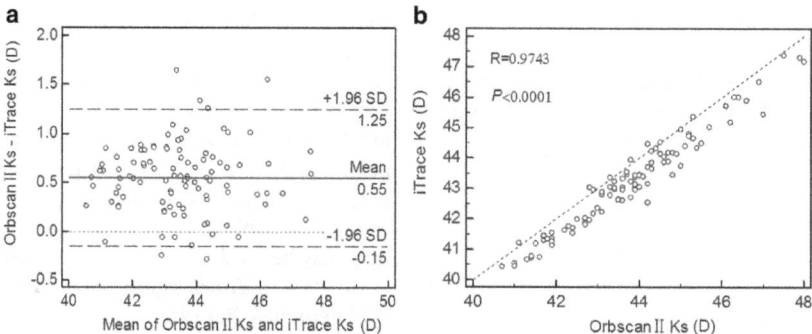

Fig. 2 Ks measurements by the Orbsan II versus the iTrace. **a** Bland-Altman plot. **b** Scatter diagram and Pearson correlation analysis

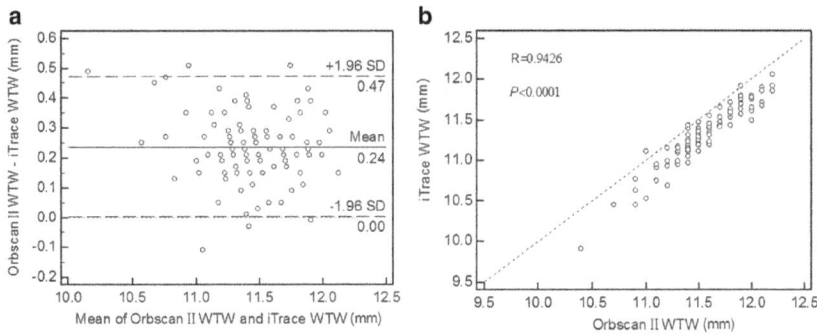

Fig. 3 The WTW distance measurements by the Orbsan II versus the iTrace. **a** Bland-Altman plot. **b** Scatter diagram and Pearson correlation analysis

Salouti et al. [30] reported that a difference ≥0.50 mm for the WTW distance was considered as clinically relevant. The results of this study show that the range of the 95 % LoA was approximately 0.5 mm (0.47 mm for all the subjects, 0.46 mm for males and 0.49 mm for females) with the Orbscan II topographer, versus the iTrace aberrometer. This difference is clinically relevant in determining an accurate lens diameter for implantation of the STAAR Surgical V4 (Version 4) ICL, because this phakic IOL's diameter should be approximately 0.5 to 1.0 mm larger than the WTW distance measurement in myopic eyes [8]. Moreover, an over- or under-sized ICL may induce unwanted complications, such as IOL rotation or decentration, pigment dispersion, pupillary block glaucoma, and cataract formation [31, 32].

The observed differences in the corneal power and WTW distance measurements between the two devices are unclear, but the use of distinct methodologies in each device might induce this tendency. For the keratometry values, both systems measure anterior corneal curvature using the Placido rings while the Orbscan II topographer can analyze the posterior surface with the help of scanning slits. The accuracy of the WTW distance measurements relies on the quality of the anterior segment images. With the Orbscan II topographer, this is composed of multiple scanning slit images, furthermore, the Orbscan II automatically rejects low-quality images. While with the iTrace aberrometer, the quality of the image is discernible by the operator. On the other hand, a longer capture time to acquire multiple images by the Orbscan II topographer might affect fixation and data accuracy, leading to a poor agreement with the data measured by the iTrace aberrometer.

There are several limitations of the present study. First, the keratometry values were calculated solely from the anterior corneal surface. Second, our comparisons were merely restricted to normal, healthy corneas from a limited age group of refractive surgery and Orthokeratology candidates, the keratometry and WTW distance scan images were of excellent quality. In hyperopic patients or older patients with cataract, the results may be different. Further studies are required to comprehensively assess the agreement of the corneal power and WTW distance measurements obtained by the two devices in such cases. Finally, our study only used one operator for each device, the interobserver repeatability of the corneal power and WTW distance measurements by the two devices deserves further investigations.

Table 2 Comparison of the corneal power and WTW distance measurements in age <19 years old and age ≥19 years old groups

groups	parameters	Orbscan II	iTrace	P Value[a]	95 % LoA
age <19	Kf (D)	42.29 ± 1.38	41.84 ± 1.45	<0.0001	−0.16,1.07
years old	Ks (D)	43.47 ± 1.65	42.95 ± 1.71	<0.0001	−0.08,1.11
(n = 40)	WTW (mm)	11.60 ± 0.29	11.37 ± 0.30	<0.0001	0.00,0.45
age ≥19	Kf (D)	42.74 ± 1.30	42.20 ± 1.26	<0.0001	−0.23,1.30
years old	Ks (D)	43.96 ± 1.51	43.39 ± 1.45	<0.0001	−0.19,1.34
(n = 60)	WTW (mm)	11.55 ± 0.36	11.30 ± 0.39	<0.0001	0.01,0.48

Data are expressed as mean ± SD; [a]paired t test <0.05 considered significant; Kf = flat axis power; Ks = steep axis power, D = diopter, LoA = limits of agreement

Table 3 Comparison of the corneal power and WTW distance measurements in male and female subjects

gender	parameters	Orbscan II	iTrace	P Value[a]	95 % LoA
Male	Kf (D)	42.12 ± 1.39	41.63 ± 1.37	<0.0001	−0.28,1.26
(n = 51)	Ks (D)	43.34 ± 1.63	42.79 ± 1.65	<0.0001	−0.17,1.26
	WTW (mm)	11.64 ± 0.32	11.40 ± 0.33	<0.0001	0.01,0.47
Female	Kf (D)	43.02 ± 1.14	42.51 ± 1.16	<0.0001	−0.13,1.16
(n = 49)	Ks (D)	44.20 ± 1.41	43.65 ± 1.36	<0.0001	−0.14,1.24
	WTW (mm)	11.49 ± 0.34	11.25 ± 0.37	<0.0001	−0.01,0.48

Data are expressed as mean ± SD; [a]paired t test <0.05 considered significant; Kf = flat axis power; Ks = steep axis power, D = diopter, LoA = limits of agreement

Conclusions

The present study demonstrated that measurements of the corneal power and WTW distance with the Orbscan II topographer were larger than those obtained with the iTrace aberrometer in the assessment of myopic eyes. The differences between the two devices were not within clinically acceptable levels, and therefore the two devices could not be used interchangeably in clinical practice.

Ethics approval and consent to participate

The ethics committee of Xiangya Hospital approved this study (No. 201408390). Adults and parents of juveniles provided the written informed consent in accordance with the Declaration of Helsinki. The trial registration was requested on August 2nd, 2014.

Consent for publication

Not applicable for this study.

Abbreviations

BCVA: best corrected distance visual acuity; D: diopter; HOAs: higher-order optical aberrations; ICL: implantable collamer lenses; IOL: intraocular lens; Kf: keratometry in the flat meridian; Ks: keratometry in the steep meridian; LoA: limits of agreement; WTW: white-to-white.

Competing interests

The authors declare that they have no competing interests.

Authors' contributions

YC and XBX participated in study concept and design. YC participated in data acquisition, data analysis, ethical form preparation and application, and prepared the manuscript. XBX participated in critical review of the manuscript. All authors read and approved the final manuscript.

Acknowledgements

We would like to acknowledge Shuang Liu and Mengjun Li for operating the instruments. Grants were provided by the Graduate Student Research Innovation Project of Hunan Province (No. 2501-71380100006), and the Natural Science Foundation of Hunan Province, China (No.12JJ3120).

References

1. Qazi MA, Cua IY, Roberts CJ, Pepose JS. Determining corneal power using Orbscan II videokeratography for intraocular lens calculation after excimer laser surgery for myopia. J Cataract Refract Surg. 2007;33:21–30.
2. Martinez CE, Klyce SD. Corneal topography in cataract surgery. Curr Opin Ophthalmol. 1996;7:31–8.
3. Olsen T. Calculation of intraocular lens power: a review. Acta Ophthalmol Scand. 2007;85:472–85.
4. Seitz B, Langenbucher A. Intraocular lens power calculation in eyes after corneal refractive surgery. J Refract Surg. 2000;16:349–61.
5. Rosa N, Capasso L, Lanza M, Borrelli M. Clinical results of a corneal radius correcting factor in calculating intraocular lens power after corneal refractive surgery. J Refract Surg. 2009;25:599–603.
6. Lovisolo CF, Reinstein DZ. Phakic intraocular lenses. Surv Ophthalmol. 2005;50:549–87.
7. Perez-Cambrodi RJ, Pinero DP, Ferrer-Blasco T, Cervino A, Brautaset R. The posterior chamber phakic refractive lens (PRL): a review. Eye (Lond). 2013;27:14–21.
8. Seo JH, Kim MK, Wee WR, Lee JH. Effects of white-to-white diameter and anterior chamber depth on implantable collamer lens vault and visual outcome. J Refract Surg. 2009;25:730–8.
9. Reinstein DZ, Lovisolo CF, Archer TJ, Gobbe M. Comparison of postoperative vault height predictability using white-to-white or sulcus diameter-based sizing for the visian implantable collamer lens. J Refract Surg. 2013;29:30–5.
10. Wang L, Auffarth GU. White-to-white corneal diameter measurements using the eyemetrics program of the Orbscan topography system. Dev Ophthalmol. 2002;34:141–6.
11. Cairns G, McGhee CN. Orbscan computerized topography: attributes, applications, and limitations. J Cataract Refract Surg. 2005;31:205–20.
12. Baumeister M, Terzi E, Ekici Y, Kohnen T. Comparison of manual and automated methods to determine horizontal corneal diameter. J Cataract Refract Surg. 2004;30:374–80.
13. Menassa N, Kaufmann C, Goggin M, Job OM, Bachmann LM, Thiel MA. Comparison and reproducibility of corneal thickness and curvature readings obtained by the Galilei and the Orbscan II analysis systems. J Cataract Refract Surg. 2008;34:1742–7.
14. Crawford AZ, Patel DV, McGhee CN. Comparison and repeatability of keratometric and corneal power measurements obtained by Orbscan II, Pentacam, and Galilei corneal tomography systems. Am J Ophthalmol. 2013;156:53–60.
15. Oliveira CM, Ferreira A, Franco S. Wavefront analysis and Zernike polynomial decomposition for evaluation of corneal optical quality. J Cataract Refract Surg. 2012;38:343–56.
16. Maeda N. Clinical applications of wavefront aberrometry - a review. Clin Experiment Ophthalmol. 2009;37:118–29.
17. Marcos S. Aberrometry: basic science and clinical applications. Bull Soc Belge Ophtalmol. 2006;197–213.
18. Jun I, Choi YJ, Kim EK, Seo KY, Kim TI. Internal spherical aberration by ray tracing-type aberrometry in multifocal pseudophakic eyes. Eye (Lond). 2012;26:1243–8.
19. Rozema JJ, Van Dyck DE, Tassignon MJ. Clinical comparison of 6 aberrometers. Part 1: Technical specifications. J Cataract Refract Surg. 2005;31:1114–27.
20. Visser N, Berendschot TT, Verbakel F, Tan AN, de Brabander J, Nuijts RM. Evaluation of the comparability and repeatability of four wavefront aberrometers. Invest Ophthalmol Vis Sci. 2011;52:1302–11.
21. Bland JM, Altman DG. Statistical methods for assessing agreement between two methods of clinical measurement. Lancet. 1986;1:307–10.
22. Alio JL, Abdelghany AA, Fernandez-Buenaga R. Enhancements after cataract surgery. Curr Opin Ophthalmol. 2015;26:50–5.
23. Gomez ML. Measuring the quality of vision after cataract surgery. Curr Opin Ophthalmol. 2014;25:3–11.
24. Norrby S. Sources of error in intraocular lens power calculation. J Cataract Refract Surg. 2008;34:368–76.
25. Olsen T. On the calculation of power from curvature of the cornea. Br J Ophthalmol. 1986;70:152–4.
26. Bland JM, Altman DG. Measuring agreement in method comparison studies. Stat Methods Med Res. 1999;8:135–60.
27. Shirayama M, Wang L, Weikert MP, Koch DD. Comparison of corneal powers obtained from 4 different devices. Am J Ophthalmol. 2009;148:528–35. e521.
28. Tajbakhsh Z, Salouti R, Nowroozzadeh MH, Aghazadeh-Amiri M, Tabatabaee S, Zamani M. Comparison of keratometry measurements using the Pentacam HR, the Orbscan IIz, and the TMS-4 topographer. Ophthalmic Physiol Opt. 2012;32:539–46.
29. Martin R, Ortiz S, Rio-Cristobal A. White-to-white corneal diameter differences in moderately and highly myopic eyes: partial coherence interferometry versus scanning-slit topography. J Cataract Refract Surg. 2013;39:585–9.
30. Salouti R, Nowroozzadeh MH, Zamani M, Ghoreyshi M, Khodaman AR. Comparison of Horizontal corneal diameter measurements using the Orbscan IIz and Pentacam HR systems. Cornea. 2013;32:1460–4.
31. Kohnen T, Kook D, Morral M, Guell JL. Phakic intraocular lenses: part 2: results and complications. J Cataract Refract Surg. 2010;36:2168–94.
32. Guell JL, Morral M, Kook D, Kohnen T. Phakic intraocular lenses part 1: historical overview, current models, selection criteria, and surgical techniques. J Cataract Refract Surg. 2010;36:1976–93.

21

Correlation between optic nerve head circulation and visual function before and after anti-VEGF therapy for central retinal vein occlusion: prospective, interventional case series

Daisuke Nagasato[1,2], Yoshinori Mitamura[3*], Kentaro Semba[3], Kei Akaiwa[3], Toshihiko Nagasawa[1,2], Yuki Yoshizumi[1], Hitoshi Tabuchi[1] and Yoshiaki Kiuchi[2]

Abstract

Background: To determine the correlation between the optic nerve head (ONH) circulation determined by laser speckle flowgraphy and the best-corrected visual acuity or retinal sensitivity before and after intravitreal bevacizumab or ranibizumab for central retinal vein occlusion.

Methods: Thirty-one eyes of 31 patients were treated with intravitreal bevacizumab or ranibizumab for macular edema due to a central retinal vein occlusion. The blood flow in the large vessels on the ONH, the best-corrected visual acuity, and retinal sensitivity were measured at the baseline, and at 1, 3, and 6 months after treatment. The arteriovenous passage time on fluorescein angiography was determined. The venous tortuosity index was calculated on color fundus photograph by dividing the length of the tortuous retinal vein by the chord length of the same segment. The blood flow was represented by the mean blur rate (MBR) determined by laser speckle flowgraphy. To exclude the influence of systemic circulation and blood flow in the ONH tissue, the corrected MBR was calculated as MBR of ONH vessel area – MBR of ONH tissue area in the affected eye divided by the vascular MBR – tissue MBR in the unaffected eye. Pearson's correlation tests were used to determine the significance of correlations between the MBR and the best-corrected visual acuity, retinal sensitivity, arteriovenous passage time, or venous tortuosity index.

Results: At the baseline, the corrected MBR was significantly correlated with the arteriovenous passage time and venous tortuosity index ($r = -0.807$, $P < 0.001$; $r = -0.716$, $P < 0.001$; respectively). The corrected MBR was significantly correlated with the best-corrected visual acuity and retinal sensitivity at the baseline, and at 1, 3, and 6 months (all $P < 0.050$). The corrected MBR at the baseline was significantly correlated with the best-corrected visual acuity at 6 months ($r = -0.651$, $P < 0.001$) and retinal sensitivity at 6 months ($r = 0.485$, $P = 0.005$).

Conclusions: The pre-treatment blood flow velocity of ONH can be used as a predictive factor for the best-corrected visual acuity and retinal sensitivity after anti-VEGF therapy for central retinal vein occlusion.

Trial registration: Trial Registration number: UMIN000009072. Date of registration: 10/15/2012.

Keywords: Anti-vascular endothelial growth factor agent, Central retinal vein occlusion, Fundus-related microperimetry, Laser speckle flowgraphy, Retinal blood flow

* Correspondence: ymitaymitaymita@yahoo.co.jp
[3]Department of Ophthalmology, Institute of Biomedical Sciences, Tokushima University Graduate School, 3-18-15 Kuramoto, Tokushima 770-8503, Japan
Full list of author information is available at the end of the article

Background

A central retinal vein occlusion (CRVO) is one of the major causes of vision reduction, and anti-vascular endothelial growth factor (VEGF) agents have been shown to significantly improve visual acuity in eyes with macular edema (ME) due to a CRVO [1].

Laser speckle flowgraphy (LSFG) is a non-invasive method of real-time measurements of the blood flow on the optic nerve head (ONH), retina, and choroid [2–6]. It can measure the relative blood flow velocity, called the mean blur rate (MBR), that has been shown to be significantly correlated with the actual blood flow rate determined by the hydrogen gas clearance method and the microspheres technique [7, 8]. It has been reported that LSFG can record the blood flow from the same location of an eye with high reproducibility especially on the ONH [9]. This then provides an accurate way to monitor the circulation changes before and after pharmacological interventions [10].

Yamada et al. reported that the MBR values in large ONH vessels measured by LSFG were correlated with the higher aqueous VEGF concentrations in eyes with CRVO [11]. Nagaoka et al. reported that a single intravitreal bevacizumab (IVB) injection did not affected the retinal microcirculation in eyes with acute branch retinal vein occlusion (BRVO) for at least 3 months after the injection [12]. However, there has been no report that compared the ocular circulation before and after anti-VEGF therapy for CRVO except for a report of 3 cases in which the statistical association between ONH circulation and visual function was not determined [13].

Thus, the purpose of this study was to examine the relationship between the retinal blood flow and visual acuity or retinal sensitivity in 31 eyes before and after IVB or intravitreal ranibizumab (IVR) for CRVO.

Methods

This was a prospective, interventional case series of 31 eyes of 31 treatment-naïve patients (20 men and 11 women) with unilateral CRVO. The patients were examined by LSFG and microperimetry at the baseline and at 1, 3, and 6 months after IVB or IVR for ME due to a CRVO. The fluorescein arteriovenous passage time was determined at the baseline. All patients were examined within 3 month of the onset of the symptoms. The age of the patients at presentation ranged from 40 to 83 years (mean, 66.9 years). All treatment-naïve patients who were diagnosed with ME due to CRVO, had a healthy fellow eye, and had IVB or IVR injections in the Department of Ophthalmology of Saneikai Tsukazaki Hospital from October 2012 through February 2015 were studied. Approval was obtained from the Institutional Review Board of Saneikai Tsukazaki Hospital prior to beginning this study, and the patients gave their written informed consent prior to their inclusion. The patients have provided permission to publish clinical data of their case in this study. This study was registered with the University hospital Medical Information Network (UMIN) clinical trials registry. The registration title is "UMIN000009072, Correlation between optic nerve head circulation and retinal sensitivity before and after anti-VEGF drug intravitreal injection for central retinal vein occlusion" (October 15, 2012). The procedures used in this study adhered to the tenets of the Declaration of Helsinki.

Patients with ME due to a CRVO, central foveal thickness of ≥250 μm in the optical coherence tomographic (OCT) images, and a decimal visual acuity from 0.01 to 0.8 were studied. Patients with a history of cerebral infarction, anti-VEGF therapy, vitrectomy, and uveitis, or other vitreoretinal diseases were excluded. In addition, patients with uncontrolled high blood pressure, diabetes, intraocular pressure (IOP) of 21 mmHg or more, or iris neovascularization were excluded.

The blood flow of the major blood vessels on the ONH was measured in all patients, and the arteriovenous passage time of the retina was determined by fluorescein angiography (FA). A previous study investigating CRVO with FA [14] showed that more than 10 disc areas of the nonperfusion areas were observed in the ischemic type of CRVO. Thus, a diagnosis of ischemic CRVO was made in eyes with more than 10 disc areas of the nonperfusion areas [11]. The venous tortuosity index was calculated on color fundus photograph.

Patients who started their treatment between October 2012 and August 2013 received IVB injections (1.25 mg/0.05 mL), and those who started treatment between September 2013 and February 2015 received IVR injections (0.5 mg/0.05 mL). After the initial treatment, the patients were examined once a month. When the central foveal thickness was ≥250 μm, or the physician determined that additional treatment was necessary, the patients received additional injections of the same anti-VEGF agent.

All patients had a standard ophthalmologic examination including IOP measurements before and after IVB or IVR. The best-corrected visual acuity (BCVA) was measured with a standard Japanese Landolt visual acuity chart, and the decimal visual acuity was converted to the logarithm of the minimal angle of resolution (logMAR) units for statistical analyses. The anterior and posterior segments were examined by slit-lamp biomicroscopy, indirect ophthalmoscopy, color fundus photography, and spectral-domain OCT (SD-OCT). The systolic blood pressure (SBP), diastolic blood pressure (DBP), and heart rate were measured. The mean arterial pressure (MAP) and the mean ocular perfusion pressure (MOPP) were calculated according to the following formulas and used for the analyses: $MAP = DBP + 1/3 (SBP - DBP)$, and $MOPP = 2/3 MAP - IOP$.

Laser speckle flowgraphy

LSFG-NAVI (Softcare, Fukuoka, Japan) was used to evaluate the ONH circulation in eyes with a CRVO (Figs. 1 and 2). The principles of LSFG have been reported in detail [15].   In brief, LSFG uses a diode laser (wavelength 830 nm) to detect the movement of the red blood cells in the blood vessels. The light scattered by the movement of the blood cells creates speckle patterns on the area where the sensor is focused, and the scattered light produces a blur in the speckle patterns. The mean blur rate, which is the change in the blur, is a quantitative value that represents the relative blood flow velocity [15–19].

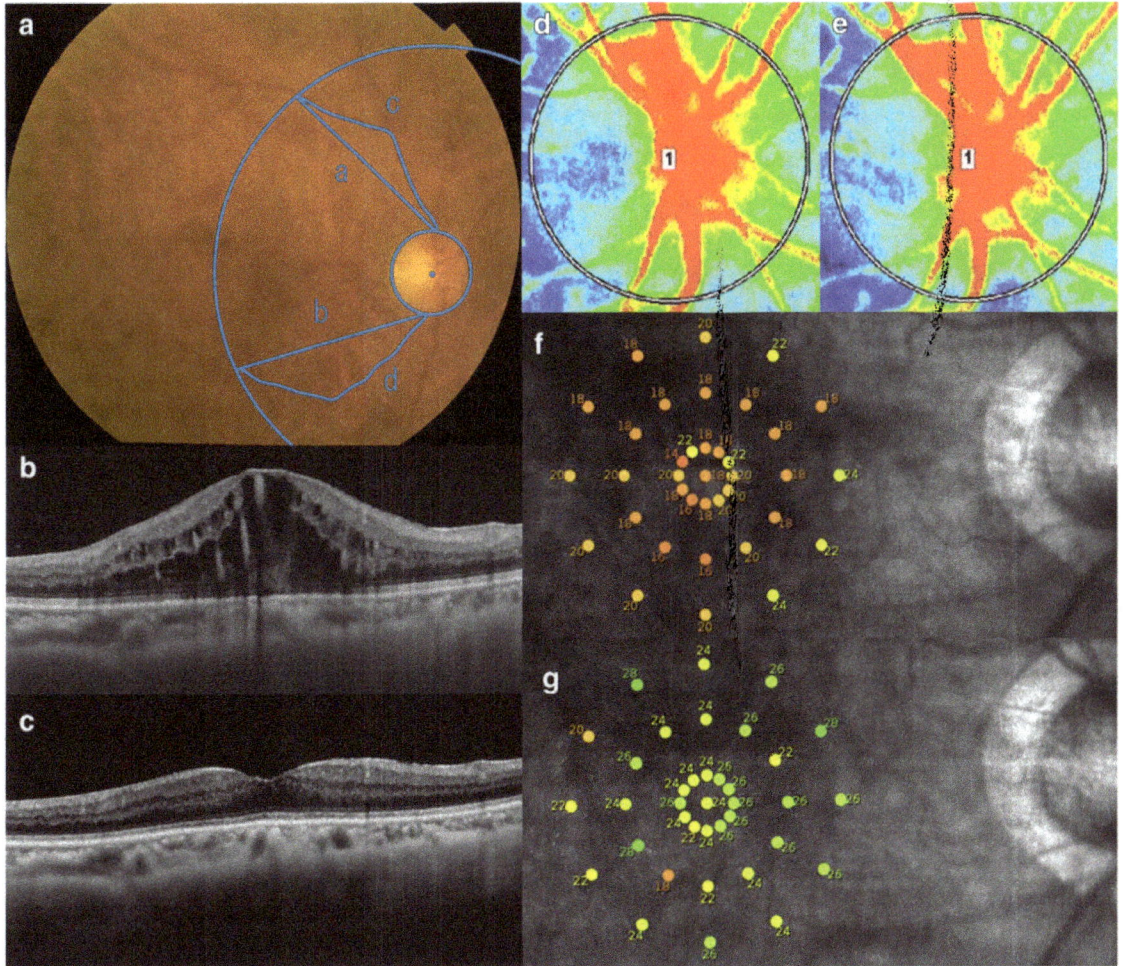

Fig. 1 Ophthalmologic examination images before and 6 months after anti-VEGF therapy for central retinal vein occlusion. Fundus photograph, spectral-domain optical coherence tomographic (SD-OCT) images, laser speckle flowgraphic (LSFG) images, and microperimetric maps before and 6 months after an initial anti-VEGF therapy of the right eye of a 66-year-old woman with cystoid macular edema (CME) due to a central retinal vein occlusion are presented. The decimal best-corrected visual acuity was 0.5 before the treatment and 1.0 at 6 months after the treatment. **a**: Fundus photograph at the baseline. The venous tortuosity index was calculated on color fundus photograph. Measurements of superior and inferior venous arcades were obtained starting from the optic disc margin to the crossing point of a circle whose diameter is the distance from the center of optic disc to the fovea. The course of the veins was traced using Photoshop (Adobe Systems, Inc. Ca, USA). NIH ImageJ software was used to measure the lengths of the tortuous vein (c and d) and chord of the vessels (a and b). The venous tortuosity was calculated by dividing the length of the tortuous retinal vein by the chord length of the same segment (c/a and d/b). The average of the venous tortuosity ((c/a + d/b)/2) was calculated to obtain the venous tortuosity index. **b**: SD-OCT image at the baseline showing CME. **c**: SD-OCT image at 6 months showing a resolution of the CME. **d**: A false-color composite map of the optic nerve head was created using the LSFG findings at the baseline. The red area indicates a faster blood flow, and the blue area indicates a slower blood flow. **e**: A false-color composite map by LSFG at 6 months. There is no obvious difference in the blood flow as compared with the LSFG map at the baseline (**d**). **f**: Microperimetric map image at the baseline. A total of 37 stimulus locations covering the central 10° field were tested. The mean retinal sensitivity at the 37 locations is 19.1 dB. **g**: Microperimetric map image at 6 months. The mean retinal sensitivity at the 37 locations is 24.5 dB

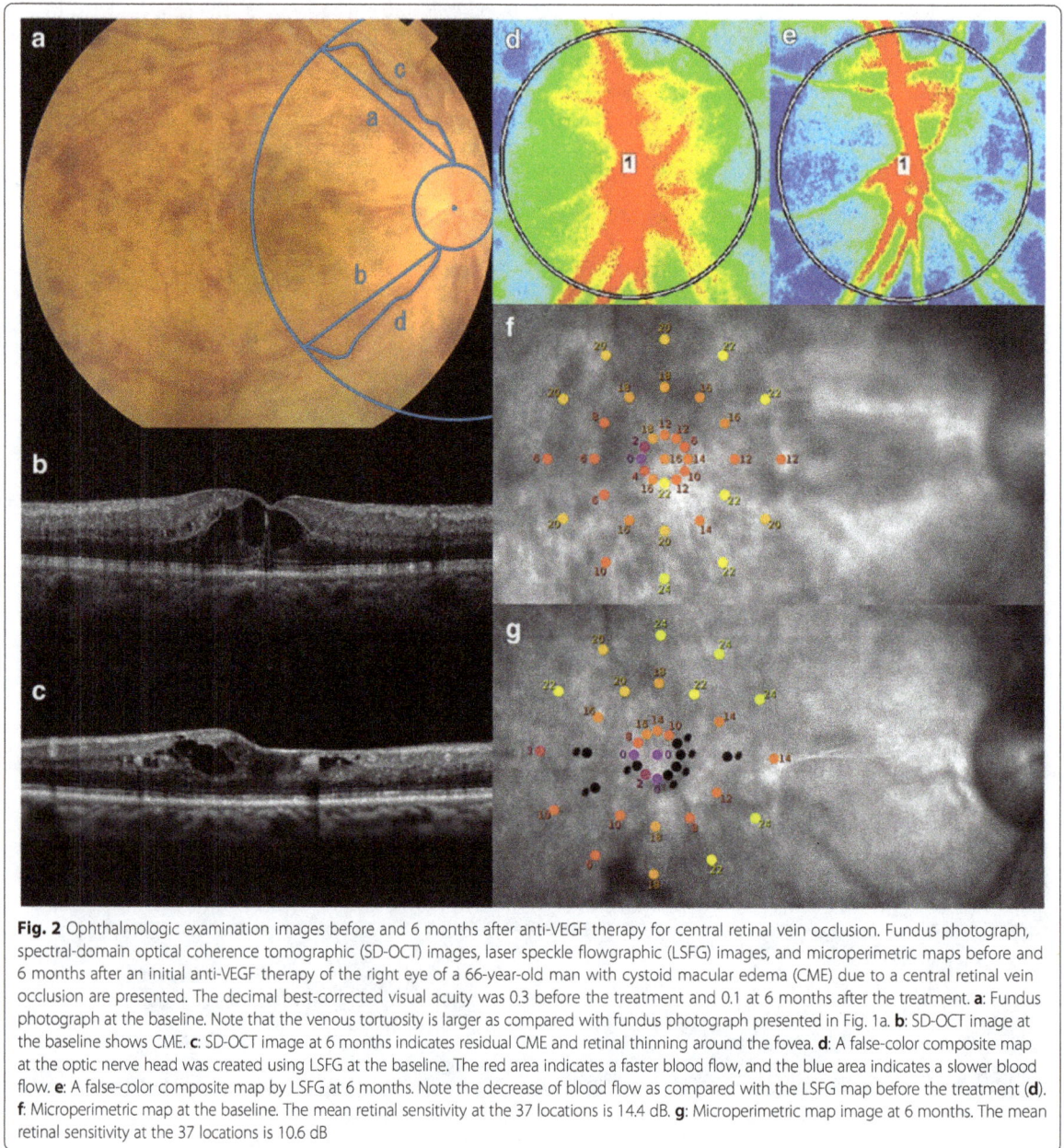

Fig. 2 Ophthalmologic examination images before and 6 months after anti-VEGF therapy for central retinal vein occlusion. Fundus photograph, spectral-domain optical coherence tomographic (SD-OCT) images, laser speckle flowgraphic (LSFG) images, and microperimetric maps before and 6 months after an initial anti-VEGF therapy of the right eye of a 66-year-old man with cystoid macular edema (CME) due to a central retinal vein occlusion are presented. The decimal best-corrected visual acuity was 0.3 before the treatment and 0.1 at 6 months after the treatment. **a**: Fundus photograph at the baseline. Note that the venous tortuosity is larger as compared with fundus photograph presented in Fig. 1a. **b**: SD-OCT image at the baseline shows CME. **c**: SD-OCT image at 6 months indicates residual CME and retinal thinning around the fovea. **d**: A false-color composite map at the optic nerve head was created using LSFG at the baseline. The red area indicates a faster blood flow, and the blue area indicates a slower blood flow. **e**: A false-color composite map by LSFG at 6 months. Note the decrease of blood flow as compared with the LSFG map before the treatment (**d**). **f**: Microperimetric map at the baseline. The mean retinal sensitivity at the 37 locations is 14.4 dB. **g**: Microperimetric map image at 6 months. The mean retinal sensitivity at the 37 locations is 10.6 dB

The patient's pupil was dilated with Mydrin P (1 % tropicamide and 2.5 % phenylephrine) 30 min prior to the LSFG examinations. During the examinations, the patients were instructed to fixate steadily on a target light while the speckle pattern on the ONH was recorded. With an auto-tracking system, the same site can be measured for several seconds. The relative blood flow velocity is represented by the MBR and displayed as a two-dimensional color map. The MBR of the vessel area is expressed as the MV and the MBR of the tissue area as the MT. The appropriate threshold between the vessel and tissue areas is automatically determined by the built-in software, and the MBR of the area of the major arteries and veins as MV and the MBR of the tissue area as MT can be calculated (Fig. 3) [9].

When measuring the retinal circulation with LSFG, the measurements are influenced by the deep choroidal circulation. Similarly, the ONH measurements are influenced by the blood flow of the ONH tissue (MT) [15, 16]. To evaluate the major arteriovenous circulation

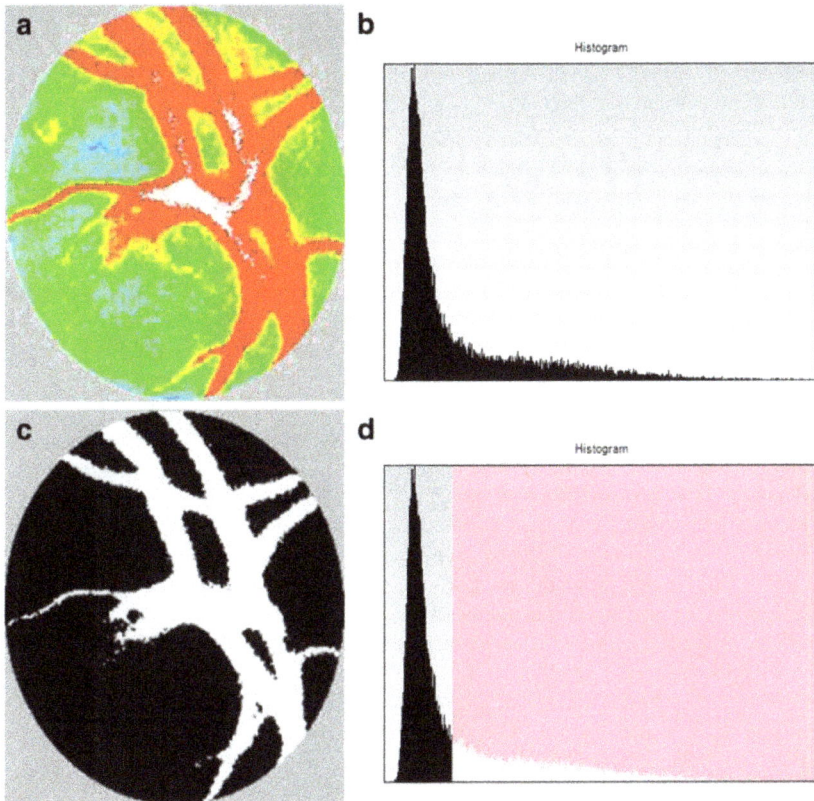

Fig. 3 Composite maps and histograms at the optic nerve head (ONH) created by laser speckle flowgraphy. **a**: A false-color composite map at the ONH. **b**: A histogramic analysis of the ONH. The vertical axis represents the number of pixels and the horizontal axis represents the mean blur rate. **c**: A binary format image for segmentation between the vessel (white area) and tissue (black area) areas. **d**: A histogram analyzed using the built-in image viewer software that uses an automated definitive threshold. The area to the left of the threshold line corresponds to the ONH tissue (black area in **c**), whereas the area to the right of the line corresponds to the ONH vessel (white area in **c**)

of the ONH excluding the blood flow of the ONH tissue, the value was obtained by subtracting the MT from the MV [11]. In addition, to exclude the influence of each patient's systemic circulation at the time of the measurements and to allow for inter-patient comparisons of the measurements, a corrected MBR value was obtained by the MBR (MV minus MT) of the affected eye divided by the MBR (MV minus MT) of the fellow eye [11]. The LSFG was measured at the baseline and at 1, 3, and 6 months after the initial treatment.

Microperimetry

The retinal sensitivity was determined by macular integrity assessment (MAIA) microperimetry (CenterVue, Padova, Italy; Figs. 1 and 2). MAIA testing was conducted in a dark room without pupil dilation. The testing conditions were similar to that described in detail in previous studies [17, 18]. Briefly, 37 loci in the 10° central macula was assessed using a 4 to 2 threshold strategy, a fixation target that consisted of a red circle with a

1° diameter, stimulus size of Goldmann III, background luminance of 4 apostilb (asb), maximum luminance of 1000 asb, and a stimulus dynamic range of 36 dB.

Calculation of venous tortuosity index

The venous tortuosity index was calculated as previously reported (Figs. 1 and 2) [20, 21]. Briefly, color fundus photographs were obtained with a Topcon fundus camera (TRC-50DX, Topcon, Tokyo, Japan). The course of the veins was traced using the Photoshop software (Adobe Systems, Inc. Ca, USA). Measurements of the superior and inferior venous arcades were obtained starting from the ONH margin to the crossing point of a circle whose diameter was the distance from the center of ONH to the fovea. NIH ImageJ software was used to measure the length of the tortuous vein and length of the chord of the vessel. The venous tortuosity was calculated by dividing the arc length of the retinal vein by the chord length of the same segment. The average of the venous tortuosity of the superior and inferior venous arcades was calculated to obtain the venous tortuosity index.

Statistical analyses

Repeated-measures analysis of variance (ANOVA) with Greenhouse-Geisser corrections was used to determine the significance of the changes in the BCVA, retinal sensitivity, corrected MBR, MV, MT, SBP, DBP, heart rate, IOP, MAP, and MOPP. The Bonferroni test was used for post hoc analysis. Pearson's correlation tests were used to determine the significance of correlations between the corrected MBR and the BCVA, retinal sensitivity, arteriovenous passage time, or venous tortuosity index. A P value of <0.05 was considered statistically significant.

Results

All patients were followed for at least 6 months after the initial injection of IVB or IVR. IVB was performed on 15 eyes and IVR on 16 eyes. The injections were administered two to five times (3.52 ± 0.88 (mean $\pm$ SD)) to each patient during the 6 months. According to the FA findings, the diagnosis of nonischemic CRVO was made in 26 eyes (Figs. 4 and 5), and the diagnosis of ischemic CRVO was made in 5 eyes. The SBP, DBP, heart rate, IOP, MAP, and MOPP were not significantly different among the baseline and 1, 3, and 6 months after the treatments ($P = 0.930$, $P = 0.958$, $P = 0.966$, $P = 0.745$, $P = 0.969$, $P = 0.886$, respectively).

At the baseline, the corrected MBR was 0.63 ± 0.26. The arteriovenous passage time on FA was 14.0 ± 5.2 s, and the venous tortuosity index on color fundus photograph was 1.113 ± 0.053. The corrected MBR was significantly correlated with the arteriovenous passage time ($r = -0.807$, $P < 0.001$; Fig. 6a) and venous tortuosity

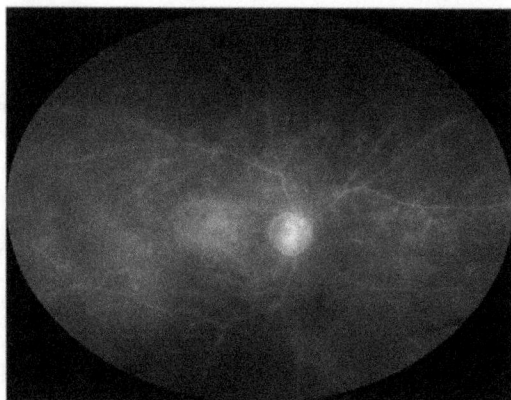

Fig. 5 Fluorescein angiography before anti-VEGF therapy for central retinal vein occlusion (CRVO). The same case presented in Fig. 2. Because there are not more than 10 disc areas of the nonperfusion areas, this case was also diagnosed with nonischemic CRVO

index ($r = -0.716$, $P < 0.001$). The corrected MBR after the first intravitreal injection was 0.60 ± 0.23 at 1 month, 0.61 ± 0.23 at 3 months, and 0.62 ± 0.28 at 6 months (Additional file 1). No significant differences were observed in the corrected MBR among the baseline and post-treatment times ($P = 0.379$). The MV in the affected eye was 34.8 ± 11.2 at the baseline, 32.0 ± 10.3 at 1 month, 31.6 ± 10.9 at 3 months, and 32.9 ± 12.2 at 6 months. No significant differences were observed in the MV among the baseline and post-treatment times ($P = 0.116$). The MT was 14.3 ± 4.6 at the baseline, 12.4 ± 3.8 at 1 month, 11.7 ± 4.0 at 3 months, and 12.3 ± 4.2 at 6 months. Significant differences were observed in the MT among the baseline and post-treatment times ($P = 0.003$). The MT at 1 and 3 months was significantly smaller than that at the baseline ($P = 0.011$, $P = 0.002$, respectively).

The mean BCVA was 0.68 ± 0.48 logMAR units at the baseline, 0.39 ± 0.36 logMAR units at 1 month after the first intravitreal injection, 0.36 ± 0.35 logMAR units at 3 months, and 0.33 ± 0.42 logMAR units at 6 months. Significant differences were observed in the BCVA among the baseline and post-treatment times ($P < 0.001$). The BCVA at 1, 3, and 6 months was significantly better than that at the baseline ($P < 0.001$, $P = 0.001$, $P = 0.007$, respectively).

The retinal sensitivity was 15.2 ± 7.5 dB at the baseline, 18.7 ± 6.6 dB at 1 month, 20.9 ± 6.0 dB at 3 months, and 20.4 ± 6.0 dB at 6 months. Significant differences were observed in the retinal sensitivity among the baseline and post-treatment times ($P < 0.001$). The retinal sensitivity at 1, 3, and 6 months was significantly better than that at the baseline ($P = 0.001$, $P < 0.001$, $P = 0.001$, respectively).

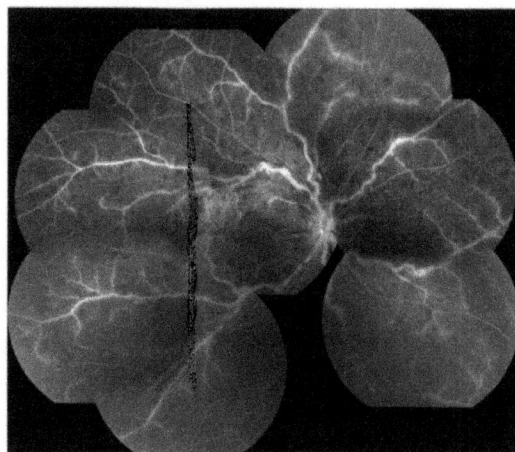

Fig. 4 Fluorescein angiography before anti-VEGF therapy for central retinal vein occlusion (CRVO). The same case presented in Fig. 1. Because there are not more than 10 disc areas of the nonperfusion areas, this case was diagnosed with nonischemic CRVO

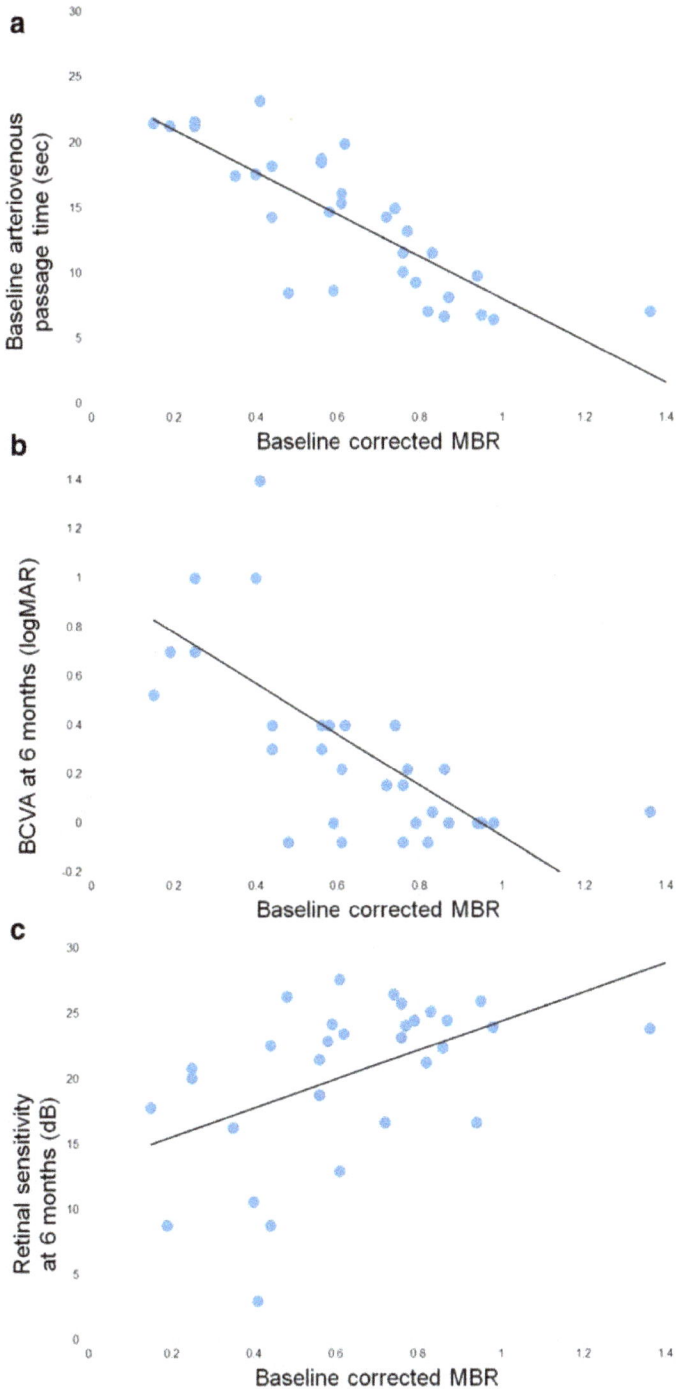

Fig. 6 (See legend on next page.)

(See figure on previous page.)
Fig. 6 Correlation between optic nerve head (ONH) circulation and arteriovenous passage time or visual function. Correlation between the baseline mean blur rate (MBR) at the ONH and the baseline arteriovenous passage time, the best-corrected visual acuity (BCVA) at 6 months, or mean retinal sensitivity at 6 months is presented. To exclude the influence of systemic circulation and blood flow of ONH tissue, the corrected MBR was calculated as; (MBR of ONH vessel area – MBR of ONH tissue area) in the affected eye ÷ (vascular MBR – tissue MBR) in the healthy fellow eye [11]. **a**: Correlation between the baseline corrected MBR at the ONH and the arteriovenous passage time at the baseline. The corrected MBR is significantly correlated with the arteriovenous passage time on fluorescein angiography ($r = -0.807$, $P <0.001$). The solid line represents the linear regression line ($y = -16.102x + 24.200$). **b**: Correlation between the baseline corrected MBR at the ONH and BCVA in logMAR units at 6 months after the initial treatment. The corrected MBR is significantly correlated with the BCVA at 6 months ($r = -0.651$, $P <0.001$). The solid line represents the linear regression line ($y = -1.036x + 0.983$). **c**: Correlation between the baseline corrected MBR at the ONH and mean retinal sensitivity at 6 months. The corrected MBR is significantly correlated with the retinal sensitivity at 6 months ($r = 0.485$, $P = 0.005$). The solid line represents the linear regression line ($y = 11.059x + 13.378$)

The MBR was significantly correlated with the BCVA (all $P <0.005$) and the retinal sensitivity (all $P <0.050$, Table 1) at all time points.

There was a significant correlation between the corrected MBR at the baseline and the BCVA at 6 months ($r = -0.651$, $P <0.001$; Fig. 6b). There was also a significant correlation between the corrected MBR at the baseline and the retinal sensitivity at 6 months ($r = 0.485$, $P = 0.005$; Fig. 6c).

Discussion

The results showed that the corrected MBR at the baseline was significantly correlated with the BCVA and retinal sensitivity at 6 months after anti-VEGF therapy. This indicates that the visual prognosis is good in patients with CRVO who have good blood flow on the ONH at the baseline. In a report on 3 cases with CRVO, Matsumoto et al. also suggested that the prognosis of CRVO may be predicted by measuring the MBR using LSFG [13]. In eyes with ME due to a BRVO, Nagaoka et al. reported that the visual prognosis was good when the retinal blood flow measured by laser Doppler velocimetry before IVB was good [12]. Taken together, these results suggest that the status of the blood flow prior to the treatment is a useful predictor of the post-treatment BCVA for both CRVO and BRVO.

Table 1 Correlations between MBR on ONH and BCVA or retinal sensitivity before and after anti-VEGF therapy

	Corrected MBR on ONH			
	Baseline	1 month	3 months	6 months
BCVA (logMAR)	$r = -0.543$	$r = -0.672$	$r = -0.546$	$r = -0.565$
	$P = 0.001$	$P < 0.001$	$P = 0.001$	$P <0.001$
Retinal sensitivity (dB)	$r = 0.572$	$r = 0.608$	$r = 0.552$	$r = 0.430$
	$P <0.001$	$P <0.001$	$P = 0.001$	$P = 0.015$

BCVA, best corrected visual acuity; Corrected MBR, (MBR of ONH vessel area – MBR of ONH tissue area) in the affected eye ÷ (vascular MBR – tissue MBR) in the unaffected eye; logMAR, logarithm of the minimum angle of resolution; MBR, mean blur rate; ONH, optic nerve head; VEGF, vascular endothelial growth factor

The measurements of the LSFG had excellent reproducibility which then permitted a non-invasive method to measure the ocular circulation. Aizawa et al. used LSFG and reported that the intra-session reproducibility of the MBR in the ONH of three continuous examinations was excellent with a coefficient of variation of 3.4 ± 2.0 and an intraclass correlation coefficient of 0.95 [9]. Aizawa et al. also reported that the MBR of the ONH tissue was strongly correlated with the visual field sensitivity in eyes with glaucoma [3]. In addition, Maekubo et al. reported that measurements of the ONH circulation by LSFG could be used for differentiating nonarteritic ischemic optic neuropathy from anterior optic neuritis [19]. Based on these findings, measuring the ONH circulation by LSFG can be considered a useful method in the clinic.

Yamada et al. measured the MBR on the ONH in eyes with untreated CRVO [11]. The corrected MBR was calculated to exclude the influence of the systemic circulation and blood flow of the ONH tissue. After obtaining the MBR values by subtracting the MT from the MV, the ONH blood flow was evaluated by taking the MBR values of the affected eye divided by the MBR values of the healthy fellow eye. The authors reported that this corrected MBR was significantly correlated with the arteriovenous passage time [11]. Similarly, a significant correlation was found between the corrected MBR and arteriovenous passage time in the present study. The strong correlation between the corrected MBR and arteriovenous passage time, which has been used as an indicator of retinal circulation, confirms that the method we used is a highly reliable way to evaluate the circulatory status of the ONH. In addition, Yamada et al. reported that the corrected MBR values in large ONH vessels were significantly correlated with the aqueous VEGF concentrations in eyes with CRVO [11].

It is sometimes difficult to distinguish the vessel and tissue areas at the ONH in eyes with CRVO, because dilatation or blood stasis of capillary vessel on ONH obscures the boundary between the large vessel and tissue on the LSFG images. Thus, the MV and MT values measured in eyes with CRVO may include a measurement error. However, the corrected MBR in the present study was significantly correlated with not only arteriovenous passage time on FA but also the venous tortuosity index on fundus photograph, which suggests that this measurement error is considered to be small.

Nitta et al. reported that there was no significant change in the MBR measured by LSFG in the retinal artery, retinal vein, or ONH after a single IVB injection in eyes with a BRVO [22]. Nagaoka et al. also reported no significant changes in the retinal blood flow measured by laser Doppler velocimetry after a single IVB injection for BRVO [12]. Consistent with these findings, our results showed no significant differences in the corrected MBR after IVB or IVR in eyes with a CRVO. On the other hand, Matsumoto et al. reported 3 cases of ME secondary to nonischemic CRVO in which the blood flow increased after IVBs [13]. In their case, the MBR increased in 3 or 4 weeks after the IVB was confirmed by LSFG, but long term changes of the MBR and exact relationship between the MBR and visual prognosis were unclear.

This study has several limitations. First, the sample size was small, and the follow-up period was short. Further studies with a larger sample size and longer follow-up periods would be required to confirm our findings. We also need to keep in mind that when using LSFG the MBR is a relative value of the blood flow velocity and not the absolute value. Therefore, when comparing the difference between eyes, we used the corrected MBR value. The other limitation is that the present study included both patients treated with IVB and those with IVR. Lastly, Mayama et al. reported that phenylephrine eye drops can depress the ONH circulation [23]. In our study, Mydrin P, tropicamide and phenylephrine, was used prior to the LSFG testing to obtain more accurate measurements of the ONH circulation with LSFG. Thus, there is a possibility that phenylephrine may have influenced the ONH circulation. However, because Mydrin P was administered to both the affected and unaffected eyes and ONH circulation was evaluated using the equation; the MBR of the affected eye/MBR of the unaffected eye, the magnitude of this influence may be small.

Conclusions

The blood flow velocity on the ONH was significantly correlated with the BCVA and retinal sensitivity before and after anti-VEGF therapy for CRVO. We suggest that the blood flow velocity of the ONH before the therapy is a predictive factor for the visual outcome after treatment for CRVO.

Ethics and consent to participate

Approval was obtained from the Institutional Review Board of Saneikai Tsukazaki Hospital prior to beginning this study, and the patients gave their written informed consent prior to their inclusion. The procedures used in this study adhered to the tenets of the Declaration of Helsinki.

Consent to publish

The patients have provided permission to publish clinical data of their case in this study.

Additional file

Additional file 1: Raw data (MBR, visual function). (DOC 68 kb)

Abbreviations
asb: apostilb; BCVA: best-corrected visual acuity; BRVO: branch retinal vein occlusion; CRVO: central retinal vein occlusion; DBP: diastolic blood pressure; FA: fluorescein angiography; IOP: intraocular pressure; IVB: intravitreal bevacizumab; IVR: intravitreal ranibizumab; LSFG: laser speckle flowgraphy; MAIA: macular integrity assessment; MAP: mean arterial pressure; MBR: mean blur rate; ME: macular edema; MOPP: mean ocular perfusion pressure; MT: mean blur rate of tissue area; MV: mean blur rate of vessel area; OCT: optical coherence tomography; ONH: optic nerve head; SBP: systolic blood pressure; SD-OCT: spectral-domain optical coherence tomography; UMIN: University hospital Medical Information Network; VEGF: vascular endothelial growth factor.

Competing interests
The authors declare that they have no competing interests.

Authors' contributions
Design of the study (YM), conduct of the study (DN, TN, YY, HT), management of the data (DN, YM, KS, KA, TN, YY, HT), analysis of the data (DN, YM, KS, KA, YK), interpretation of the data (DN, YM, KS, KA, YK), preparation of the manuscript (DN, YM) and overall coordination (YK). All authors read and approved the final manuscript.

Acknowledgements
This work was supported in part by Grants-in-Aid 25462717 (to YM) from the Ministry of Education, Culture, Sports, Science and Technology, Japan. The funding agencies had no role in the study design, data collection and analysis, decision to publish, or preparation of the manuscript. The authors thank Professor Emeritus Duco Hamasaki of the Bascom Palmer Eye Institute of the University of Miami for providing critical discussions and suggestions for our study and revision of the final manuscript.

Author details
¹Department of Ophthalmology, Saneikai Tsukazaki Hospital, Himeji, Japan. ²Department of Ophthalmology and Visual Sciences, Graduate School of Biomedical Sciences, Hiroshima University, Hiroshima, Japan. ³Department of Ophthalmology, Institute of Biomedical Sciences, Tokushima University Graduate School, 3-18-15 Kuramoto, Tokushima 770-8503, Japan.

References
1.   Yeh S, Kim SJ, Ho AC, Schoenberger SD, Bakri SJ, Ehlers JP, et al. Therapies for macular edema associated with central retinal vein occlusion: a report by the American Academy of Ophthalmology. Ophthalmology. 2015;122(4):769–78.
2.   Sugiyama T, Araie M, Riva CE, Schmetterer L, Orgul S. Use of laser speckle flowgraphy in ocular blood flow research. Acta Ophthalmol. 2010;88(7):723–9.
3.   Aizawa N, Kunikata H, Yokoyama Y, Nakazawa T. Correlation between optic disc microcirculation in glaucoma measured with laser speckle flowgraphy

and fluorescein angiography, and the correlation with mean deviation. Clin Exp Ophthalmol. 2014;42(3):293–4.

4. Iwase T, Ra E, Yamamoto K, Kaneko H, Ito Y, Terasaki H. Differences of retinal blood flow between arteries and veins determined by laser speckle flowgraphy in healthy subjects. Medicine (Baltimore). 2015;94(33):e1256.

5. Yanagida K, Iwase T, Yamamoto K, Ra E, Kaneko H, Murotani K, et al. Sex-related differences in ocular blood flow of healthy subjects using laser speckle flowgraphy. Invest Ophthalmol Vis Sci. 2015;56(8):4880–90.

6. Iwase T, Yamamoto K, Ra E, Murotani K, Matsui S, Terasaki H. Diurnal variations in blood flow at optic nerve head and choroid in healthy eyes: diurnal variations in blood flow. Medicine (Baltimore). 2015;94(6):e519.

7. Takahashi H, Sugiyama T, Tokushige H, Maeno T, Nakazawa T, Ikeda T, et al. Comparison of CCD-equipped laser speckle flowgraphy with hydrogen gas clearance method in the measurement of optic nerve head microcirculation in rabbits. Exp Eye Res. 2013;108:10–5.

8. Wang L, Cull GA, Piper C, Burgoyne CF, Fortune B. Anterior and posterior optic nerve head blood flow in nonhuman primate experimental glaucoma model measured by laser speckle imaging technique and microsphere method. Invest Ophthalmol Vis Sci. 2012;53(13):8303–9.

9. Aizawa N, Yokoyama Y, Chiba N, Omodaka K, Yasuda M, Otomo T, et al. Reproducibility of retinal circulation measurements obtained using laser speckle flowgraphy-NAVI in patients with glaucoma. Clin Ophthalmol. 2011;5:1171–6.

10. Sugiyama T, Kojima S, Ishida O, Ikeda T. Changes in optic nerve head blood flow induced by the combined therapy of latanoprost and beta blockers. Acta Ophthalmol. 2009;87(7):797–800.

11. Yamada Y, Suzuma K, Matsumoto M, Tsuiki E, Fujikawa A, Harada T, et al. Retinal blood flow correlates to aqueous vascular endothelial growth factor in central retinal vein occlusion. Retina. 2015;35(10):2037–42.

12. Nagaoka T, Sogawa K, Yoshida A. Changes in retinal blood flow in patients with macular edema secondary to branch retinal vein occlusion before and after intravitreal injection of bevacizumab. Retina. 2014;34(10):2037–43.

13. Matsumoto M, Suzuma K, Fukazawa Y, Yamada Y, Tsuiki E, Fujikawa A, et al. Retinal blood flow levels measured by laser speckle flowgraphy in patients who received intravitreal bevacizumab injection for macular edema secondary to central retinal vein occlusion. Retin Cases Brief Rep. 2014;8(1):60–6.

14. Group CVOS. Natural history and clinical management of central retinal vein occlusion. The Central Vein Occlusion Study Group. Arch Ophthalmol. 1997;115(4):486–91.

15. Isono H, Kishi S, Kimura Y, Hagiwara N, Konishi N, Fujii H. Observation of choroidal circulation using index of erythrocytic velocity. Arch Ophthalmol. 2003;121(2):225–31.

16. Nagahara M, Tamaki Y, Tomidokoro A, Araie M. In vivo measurement of blood velocity in human major retinal vessels using the laser speckle method. Invest Ophthalmol Vis Sci. 2011;52(1):87–92.

17. Sato S, Hirooka K, Baba T, Tenkumo K, Nitta E, Shiraga F. Correlation between the ganglion cell-inner plexiform layer thickness measured with cirrus HD-OCT and macular visual field sensitivity measured with microperimetry. Invest Ophthalmol Vis Sci. 2013;54(4):3046–51.

18. Roisman L, Ribeiro JC, Fechine FV, Lavinsky D, Moraes N, Campos M, et al. Does microperimetry have a prognostic value in central serous chorioretinopathy? Retina. 2014;34(4):713–8.

19. Maekubo T, Chuman H, Nao-I N. Laser speckle flowgraphy for differentiating between nonarteritic ischemic optic neuropathy and anterior optic neuritis. Jpn J Ophthalmol. 2013;57(4):385–90.

20. Ferrara DC, Koizumi H, Spaide RF. Early bevacizumab treatment of central retinal vein occlusion. Am J Ophthalmol. 2007;144(6):864–71.

21. Yasuda S, Kachi S, Kondo M, Ueno S, Kaneko H, Terasaki H. Significant correlation between retinal venous tortuosity and aqueous vascular endothelial growth factor concentration in eyes with central retinal vein occlusion. PLoS One. 2015;10(7):e0134267.

22. Nitta F, Kunikata H, Aizawa N, Omodaka K, Shiga Y, Yasuda M, et al. The effect of intravitreal bevacizumab on ocular blood flow in diabetic retinopathy and branch retinal vein occlusion as measured by laser speckle flowgraphy. Clin Ophthalmol. 2014;8:1119–27.

23. Mayama C, Ishii K, Saeki T, Ota T, Tomidokoro A, Araie M. Effects of topical phenylephrine and tafluprost on optic nerve head circulation in monkeys with unilateral experimental glaucoma. Invest Ophthalmol Vis Sci. 2010;51(8):4117–24.

22

Peripapillary choroidal thickness after intravitreal ranibizumab injections in eyes with neovascular age-related macular degeneration

Cheolmin Yun[1], Jaeryung Oh[1*], Kwang-Eon Choi[1], Soon-Young Hwang[2], Seong-Woo Kim[1] and Kuhl Huh[1]

Abstract

Background: The purpose of this study was to investigate peripapillary choroidal thickness (CT) in eyes with neovascular age-related macular degeneration (AMD) and to assess whether peripapillary CT is affected by intravitreal injection of ranibizumab (IVR) in eyes with neovascular AMD.

Methods: Peripapillary and subfoveal CT were measured in spectral domain optical coherence tomography images from 39 eyes of neovascular AMD patients and 39 eyes of age-matched controls retrospectively. The patients were treated with 0.5 mg IVR monthly for 3 months and retreated as needed. Peripapillary CT at baseline, 3 months and 6 months was measured at four locations (superior, nasal, inferior and temporal areas).

Results: The mean peripapillary and subfoveal baseline CTs of the eyes with neovascular AMD (153.3 ± 45.3 μm and 228.6 ± 78.6 μm) were not different from those of the controls (149.0 ± 42.3 μm and 221.4 ± 54.1 μm; $P = 0.665$ and $P = 0.639$, respectively). Subfoveal CT decreased at 3 months (213.8 ± 75.8 μm, $P < 0.001$) and 6 months (215.1 ± 72.8 μm, $P = 0.002$) following IVR treatment. Mean peripapillary CT did not show significant changes at 3 months (149.6 ± 43.8 μm, $P = 0.156$) or 6 months (150.0 ± 43.4 μm, $P = 0.187$). Subanalysis revealed that only temporal peripapillary CT decreased from baseline (167.1 ± 54.5 μm) to 3 months (159.4 ± 50.8 μm, $P = 0.010$) and was sustained at 6 months (160.6 ± 49.6, $P = 0.026$). However, superior, nasal and inferior peripapillary CT did not show significant changes after IVR.

Conclusions: Changes in peripapillary CT after IVR were limited to the macular area. This result may suggest that IVR does not affect CT outside of the macula in the eyes of patients with neovascular AMD.

Keywords: Age-related macular degeneration, Choroidal thickness, Optical coherence tomography, Peripapillary choroidal thickness, Ranibizumab

Background

Age-related macular degeneration (AMD) is a leading cause of vision loss in the elderly worldwide [1]. With the development and introduction of anti-vascular endothelial growth factor (VEGF) therapy, the functional outcomes of neovascular AMD have been markedly improved [2–4]. Ranibizumab (Lucentis; Genentech, Inc., San Francisco, CA; co-developed by Genentech, Inc and Novartis), is an

FDA approved VEGF-A inhibitor that is commonly used for the treatment of AMD [5].

Previous studies have suggested that AMD may be a vascular disorder associated with altered blood flow in the choroid [6, 7]. Because abnormalities in choroidal circulation and structure are thought to be associated with the pathogenesis of AMD [8, 9], there have been many studies on choroidal thickness (CT) in AMD [10–13]. Recently, some studies have suggested that the CT in patients with neovascular AMD may be affected by intravitreal injection of ranibizumab (IVR) [14, 15]. Because VEGF is known to be associated with the maintenance of choriocapillaries and ocular blood flow, there have been concerns regarding

* Correspondence: ojr4991@yahoo.co.kr
[1]Department of Ophthalmology, Korea University College of Medicine, 126-1 Anam-dong 5-ga, Sungbuk-gu, Seoul 136-705, South Korea
Full list of author information is available at the end of the article

potential undesired effects of anti-VEGF therapy on the choroid [16, 17]. However, recent studies found that CT changes following IVR treatment for neovascular AMD were limited to the choroid of the macular region [14, 15]. It is not certain whether CT outside the macula is affected by IVR, and the effect of anti-VEGF therapy on CT of normal choroid without overlying retinal pathology remains unclear [18].

The choroid is a highly vascular tissue of the eye that supplies blood to the outer retina, retinal pigment epithelium (RPE), and possibly the optic nerve head [19]. The choroid is supplied by various ciliary arteries that originate from the ophthalmic arteries [20]. The branches of the posterior ciliary artery (PCA) consist of long PCAs and short PCAs [20]. The posterior choriocapillaries in the peripapillary and submacular region are supplied by the short PCAs. These arteries have strictly segmental blood flow without anastomosis and supply a well-defined sector of the choroid [21]. The medial PCA supplies the nasal choroid, while the lateral PCA supplies the area of the choroid not supplied by the medial PCA [20]. Therefore, blood flow to the nasal peripapillary choroid could differ from the flow to the temporal peripapillary and subfoveal choroid. Recently, several studies on the choroid outside of the macula in retinal disease have focused on the peripapillary choroid and the nasal peripapillary choroid represented the choroid outside of macula [22–24]. We hypothesized that the change in CT after IVR would differ between the macula and areas outside of the macula. We also investigated the peripapillary and subfoveal CT in neovascular AMD and the change in CT after IVR treatment.

Methods

The Institutional Review Board of Korea University Medical center approved this study (IRB No. ED14121), and all research and data collection was conducted in accordance with the tenets of the Declaration of Helsinki. We performed a retrospective case–control study of patients 50 years of age or older who were diagnosed with neovascular AMD between February 2011 and March 2013 at Korea University Medical Center. We included patients who underwent IVR for neovascular AMD. Age-matched controls were selected from the spectral domain optical coherence tomography (SD-OCT) database based on classification of normal eyes. Patients with a primary diagnosis of AMD, a history of laser photocoagulation of the macula, serous detachment of the macula, rhegmatogenous or tractional retinal detachment, high myopia, tapetoretinal degeneration, optic disc abnormalities such as glaucoma, beta zone peripapillary atrophy, or neurologic deficits were excluded from the control group.

Neovascular AMD was diagnosed in patients who were older than 50 and showed exudative changes from choroidal neovascularization (CNV) on fluorescein angiography (FA) and SD-OCT. This study excluded cases of polypoidal choroidal vasculopathy (PCV). PCV was diagnosed based on the presence of CNV on FA with characteristic findings on SD-OCT and if any one of the following criteria were met: 1) branching vascular networks underneath the RPE and focal hyperfluorescent polyps were present on indocyanine green angiography, 2) recurrent hemorrhagic or serous pigmented epithelial detachments were detected, or 3) the existence of an elevated reddish-orange lesion protruding from the choroid on fundus examination [25–28]. Neovascular lesions were classified into type 1 (sub-RPE), type 2 (subretinal) or type 3 (intraretinal) according to the MPS criteria and to the guidelines provided by Freund and colleagues based on angiographic and OCT features [29–31]. Classifications were independently determined by two retina specialists (C.Y. and J.A.). Disagreements were resolved upon further review by two observers. Cases with refractive errors ≤ -6.0 diopters or axial length ≥ 26.0 mm and cases with a history of cataract surgery within the past 6 months, refractive surgery or vitreoretinal surgery were also excluded from this study. Patients with a history of glaucoma, optic nerve disorder, beta zone peripapillary atrophy, retinal or choroidal disorder including vascular disease or uveitis and previous treatment with photodynamic therapy or other intravitreal anti-VEGF injection were also excluded from this study. Images were excluded if they were found to be low quality with a signal strength indicator (Q-factor) value < 45 or if the choroidal layer was not visible due to severe subfoveal hemorrhage. Data were collected at baseline, 3 months and 6 months after IVR.

Intravitreal injection of ranibizumab

A single surgeon (JO) performed all injections. Before intravitreal injection, local anesthesia was induced with proxymetacaine hydrochloride drops (Alcaine 0.5 %; Alcon, Fort Worth, TX, USA). After the periocular disinfection procedure, the patient was draped. With lid speculum insertion, 5 % povidone iodine was introduced on the conjunctiva for 30 s. After injection of 0.05 ml ranibizumab into the eye 3.5 mm from the limbus, antibiotic eye drops were administered. After three monthly injections of IVRs, patients were followed up every month, and retreatment was considered if any of the following changes were observed: (1) visual acuity loss with the presence of fluid in the macula detected by OCT, (2) OCT central retinal thickness (CRT) increased by at least 100 μm, (3) new macular hemorrhage, or (4) persistent fluid on OCT at least 1 month after the previous IVR [32]. Responders were defined as patients with a disappearance of subretinal fluid or macular edema or those with a decrease in CRT of more than 100 μm on OCT 3 months after IVR as compared to the initial visit. Non-responders were defined as those with no change in subretinal fluid or macular edema or with a decrease in CRT of less than 100 μm on OCT when compared to the initial visit.

Spectral domain optical coherence tomography
This study used a SD-OCT (3D OCT-1000 Mark II, software version 6.21; Topcon Corp., Tokyo, Japan) with a wavelength of 840 nm, a horizontal resolution of less than 20 μm, and an axial resolution of up to 5 μm. Choroidal mode was used to capture choroidal layer images. Horizontal 6-mm line-scans centered on the fovea and circle scans in a 3.4-mm zone around the optic disc were obtained. The line scan and circle scan consisted of 1024 A-scans, and circle scan images were scanned four times. All images were averaged to improve the signal-to-noise ratio.

Measurement of peripapillary choroidal thickness
Peripapillary CT was measured in a 3.4-mm diameter circle scan performed around the optic disc. The circle scan was performed using a standard protocol for retinal nerve fiber layer (RNFL) assessment, and the retinal thickness (RT) and RNFL thickness was assessed in four sectors (superior, nasal, inferior and temporal) around the disc. The thickness value represents the mean thickness of the layers within each sector. Peripapillary RT and RNFL thickness were obtained through automatic segmentation using the OCT viewer software after confirmation of appropriately placed segmentation lines. In cases with abnormal segmentation of the RPE or NFL due to drusen ($n = 1$) or posterior hyaloid membranes ($n = 3$), the segmentation errors were modified. Peripapillary CT was measured using a previously reported method [22, 24, 33]. Briefly, the modification tool in the SD-OCT image viewer program was used to move the segmentation line indicating RPE to the chorioscleral junction. With this modification, we obtained the chorioretinal thickness between the ILM and chorioscleral junction. Peripapillary CT was calculated by subtracting RT from the chorioretinal thickness in each sector (Fig. 1). All measurements were performed by two independent blinded examiners (CY and KC), and the mean value from the two observers was used for analysis.

Measurement of subfoveal choroidal thickness
Choroidal layer images of the macula were obtained using choroidal mode within the OCT with a 6-mm line scan image centered on the fovea [12, 34]. CT measurement was performed manually with a caliper tool built in the image viewer program of SD-OCT. CT was defined as the length between the outer surface of a hyper-reflective line of the RPE and the inner margin of the

chorioscleral junction perpendicularly (Fig. 1). All measurements were performed by two independent, blinded examiners (CY and KC). The mean value from the two observers was used for analysis.

Statistical methods
Controls were selected from the hospital OCT database and frequency-matched to the age distribution of AMD cases with a statistician's assistance. If a patient had neovascular AMD in both eyes, the right eye was selected for analysis, and age matching was based on the statistician's discretion.

A Kolmogorov-Smirnov test was performed to determine whether the variables demonstrated a normal distribution. The student t-test, chi-square test and Fisher's exact test were used to compare the parameters between AMD patients and the controls. A paired t-test was used to analyze the difference between the peripapillary CT, RT and RNFL thickness means in each sector and the macular CT during each visit. The Pearson's correlation test was used to analyze the relationships between parameters.

By comparing CT before and after IVR, the proportional change in CT was calculated as the difference in CT (CT at 3 months – CT at baseline) divided by CT at baseline. The control group parameters included mean refractive error, RT, RNFL thickness and CT of the right eye. Statistical analyses were performed using SPSS software version 20.0 for Windows (IBM Corp., Armonk, NY, USA). Results were considered statistically significant at P values < 0.05.

Results
After reviewing the medical records of 79 patients who were diagnosed with neovascular AMD, we excluded 23 cases of PCV, two cases of high myopia, one case of history of vitreoretinal surgery, three cases of low quality image, six cases of glaucoma, five cases of beta zone peripapillary atrophy. In a total of 39 eyes of 39 patients with neovascular AMD and an equal number of controls eyes were included in this study. Mean age at diagnosis in the neovascular AMD group was not different from that of the control group (Table 1). There were no differences in sex or lens status between the two groups. The mean number of IVRs within the 6-month period was 4.4 ± 0.9 (range, 3–6). Mean BCVA (LogMAR) of the 39 patients was 0.73 ± 0.45 at baseline, 0.50 ± 0.38 at 3 months, and 0.51 ± 0.44 at 6 months. Mean BCVA values at 3 months and 6 months were significantly improved when compared to baseline (all, $P < 0.001$). At baseline, the neovascular lesions were categorized as type 2 (35 eyes, 89.7 %) and type 3 (4 eyes, 10.3 %).

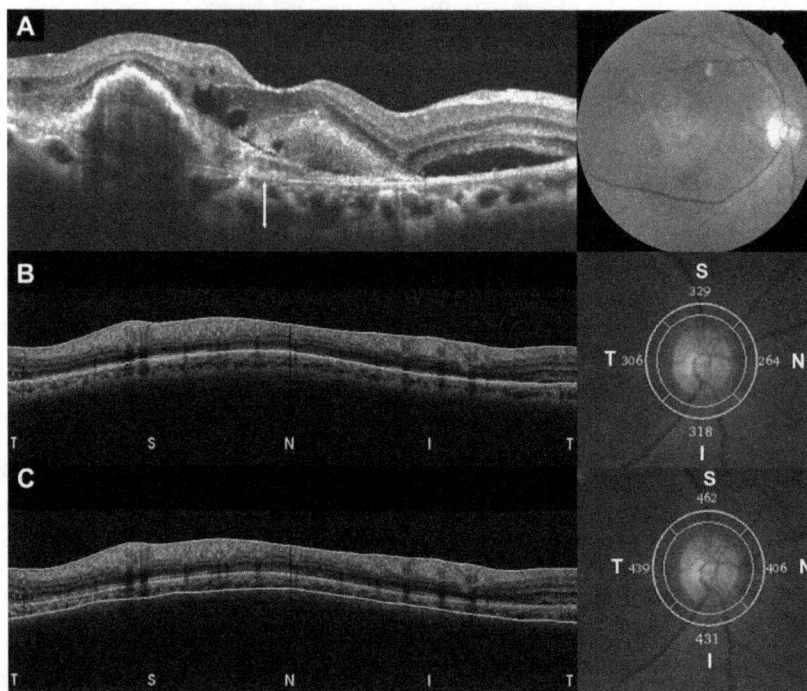

Fig. 1 Measurement of subfoveal and peripapillary choroidal thickness (CT). Subfoveal CT (white arrow) was measured perpendicularly from the outer surface of the line corresponding to the retinal pigment epithelium (RPE) to the inner chorioscleral junction (**a**). A 360°, 3.4-mm-diameter circle scan provided retinal thickness (RT) and retinal nerve fiber layer (RNFL) thickness from four sectors around the optic disc. The thickness value of each sector represents the mean thickness of the layers within each sector (**b**). The RT of each sector was determined between two segmentation lines of the internal limiting membrane (ILM) and RPE. The segmentation line of the RPE was then modified to the chorioscleral junction by the examiner using the modification tool in the optical coherence tomography image viewer program (**c**). Chorioretinal thickness between the ILM and chorioscleral junction was obtained, and CT was calculated by subtracting the RT from the chorioretinal thickness of each sector. T, temporal; S, superior; I, inferior; N, nasal

Comparison of baseline choroidal thickness in AMD eyes and controls

The mean peripapillary CT of the eyes in the AMD group was not significantly different from that of the control group (Table 2). In the control group, the mean peripapillary CT correlated with age ($r = -0.415$, $P = 0.009$), but the mean peripapillary CT of the AMD group did not correlate with age ($r = -0.169$, $P = 0.303$).

The mean subfoveal CT of the AMD group was not significantly different from that of the control group (Table 2). In the control group, subfoveal CT correlated with age ($r = -0.386$, $P = 0.015$), but subfoveal CT in the AMD group did not correlate with age ($r = -0.162$, $P = 0.324$).

Choroidal thickness after intravitreal injection of ranibizumab

The mean peripapillary CT at baseline in the AMD group decreased after IVR, but this was not a statistically significant difference at 3 months or 6 months (Table 3). Among the four sectors of the peripapillary area, only the temporal

Table 1 Baseline characteristics of patients with age-related macular degeneration and age-matched controls

	AMD group (n = 39)	Control group (n = 39)	P value
Mean age at diagnosis (years)	68.8 ± 6.5	68.3 ± 6.5	0.755*
Sex (M : F)	18 : 21	16 : 23	0.648**
Lens (Phakia : Pseudophakia)	37 : 2	35 : 4	0.675**
Refractive error (D)[a]	0.46 ± 1.43	0.34 ± 1.64	0.734*
Type of neovascularization, eyes (%)			
Type 2	35 (89.7 %)		
Type 3	4 (10.3 %)		

Continuous variables are expressed as mean ± standard deviation
*P value based on student t-test
**P value based on Chi-square test or Fisher's exact test for categorical variables
[a]Refractive errors were obtained from 37 eyes in the AMD group and 35 eyes in the control group, which included all eyes except two eyes exhibiting pseudophakia in the AMD group and four eyes exhibiting pseudophakia in the control group
AMD age-related macular degeneration, M Male, F female, D diopters

Table 2 Comparison of choroidal thickness between patients with neovascular age-related macular degeneration and age-matched controls

	AMD group (n = 39)	Control group (n = 39)	P value*
Subfoveal CT (μm)	228.6 ± 78.6	224.2 ± 54.7	0.775
Peripapillary CT (μm)			
Mean	153.2 ± 45.3	148.2 ± 38.8	0.600
Superior	165.2 ± 49.5	160.3 ± 42.6	0.637
Nasal	153.2 ± 43.0	148.3 ± 36.5	0.591
Inferior	127.3 ± 40.0	122.7 ± 32.5	0.577
Temporal	167.1 ± 54.5	161.4 ± 49.8	0.635

Continuous variables are expressed as mean ± standard deviation
*Comparison of baseline parameters between the control group and AMD group, P value was based on the student t-test
AMD age-related macular degeneration, CT choroidal thickness

peripapillary CT decreased at both 3 and 6 months, while other areas showed no significant changes. Mean subfoveal CT at baseline in the AMD group was significantly reduced at 3 months and at 6 months (Table 3) (Figs. 2 and 3). The difference in value or proportion of subfoveal and mean peripapillary CT at 6 months was not associated with the number of IVRs received (Pearson's correlation test, all, $P > 0.05$). Mean subfoveal CT and peripapillary CT

at both 3 and 6 months showed no significant differences when compared with the baseline values of the normal controls. An additional file shows this in more detail [Additional file 1].

By neovascularization type, the type 2 group showed decreased subfoveal CT at both 3 and 6 months (all, $P < 0.05$), while the mean peripapillary CT showed no changes (all, $P > 0.05$) (Table 4). The type 3 group showed a tendency toward decreased subfoveal CT, but this was not seen in mean peripapillary CT. Because of the small number of type 3 cases, the statistical power was not available.

Thirty eyes (76.9 %) showed treatment response and nine eyes (23.1 %) showed non-response. In univariate analysis, a decreased proportion of both subfoveal CT and temporal peripapillary CT were associated with treatment response (Table 5). In multivariate analysis, only a decreased proportion of subfoveal CT was associated with treatment response (Table 6).

Retinal thickness and retinal nerve fiber layer thickness

CRT and temporal peripapillary RT of the AMD group decreased at 3 months and at 6 months when compared with the baseline values, while the mean RNFL thickness showed no significant change 3 months or 6 months after IVR (Table 3).

Table 3 Changes in choroidal thickness, retinal thickness and retinal nerve fiber layer thickness during ranibizumab treatment

	Baseline	3 months	P value*	6 months	P value*
Subfoveal CT (μm)	228.6 ± 78.6	213.8 ± 75.5	<0.001	214.1 ± 72.8	<0.001
Peripapillary CT (μm)					
Mean	153.2 ± 45.3	149.6 ± 43.8	0.156	150.0 ± 43.4	0.187
Superior	165.2 ± 49.5	162.2 ± 48.7	0.252	162.6 ± 47.8	0.330
Nasal	153.2 ± 43.0	151.6 ± 43.3	0.532	150.8 ± 42.7	0.378
Inferior	127.3 ± 40.0	125.1 ± 38.3	0.321	125.9 ± 37.5	0.555
Temporal	167.1 ± 54.5	159.4 ± 50.8	0.010	160.6 ± 49.6	0.011
Central RT (μm)	300.4 ± 93.0	233.6 ± 62.0	0.001	232.9 ± 61.9	0.001
Peripapillary RT (μm)					
Mean	282.8 ± 19.7	279.9 ± 22.1	0.009	279.8 ± 20.2	0.033
Superior	303.0 ± 28.3	301.6 ± 30.1	0.169	300.7 ± 26.9	0.171
Nasal	250.4 ± 22.1	251.0 ± 26.7	0.732	251.0 ± 22.9	0.812
Inferior	300.4 ± 22.0	300.2 ± 24.8	0.829	298.2 ± 22.7	0.246
Temporal	276.8 ± 21.2	267.0 ± 20.1	<0.001	269.3 ± 21.9	0.015
RNFL thickness (μm)					
Mean	111.7 ± 11.4	112.9 ± 10.6	0.666	113.1 ± 11.9	0.611
Superior	130.4 ± 17.5	131.8 ± 16.3	0.736	134.0 ± 16.4	0.373
Nasal	89.3 ± 15.8	92.2 ± 18.9	0.478	90.4 ± 19.3	0.790
Inferior	135.1 ± 16.9	137.9 ± 17.0	0.439	138.6 ± 18.9	0.350
Temporal	92.1 ± 16.2	89.4 ± 13.4	0.379	89.4 ± 16.0	0.385

Continuous variables are expressed as mean ± standard deviation
*Comparison of the parameters in each AMD group visit; P value was based on the paired t-test
CT choroidal thickness, RT retinal thickness, RNFL retinal nerve fiber layer

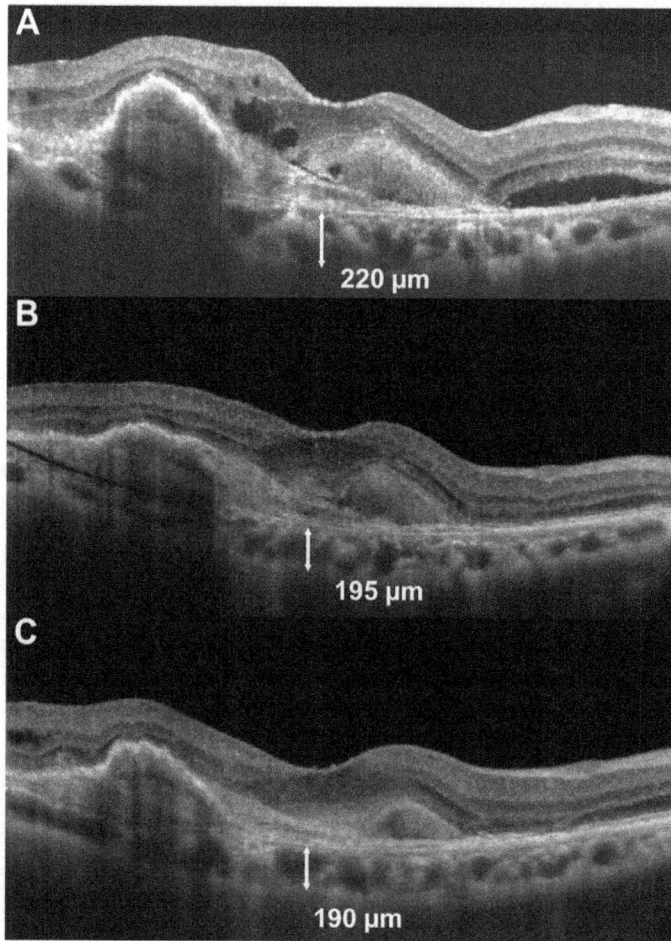

Fig. 2 Changes in subfoveal choroidal thickness (SFCT) in a 74-year-old woman with neovascular age-related macular degeneration. SD-OCT image at baseline (**a**) showed subretinal fluid accumulation in the macula. After three consecutive monthly injections of ranibizumab, the subretinal fluid disappeared, and the SFCT decreased as compared with the baseline (**b**). At 6 months, the SFCT was still lower compared with baseline (**c**)

Interobserver reliability

Interobserver reliability was assessed by analysis of intra-class correlation coefficients. The intraclass correlation coefficients ranged from 0.940 to 0.984. An additional file shows this in more detail [Additional file 2].

Discussion

In this study, macular and peripapillary CT in the AMD group did not differ from those in the control group at baseline. The macular CT results in AMD patients and normal controls are consistent with those found in previous studies, which revealed no significant differences between AMD eyes and normal eyes [11–13]. Because it has been suggested that AMD is a vascular disorder associated with altered blood flow in the choroid [6, 7], we wondered if there were regional differences in CT between the macula and outside of the macula. However,

we found no such difference in CT between the macula and outside of the macula in the neovascular AMD and control groups.

Peripapillary CT outside of the macula did not change after IVR at 6 months. These findings differed from the subfoveal choroid results. In this study, both subfoveal CT and temporal peripapillary CT decreased after three monthly IVRs, and the reduction in CT was sustained for 6 months. CT outside of the macula, including superior, nasal and inferior peripapillary CT, was not affected by IVR. Even though there was a trend toward a reduction in PCT in all sectors, these differences were not statistically significant. This may indicate that ranibizumab affects the choroid under and around the macula but not the choroid outside of the macula. We did not investigate the change in CT in AMD eyes without treatment. Therefore, the results of our study could not confirm

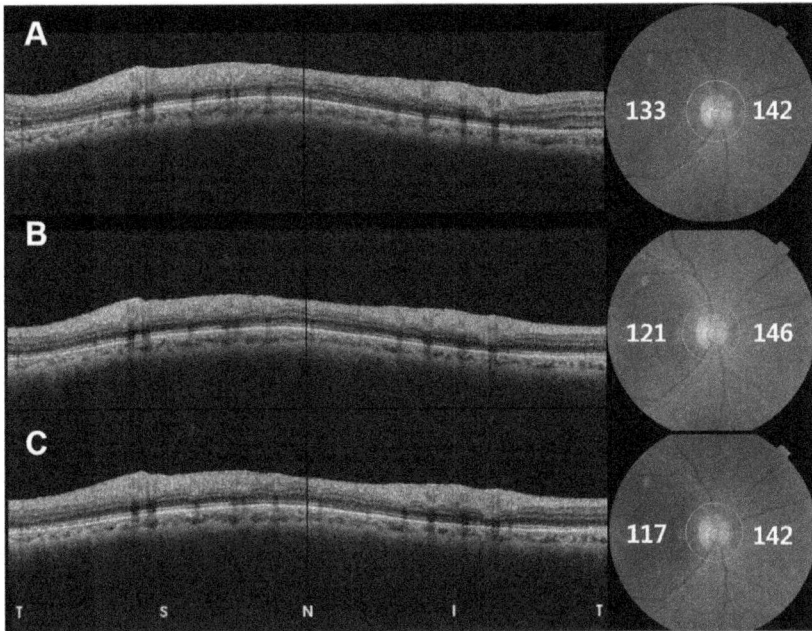

Fig. 3 Changes in peripapillary choroidal thickness (PCT) of the patient shown in Fig. 2. Peripapillary circle scans at baseline (**a**), 3 months (**b**) and 6 months after the intravitreal injection of ranibizumab (**c**). Nasal PCT at baseline (142 μm) was not changed at 3 months (146 μm) and 6 months (142 μm), while temporal PCT at baseline (133 μm) decreased at 3 months (121 μm) and 6 months (117 μm). T, temporal; S, superior; I, inferior; N, nasal

if choroidal thinning of the subfoveal area is directly induced by the IVR or by the disease course of AMD. However, the results of the current study may suggest that the CT outside of the macula is not involved in the change in CT after IVR in eyes with AMD.

In the current study, subfoveal CT decreased after IVR, a result consistent with previous studies [14, 15]. Yamazaki et al. suggested that IVR may have a pharmacologic effect on the choroid underneath the CNV lesion [15]. Changes in CT associated with IVR may be explained by two possible

Table 4 Changes in choroidal thickness during ranibizumab treatment according to neovascularization type

		Baseline	3 months	P value*	6 months	P value*
Type 2	Subfoveal CT (μm)	238.7 ± 75.8	223.4 ± 72.4	<0.001	224.0 ± 68.5	0.002
(n = 35)	Peripapillary CT (μm)					
	Mean	157.3 ± 45.1	153.3 ± 43.1	0.154	153.4 ± 42.6	0.163
	Superior	168.8 ± 47.9	165.6 ± 46.3	0.266	165.9 ± 45.3	0.313
	Nasal	155.9 ± 43.7	154.1 ± 43.5	0.511	153.2 ± 42.4	0.340
	Inferior	131.7 ± 39.8	129.2 ± 38.1	0.285	129.9 ± 38.3	0.456
	Temporal	172.5 ± 53.6	164.4 ± 49.4	0.011	164.5 ± 49.2	0.010
Type 3	Subfoveal CT (μm)	145.0 (102.8, 171.2)	124.0 (89.5, 175.8)	N/A	117.0 (83.4, 182.5)	N/A
(n = 4)	Peripapillary CT (μm)					
	Mean	112.6 (89.3, 150.8)	117.0 (80.0, 152.5)	N/A	117.0 (83.8, 182.5)	N/A
	Superior	125.0 (82.5, 193.8)	129.0 (72.8, 194.3)	N/A	131.0 (75.0, 195.3)	N/A
	Nasal	132.5 (98.5, 156.0)	129.5 (91.0, 167.3)	N/A	128.0 (87.5, 173.0)	N/A
	Inferior	88.5 (83.0, 93.3)	84.5 (77.8, 104.0)	N/A	84.5 (77.8, 110.0)	N/A
	Temporal	112.5 (84.0, 161.3)	116.5 (71.5, 160.0)	N/A	117.0 (71.3, 162.8)	N/A

Continuous variables are expressed as mean ± standard deviation or median (interquartile range)
*Comparison of parameters in each AMD group visit; P value was based on paired t-test
CT choroidal thickness, N/A not applicable

Table 5 Univariate analysis for estimating factors associated with a 3-month response after intravitreal injection of ranibizumab

Variables	P value*	OR (95 % CI)
Sex (male)	0.521	1.635 (0.365–7.326)
Age (years)	0.945	1.004 (0.894–1.128)
Eye (OD)	0.237	0.400 (0.088–1.826)
Lens status (phakic eye)	1.000	N/A
Baseline subfoveal CT (μm)	0.296	0.994 (0.984–1.005)
Baseline mean peripapillary CT (μm)	0.789	0.998 (0.981–1.015)
Decreased amount of subfoveal CT (μm)	0.097	1.030 (0.995–1.066)
Decreased proportion of subfoveal CT (%)	0.007	1.124 (1.033–1.223)
Decreased amount of mean peripapillary CT (μm)	0.094	1.041 (0.993–1.092)
Decreased proportion of mean peripapillary CT (%)	0.077	1.055 (0.994–1.120)
Decreased amount of mean temporal peripapillary CT (μm)	0.061	1.043 (0.998–1.090)
Decreased proportion of mean temporal peripapillary CT (%)	0.029	1.070 (1.007–1.137)

*P value based on logistic regression analysis
OD oculus dexter, CT choroidal thickness, N/A not applicable

mechanisms. First, decreased intraocular VEGF after IVR might affect the CT. VEGF is known to be associated with vasculogenesis and blood vessel hyperpermeability [35–37]. Hypoxia and ischemia of RPE from inadequate choroidal perfusion might produce VEGF, which may lead to neovascular AMD [38]. Both the subfoveal choroid and the peripapillary choroid may be affected by increased VEGF. Although the natural course of CT in neovascular AMD is unknown, vasodilatation may be expected in the choroid of neovascular AMD eyes, as VEGF is associated with vascular permeability [36, 37]. After a decrease in intraocular VEGF levels due to IVR, changes in vascular permeability and CT in both the macular and peripapillary region may follow. In this study, the changes in macular and temporal peripapillary CT were significant while CT outside of macula showed no significant changes. This might suggest that IVR mainly affects the abnormal CNV and the hyperpermeability associated with the CNV under and around the macula. In addition, vasoconstriction of the choroid after IVR may affect CT. Although the effect of VEGF on choroidal structure, thickness and large vessels is not clearly defined, VEGF is known to be essential for the development of the

choroid and maintenance of the choriocapillaries [39, 40]. Furthermore, the vasoconstrictive effect of ranibizumab might affect the choroidal vessels and thickness [41, 42]. In this study, a significant change in CT was observed only in the macular and temporal peripapillary areas. Thus, even though we cannot exclude the vasoconstrictive effect of IVR on the macula, IVR does not result in a change of CT outside of the macula.

In this study, decreased proportions of subfoveal and temporal peripapillary CT were associated with treatment response after three monthly doses of ranibizumab. However, in multivariate analysis, a decreased proportion of subfoveal CT was a factor associated with treatment response, which might result from the positive correlation between a decreased proportion of subfoveal CT and temporal peripapillary CT. This may suggest that decreased hyperpermeability or vasoconstriction and regression of CNV after IVR change the choroid under and around the macula. However, we cannot conclude whether decreased CT is a preceding factor associated with treatment response or if decreased CT is a result of treatment response, as the decreased ratio of CT is not a preoperative finding but rather a parameter that is calculated from CT before and after IVR.

However, the observed decrease in CT is insufficient to limit the clinical use of ranibizumab. In the present study, although macular and temporal peripapillary CT were decreased at 3 and 6 months after IVR when compared to the initial CT, the reduction in CT was relatively small, and was not associated with a loss of BCVA. In addition, CT after IVR at 3 and 6 months was not different from that of the normal controls. In addition, the non-significant changes in CT outside of the macula suggest that the effect of IVRs outside of the macula is minimal. IVRs decreased temporal peripapillary RT, but

Table 6 Multivariate analysis for estimating factors associated with a 3-month response after intravitreal injection of ranibizumab

Variables	P value*	OR (95 % CI)
Sex (male)	0.511	1.879 (0.287–12.306)
Age (years)	0.602	1.038 (0.903–1.193)
Decreased proportion of subfoveal CT	0.042	1.362 (1.016–1.825)
Decreased proportion of mean temporal peripapillary CT	0.166	0.861 (0.696–1.064)

*P value based on logistic regression analysis
CT choroidal thickness

may be associated with a decrease in CRT. The RT of other peripapillary areas and RNFL thickness were not affected by IVRs.

In the control group, the subfoveal CT and peripapillary CT showed a negative relationship with age. Previous studies have demonstrated that the subfoveal CT of normal controls and patients with dry AMD are correlated with age, but the eyes with neovascular AMD demonstrated a weaker correlation between subfoveal CT and age [13, 34]. The peripapillary CT was also related to age and had a negative correlation with the results from our previously reported study [33]. In this study, the normal control group showed a negative correlation between subfoveal and peripapillary CT and age, but the neovascular AMD group showed no correlation between subfoveal and peripapillary CT and age. This absent relationship between subfoveal CT and age might suggest an alteration in the choroid of the macula in neovascular AMD and may provide additional insight into the pathogenesis of neovascular AMD [15].

This study has several limitations. First, because it is a retrospective study with short-term results and contains a small number of cases, our study may have limited generalizability. We could not see a short-term change in CT 1 month after IVR, and it is insufficient to draw conclusions on the long-term effect of IVR on the choroid based on the short follow-up period. Further studies with larger sample sizes and longer study periods are needed. Second, because of the retrospective nature of this study, diurnal variation of CT was not considered. Mean diurnal variation of subfoveal CT in healthy individuals is about 33.7 μm and the diurnal variation of the peripapillary CT remains unclear [43]. The changes in the mean macular and peripapillary CT in this study were relatively small, and the changes in macular CT were less than those expected from diurnal variation. Although most patients visited the outpatient clinic during the day, this study did not adjust for diurnal changes in CT. Third, we could not obtain information about refractive error and axial length in all patients. Two patients in the AMD group and four patients in the control group with pseudophakia had no information available on refractive error, although the axial length in all of these patients was less than 26.0 mm. Because axial length and refractive error are known to be associated with subfoveal CT and peripapillary CT, the lack of this information in the analysis is a shortcoming of this study. Fourth, although CT measurements were performed by two independent examiners, the method was manual as no automated method exists. Fifth, we only matched patients by age, but not by sex. Although there were no differences in these characteristics between the two patient groups, the results may still be affected. Sixth, we only measured CT of the peripapillary or macular region. It could not represent CT beyond the posterior pole. Finally, because

the treatment was based on monthly dosing and a PRN schedule, the number of injections received at 6 months differed among patients. However, there was no significant correlation between the difference in subfoveal or peripapillary CT at 6 months and the number of injections.

Conclusions

The mean peripapillary CT of the AMD group was not significantly different from that of the age-matched controls. Apart from the CT in the macular area, the mean peripapillary CT and peripapillary CT outside of the macula did not change 6 months after IVR. This result may suggest that the change in CT after IVR may be limited to the macula in eyes with neovascular AMD.

Additional files

> **Additional file 1:** Comparison of choroidal thickness between neovascular AMD eyes at 3 and 6 months and normal controls. Mean subfoveal CT and peripapillary CT at both 3 and 6 months showed no significant differences when compared with the baseline values of the normal controls. (PDF 11 kb)
>
> **Additional file 2:** Interobserver measurement reliability of the choroidal thickness. Interobserver reliability was assessed by analysis of intraclass correlation coefficients. The intraclass correlation coefficients indicated good agreement. (PDF 60 kb)

Abbreviations
CT: Choroidal thickness; AMD: Age-related macular degeneration; IVR: Intravitreal ranibizumab injections; VEGF: Vascular endothelial growth factor; RPE: Retinal pigment epithelium; PCA: Posterior ciliary artery; OCT: Optical coherence tomography; CRT: Central retinal thickness; RNFL: Retinal nerve fiber layer; RT: Retinal thickness.

Competing interests
The authors declare that they have no competing interests.

Authors' contributions
CY: Research design, data acquisition, data analysis and interpretation and manuscript preparation. JO: Research design, data analysis and interpretation and manuscript preparation. KC: Data acquisition and data analysis. SH: Data analysis, interpretation and manuscript preparation. SK: Data analysis, interpretation and manuscript preparation. KH: Data analysis, interpretation and manuscript preparation. All authors read and approved the final manuscript.

Acknowledgements
This study is supported by a grant from Korea University (K1421461).

Author details
[1]Department of Ophthalmology, Korea University College of Medicine, 126-1 Anam-dong 5-ga, Sungbuk-gu, Seoul 136-705, South Korea. [2]Department of Biostatistics, Korea University College of Medicine, Seoul, South Korea.

References
1. Lim LS, Mitchell P, Seddon JM, Holz FG, Wong TY. Age-related macular degeneration. Lancet. 2012;379:1728–38.
2. Belkin M, Kalter-Leibovici O, Chetrit A, Skaat A. Time trends in the incidence and causes of blindness in Israel. Am J Ophthalmol. 2013;155:404.
3. Bloch SB, Larsen M, Munch IC. Incidence of legal blindness from age-related macular degeneration in denmark: year 2000 to 2010. Am J Ophthalmol. 2012;153:209–13. e202.

4. Campbell JP, Bressler SB, Bressler NM. Impact of availability of anti-vascular endothelial growth factor therapy on visual impairment and blindness due to neovascular age-related macular degeneration. Arch Ophthalmol. 2012;130:794–5.
5. Mitchell P, Korobelnik JF, Lanzetta P, Holz FG, Prünte C, Schmidt-Erfurth U, et al. Ranibizumab (Lucentis) in neovascular age-related macular degeneration: evidence from clinical trials. Br J Ophthalmol. 2010;94:2–13.
6. Ciulla TA, Harris A, Martin BJ. Ocular perfusion and age-related macular degeneration. Acta Ophthalmol Scand. 2001;79:108–15.
7. Friedman E. A hemodynamic model of the pathogenesis of age-related macular degeneration. Am J Ophthalmol. 1997;124:677–82.
8. Berenberg TL, Metelitsina TI, Madow B, Dai Y, Ying GS, Dupont JC, et al. The association between drusen extent and foveolar choroidal blood flow in age-related macular degeneration. Retina. 2012;32:25–31.
9. Grunwald JE, Hariprasad SM, DuPont J, Maguire MG, Fine SL, Brucker AJ, et al. Foveolar choroidal blood flow in age-related macular degeneration. Invest Ophthalmol Vis Sci. 1998;39:385–90.
10. Chung SE, Kang SW, Lee JH, Kim YT. Choroidal thickness in polypoidal choroidal vasculopathy and exudative age-related macular degeneration. Ophthalmology. 2011;118:840–5.
11. Jonas JB, Forster TM, Steinmetz P, Schlichtenbrede FC, Harder BC. Choroidal thickness in age-related macular degeneration. Retina. 2014;34:1149–55.
12. Kim SW, Oh J, Kwon SS, Yoo J, Huh K. Comparison of choroidal thickness among patients with healthy eyes, early age-related maculopathy, neovascular age-related macular degeneration, central serous chorioretinopathy, and polypoidal choroidal vasculopathy. Retina. 2011;31:1904–11.
13. Manjunath V, Goren J, Fujimoto JG, Duker JS. Analysis of choroidal thickness in age-related macular degeneration using spectral-domain optical coherence tomography. Am J Ophthalmol. 2011;152:663–8.
14. Branchini L, Regatieri C, Adhi M, Flores-Moreno I, Manjunath V, Fujimoto JG, et al. Effect of intravitreous anti-vascular endothelial growth factor therapy on choroidal thickness in neovascular age-related macular degeneration using spectral-domain optical coherence tomography. JAMA Ophthalmol. 2013;131:693–4.
15. Yamazaki T, Koizumi H, Yamagishi T, Kinoshita S. Subfoveal choroidal thickness after ranibizumab therapy for neovascular age-related macular degeneration: 12-month results. Ophthalmology. 2012;119:1621–7.
16. Blaauwgeers HG, Holtkamp GM, Rutten H, Witmer AN, Koolwijk P, Partanen TA, et al. Polarized vascular endothelial growth factor secretion by human retinal pigment epithelium and localization of vascular endothelial growth factor receptors on the inner choriocapillaris. Evidence for a trophic paracrine relation. Am J Pathol. 1999;155:421–8.
17. Pournaras CJ, Rungger-Brandle E, Riva CE, Hardarson SH, Stefansson E. Regulation of retinal blood flow in health and disease. Prog Retin Eye Res. 2008;27:284–330.
18. Mathis U, Ziemssen F, Schaeffel F. Effects of a human VEGF antibody (Bevacizumab) on deprivation myopia and choroidal thickness in the chicken. Exp Eye Res. 2014;127:161–9.
19. Hayreh SS. The blood supply of the optic nerve head and the evaluation of it - myth and reality. Prog Retin Eye Res. 2001;20:563–93.
20. Hayreh SS. Posterior ciliary artery circulation in health and disease: the Weisenfeld lecture. Invest Ophthalmol Vis Sci. 2004;45:749–57. 748.
21. Hayreh SS. In vivo choroidal circulation and its watershed zones. Eye. 1990;4:273–89.
22. Yun C, Oh J, Ahn SE, Hwang SY, Kim SW, Huh K. Peripapillary choroidal thickness in patients with early age-related macular degeneration and reticular pseudodrusen. Graefes Arch Clin Exp Ophthalmol. 2015; DOI 10.1007/s00417-015-3054-7.
23. Vujosevic S, Martini F, Cavarzeran F, Pilotto E, Midena E. Macular and peripapillary choroidal thickness in diabetic patients. Retina. 2012;32:1781–90.
24. Yun C, Oh J, Han JY, Hwang SY, Moon SW, Huh K. Peripapillary choroidal thickness in central serous chorioretinopathy : Is choroid outside the macula also thick? Retina. 2015; doi:10.1097/IAE.0000000000000539.
25. Koh AH, Expert PCVP, Chen LJ, Chen SJ, Chen Y, Giridhar A, et al. Polypoidal choroidal vasculopathy: evidence-based guidelines for clinical diagnosis and treatment. Retina. 2013;33:686–716.
26. Sengupta S, Surti R, Vasavada D. Sensitivity and specificity of spectral-domain optical coherence tomography in detecting idiopathic polypoidal choroidal vasculopathy. Am J Ophthalmol. 2015;160:203–4.
27. Ahuja RM, Stanga PE, Vingerling JR, Reck AC, Bird AC. Polypoidal choroidal vasculopathy in exudative and haemorrhagic pigment epithelial detachments. Br J Ophthalmol. 2000;84:479–84.
28. Perkovich BT, Zakov ZN, Berlin LA, Weidenthal D, Avins LR. An update on multiple recurrent serosanguineous retinal pigment epithelial detachments in black women. Retina. 1990;10:18–26.
29. Macular Photocoagulation Study Group. Subfoveal neovascular lesions in age-related macular degeneration. Guidelines for evaluation and treatment in the macular photocoagulation study. Arch Ophthalmol. 1991;109:1242–57.
30. Freund KB, Zweifel SA, Engelbert M. Do we need a new classification for choroidal neovascularization in age-related macular degeneration? Retina. 2010;30:1333–49.
31. Freund KB, Ho IV, Barbazetto IA, Koizumi H, Laud K, Ferrara D, et al. Type 3 neovascularization: the expanded spectrum of retinal angiomatous proliferation. Retina. 2008;28:201–11.
32. Fung AE, Lalwani GA, Rosenfeld PJ, Dubovy SR, Michels S, Feuer WJ, et al. An optical coherence tomography-guided, variable dosing regimen with intravitreal ranibizumab (Lucentis) for neovascular age-related macular degeneration. Am J Ophthalmol. 2007;143:566–83.
33. Oh J, Yoo C, Yun CM, Yang KS, Kim SW, Huh K. Simplified method to measure the peripapillary choroidal thickness using three-dimensional optical coherence tomography. Korean J Ophthalmol. 2013;27:172–7.
34. Margolis R, Spaide RF. A pilot study of enhanced depth imaging optical coherence tomography of the choroid in normal eyes. Am J Ophthalmol. 2009;147:811–5.
35. Liang D, Chang JR, Chin AJ, Smith A, Kelly C, Weinberg ES, et al. The role of vascular endothelial growth factor (VEGF) in vasculogenesis, angiogenesis, and hematopoiesis in zebrafish development. Mech Dev. 2001;108:29–43.
36. Roberts WG, Palade GE. Increased microvascular permeability and endothelial fenestration induced by vascular endothelial growth factor. J Cell Sci. 1995;108:2369–79.
37. Weis SM, Cheresh DA. Pathophysiological consequences of VEGF-induced vascular permeability. Nature. 2005;437:497–504.
38. Grossniklaus HE, Green WR. Choroidal neovascularization. Am J Ophthalmol. 2004;137:496–503.
39. Saint-Geniez M, Kurihara T, Sekiyama E, Maldonado AE, D'Amore PA. An essential role for RPE-derived soluble VEGF in the maintenance of the choriocapillaris. Proc Natl Acad Sci U S A. 2009;106:18751–6.
40. Saint-Geniez M, Maldonado AE, D'Amore PA. VEGF expression and receptor activation in the choroid during development and in the adult. Invest Ophthalmol Vis Sci. 2006;47:3135–42.
41. Sacu S, Pemp B, Weigert G, Matt G, Garhofer G, Pruente C, et al. Response of retinal vessels and retrobulbar hemodynamics to intravitreal anti-VEGF treatment in eyes with branch retinal vein occlusion. Invest Ophthalmol Vis Sci. 2011;52:3046–50.
42. Yokoyama K, Choshi T, Kimoto K, Shinoda K, Nakatsuka K. Retinal circulatory disturbances following intracameral injection of bevacizumab for neovascular glaucoma. Acta Ophthalmol. 2008;86:927–8.
43. Tan CS, Ouyang Y, Ruiz H, Sadda SR. Diurnal variation of choroidal thickness in normal, healthy subjects measured by spectral domain optical coherence tomography. Invest Ophthalmol Vis Sci. 2012;53:261–6.

23

Corneal permeability changes in dry eye disease

Kenji Fujitani*, Neha Gadaria, Kyu-In Lee, Brendan Barry and Penny Asbell

Abstract

Background: Diagnostic tests for dry eye disease (DED), including ocular surface disease index (OSDI), tear breakup time (TBUT), corneal fluorescein staining, and lissamine staining, have great deal of variability. We investigated whether fluorophotometry correlated with previously established DED diagnostic tests and whether it could serve as a novel objective metric to evaluate DED.

Methods: Dry eye patients who have had established signs or symptoms for at least 6 months were included in this observational study. Normal subjects with no symptoms of dry eyes served as controls. Each eye had a baseline fluorescein scan prior to any fluorescein dye. Fluorescein dye was then placed into both eyes, rinsed with saline solution, and scanned at 5, 10, 15, and 30 min. Patients were administered the following diagnostic tests to correlate with fluorophotometry: OSDI, TBUT, fluorescein, and lissamine. Standard protocols were used. $P < 0.05$ was considered significant.

Results: Fifty eyes from 25 patients (DED = 22 eyes, 11 patients; Normal = 28 eyes, 14 patients) were included. Baseline scans of the dry eye and control groups did not show any statistical difference ($p = 0.84$). Fluorescein concentration of DED and normal patients showed statistical significance at all time intervals ($p < 10^{-5}$, 0.001, 0.002, 0.049 for 5, 10, 15, & 30 min respectively). Fluorophotometry values converged towards baseline as time elapsed, but both groups were still statistically different at 30 min ($p < 0.01$). We used four fluorophotometry scoring methods and correlated them with OSDI, TBUT, fluorescein, and lissamine along with adjusted and aggregate scores. The four scoring schemes did not show any significant correlations with the other tests, except for correlations seen with lissamine and 10 ($p = 0.045$, 0.034) and 15 min ($p = 0.013$, 0.012), and with aggregate scores and 15 min ($p = 0.042$, 0.017).

Conclusions: Fluorophotometry generally did not correlate with any other DED tests, even though it showed capability of differentiating between DED and normal eyes up to 30 min after fluorescein dye instillation. There may be an aspect of DED that is missed in the current regimen of DED tests and only captured with fluorophotometry. Adding fluorophotometry may be useful in screening, diagnosing, and monitoring patients with DED.

Keywords: Fluorophotometry, Dry eye, Keratoconjunctivitis sicca, Ocular surface disease, Corneal permeability

Background

Keratoconjunctivitis sicca or dry eye disease (DED) is one of the most common ocular conditions that patients seek care for and affects as many as 11.4 % of men and 16.7 % of women [1]. Current treatment options range from artificial tears to anti-inflammatory and immunosuppressant agents, and treatment has shown to drastically improve quality of life and prevent damage to the ocular surface [2]. The most common methods to diagnose DED include a comprehensive eye exam, symptom survey with Ocular Surface Disease Index (OSDI), tear breakup time (TBUT), lissamine green staining (lissamine), Schirmer's, and corneal fluorescein staining (fluorescein), but these diagnostic tests have a great deal of variability and potential for bias, making objective and accurate DED diagnosis and management difficult [3].

* Correspondence: kenji.fujitani@icahn.mssm.edu; kenji.fujitani@mssm.edu
Department of Ophthalmology, Icahn School of Medicine at Mount Sinai,
New York, NY 10029, USA

Miyata et al. suggested that a fluorophotometer could measure corneal epithelial permeability due to the correlation between fluorescein concentrations in the cornea and corneal damage [4]. Specifically, fluorophotometry could evaluate ocular surface epithelium barrier function [5]. Although some degree of corneal staining is inevitable and found on 79 % of corneas, the majority of the dye should remain in the tear film on the surface of the eye and not adhere to the eyes as the corneal epithelium protects the underlying layers of the cornea under normal conditions [6, 7].

Using the Fluorotron Master fluorophotometer (Ocumetrics, Mountain View, CA), we showed in our previous study that differentiating between DED and normal patients depending on the fluorescein concentration in the cornea at certain time intervals was possible [8]. This study aims to test the capability of the fluorophotometer further: we investigated whether fluorophotometry correlated with already established diagnostic tests for dry eye disease and whether it could serve as a minimally invasive objective metric to evaluate dry eye disease.

Methods

After receiving approval from Icahn School of Medicine at Mount Sinai's Institutional Review Board, prospective patients were recruited for this observational study. Informed consent was obtained from all subjects. The study was carried out with patients who visited the Faculty Practice of Department of Ophthalmology at Icahn School of Medicine at Mount Sinai in New York, NY.

Data were collected from normal and dry eye patients, who were followed for DED by an ophthalmologist prior to the study for 6 months or more. Patients were classified as normal or DED according to their clinical diagnosis. DED patients must have had at least 2 signs and/or symptoms of dry eyes such as foreign body sensation, ocular irritation, light sensitivity, burning and grittiness, itchiness, edema of lid, conjunctiva and cornea, or hyperemia in order to be included in the study. Normal subjects who had no signs or symptoms of dry eyes or other ocular problems except for refractive error served as controls. Patients with any conditions that limited their ability to understand the consent were excluded from the study. Pregnant patients, those under 18 years of age, patients with acute or sub-acute inflammation/infection of the anterior segment of the eye, and those with history of allergy to fluorescein were also excluded from the study.

All fluorophotometry of the cornea was performed with the Fluorotron Master flurophotometer (Ocumetrics, Mountain View, CA) in accordance to the manufacturer's instructions and the provided scanning software. Each eye had a baseline fluorescein scan performed prior to any introduction of fluorescein dye to measure each eye's intrinsic fluorescence. 50 μl of 1 % sodium fluorescein dye was then placed into both eyes. Two minutes later, the fluorescein was thoroughly rinsed with 100 μl of non-preserved normal balanced saline solution. Fluorescein scans were started immediately after washing and recorded at 5, 10, 15, and 30 min thereafter, beginning with the OD eye. The fluorescein scan involved no direct contact between the eye and the device. The corneal peak values of fluorescein concentration were recorded. The following diagnostic tests were also administered to patients with DED to correlate with fluorophotometry results: OSDI, TBUT, fluorescein, and lissamine. Standard protocols were used for the DED diagnostic exams. TBUT was observed under cobalt blue illumination, once per eye. We used the National Eye Institute scale for grading fluorescein corneal staining and the Van Bijsterveld scale for grading lissamine green staining of the conjunctiva.

Corneal fluorescein levels at multiple time points in both eyes were recorded into Microsoft Excel (Microsoft, Redmond, Washington). Spearman's correlations were used to detect any correlations between fluorophotometry and other DED diagnostic tests. Microsoft Excel and SPSS version 20.0 (SPSS Inc., Chicago, IL) were used for statistical analysis. $P < 0.05$ (two-tailed) was considered significant.

Results

We included 50 eyes from 25 patients (DED = 22 eyes, 11 patients; Normal = 28 eyes, 14 patients). Baseline scans of the dry eye (22.19 ± 8.05 ng/ml) and control (21.81 ± 5.17 ng/ml) did not show any statistical difference ($p = 0.84$). Figure 1 shows the amount of increase in fluorescein concentration relative to baseline at multiple time intervals (5, 10, 15, and 30 min). Fluorescein concentration of DED and control groups showed statistical significance at all time intervals ($p < 10^{-5}$, 0.001, 0.002, 0.049 for 5, 10, 15, & 30 min, respectively). DED always had higher fluorescein concentrations than controls. Fluorescein concentrations in both groups converged towards their baseline as time elapsed, but were still statistically different from their baseline at 30 min ($p < 0.01$).

Fluorophotometry values in DED group were categorized into 4 major schemes, which most clearly illustrated the change in fluorophotometry values: 1) increases in fluorescein concentration relative to its baseline at multiple time intervals (5, 10, 15, and 30 min) were labeled as 'DIFF X' where X represented the minutes. For instance, DIFF 10 was defined as the fluorescein concentration 10 min after washout of fluorescein dye minus the baseline fluorescein concentration of that patient. 2) log values of 'DIFF X' were taken and labeled as 'LOGDIFF X.' 3) similar to the 'DIFF X' scoring, percent changes in fluorescein concentration relative to its baseline at multiple time

Fluorescein Concentration

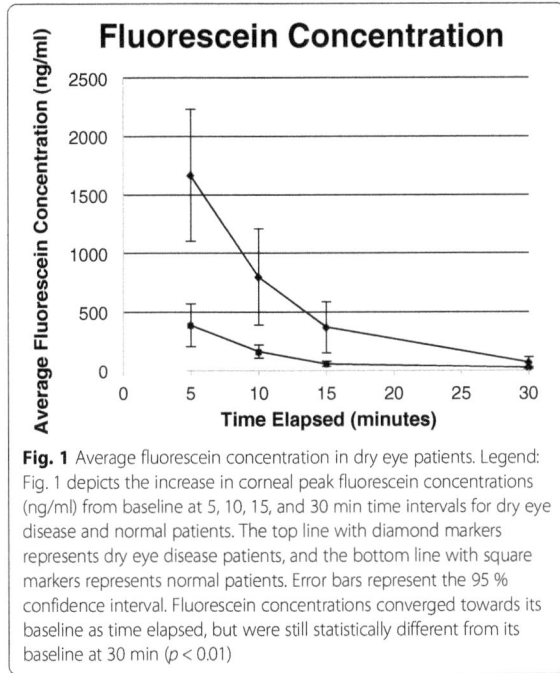

Fig. 1 Average fluorescein concentration in dry eye patients. Legend: Fig. 1 depicts the increase in corneal peak fluorescein concentrations (ng/ml) from baseline at 5, 10, 15, and 30 min time intervals for dry eye disease and normal patients. The top line with diamond markers represents dry eye disease patients, and the bottom line with square markers represents normal patients. Error bars represent the 95 % confidence interval. Fluorescein concentrations converged towards its baseline as time elapsed, but were still statistically different from its baseline at 30 min ($p < 0.01$)

intervals (5, 10, 15, and 30 min) were labeled as 'PERC X' where X represented the minutes. 4) log values of 'PERC X' were taken and labeled as 'LOGPERC X'.

To determine how fluorophotometry reflected the results of other DED diagnostic methods, we correlated the four fluorophotometry scoring schemes with OSDI, TBUT, fluorescein, and lissamine (Table 1). OSDI scores were adjusted into quartiles (0–25 = score of 1, 26–50 = score of 2, 51–75 = score of 3, 76–100 = score of 4) named 'OSDI Quartiles' to create a score that was more similar to scores of other tests. The double-digit OSDI scores were adjusted to fit with the single digit scores of other diagnostic tests. Using this, we created an aggregate score that added OSDI Quartiles, TBUT, Fluorescein, and Lissamine (Aggregate score = OSDI Quartile + TBUT + fluorescein + lissamine).

After correlation to other DED diagnostic tests, the four fluorophotometry scoring schemes generally did not show any significant correlations with OSDI, OSDI Quartiles, TBUT, fluorescein, and lissamine tests. Significant correlations were seen with lissamine scores and LOGDIFF 10 ($p = 0.045$), LOGDIFF 15 ($p = 0.013$), LOGPERC 10 ($p = 0.034$), and LOGPERC 15 ($p = 0.012$) and with aggregate scores and LOGDIFF 15 ($p = 0.042$) and LOGPERC 15 ($p = 0.017$).

Discussion

DED affects a significant number of people, with prevalence ranging from 7 % in the United States to 33 % in Taiwan and Japan, but DED is difficult to diagnose and

no clear gold standard to evaluate DED exists [9, 10]. Clinicians often rely on multitude of tests, including symptoms or signs and a battery of diagnostic tests, including TBUT, fluorescein, and lissamine. We strove to determine if fluorophotometry could fill that void through correlation with other established tests and better classify DED according to severity.

Past studies by Kinoshita et al. and Yokoi have found that the fluorophotometer could evaluate ocular surface epithelium barrier function using a similar methodology to our study [5, 11–13]. In one of their studies, they showed that in accordance with severity, fluorescein uptake in dry eye patients showed significant increase, and that with treatment with hyaluronan eye drops, there was significant barrier function improvement after 2 weeks [12, 13]. In our study, we evaluated not only fluorophotometry's ability to differentiate between dry eye and normal eyes, but also the correlations of its results with different diagnostic techniques of dry eye. Among the multitude of tests available, we aimed to investigate whether fluorophotometry could outperform any diagnostic tests, combine 2–3 diagnostic tests, or become another test that measures an aspect of dry eye that is not yet captured by any of the diagnostic tests for DED.

Consistent with our previous study, this study showed that fluorophotometry could differentiate between DED and normal eyes up to 30 min post fluorescein dye instillation [8]. However, except for minor correlations with lissamine and aggregate scores at 10 and 15 min, fluorophotometry in our current study did not show any significant correlations with other DED diagnostic tests, such as OSDI, TBUT, fluorescein, and lissamine. These differences could arise because fluorophotometry encompasses a larger view of DED, taking into account the overall increased permeability of the cornea in ocular surface disease patients rather than focusing on one aspect of DED. For instance, TBUT takes into account tear production and evaporation, but fluorophotometry includes all factors that damage the corneal epithelium, and utilizes tear break up as only one component of many factors that contribute to DED.

Another possible function for fluorophotometry is to measure aspects of DED not captured by other diagnostic tests, which are somewhat imperfect themselves and thus contribute to the difficulty of objectively diagnosing DED. Dry eye patients have ocular surface disease that increase corneal permeability to fluorescein, but the amount of change as we measured it did not correlate with other tests. Fluorophotometry may include a component not yet detected with current diagnostic tests and thus could be done to rule out DED when DED is suspected, but other diagnostic tests are normal. Due to its unique position relative to other tests, adding fluorophotometry as one of

Table 1 Comparison of four fluorophotometry scoring schemes with other dry eye diagnostic tests

		OSDI	OSDI Quartiles	TBUT	Fluorescein	Lissamine	Aggregate score
DIFF5	Correlation Coefficient	.172	.056	.213	−.086	−.075	.030
	Significance	.444	.805	.340	.703	.739	.895
DIFF10	Correlation Coefficient	.118	−.030	.050	−.163	−.274	−.186
	Significance	.602	.895	.826	.468	.216	.408
DIFF15	Correlation Coefficient	.093	−.046	−.031	−.174	−.357	−.259
	Significance	.681	.837	.891	.439	.102	.245
DIFF30	Correlation Coefficient	.276	.256	−.118	−.037	.163	−.028
	Significance	.213	.250	.602	.870	.469	.903
LOGDIFF5	Correlation Coefficient	.172	.056	.213	−.086	−.075	.030
	Significance	.444	.805	.340	.703	.739	.895
LOGDIFF10	Correlation Coefficient	−.013	−.137	−.028	−.296	**−.442***	−.364
	Significance	.955	.552	.904	.192	**.045**	.105
LOGDIFF15	Correlation Coefficient	−.040	−.156	−.120	−.307	**−.534***	**−.448***
	Significance	.864	.500	.605	.176	**.013**	**.042**
LOGDIFF30	Correlation Coefficient	.084	.079	−.127	−.187	−.100	−.211
	Significance	.726	.740	.592	.430	.673	.372
PERC5	Correlation Coefficient	0.000	−.105	.228	−.044	−.062	.013
	Significance	1.000	.642	.308	.845	.783	.954
PERC10	Correlation Coefficient	0.000	−.129	.071	−.107	−.296	−.188
	Significance	1.000	.568	.752	.636	.181	.402
PERC15	Correlation Coefficient	−.034	−.186	.012	−.225	−.361	−.316
	Significance	.881	.408	.958	.315	.099	.152
PERC30	Correlation Coefficient	.190	.179	−.119	.028	.252	−.003
	Significance	.396	.426	.596	.903	.258	.990
LOGPERC5	Correlation Coefficient	0.000	−.105	.228	−.044	−.062	.013
	Significance	1.000	.642	.308	.845	.783	.954
LOGPERC10	Correlation Coefficient	−.149	−.246	−.007	−.234	**−.464***	−.367
	Significance	.521	.282	.975	.308	**.034**	.102
LOGPERC15	Correlation Coefficient	−.186	−.312	−.076	−.363	**−.537***	**−.514***
	Significance	.420	.169	.745	.105	**.012**	**.017**
LOGPERC30	Correlation Coefficient	−.019	−.017	−.114	−.096	.016	−.166
	Significance	.937	.942	.633	.688	.947	.485

Fluorophotometry values are categorized into 4 major schemes. 1) Increases in fluorescein concentration relative to its baseline at multiple time intervals (5, 10, 15, and 30 min) are labeled 'DIFF X' where X represents the minutes. 2) Log values of 'DIFF X' are labeled 'LOGDIFF X.' 3) Percent changes in fluorescein concentration relative to its baseline at multiple time intervals (5, 10, 15, and 30 min) are labeled 'PERC X.' 4) Log values of 'PERC X' are labeled 'LOGPERC X.' Fluorophotometry scoring schemes are compared with Ocular Surface Disease Index (OSDI), tear break up time (TBUT), fluorescein, and lissamine. OSDI scores were adjusted into quartiles (0–25 = score of 1, 26–50 = score of 2, 51–75 = score of 3, 76–100 = score of 4) and called 'OSDI Quartiles.' An aggregate score was calculated by adding OSDI quartiles, TBUT, fluorescein, and lissamine

All significance (p-value) are two-tailed, and p < 0.05 was considered statistically significant. Correlation coefficients and significance are bolded with asterisks* if less than 0.05

its basic tests when evaluating DED may aid in diagnosing DED or in research settings studying DED. Continued research in this area could clarify this mismatch.

Fluorophotometry also did not correlate with clinical symptoms as measured by OSDI. Although there is some evidence showing OSDI can measure the severity of dry eye, the non-correlation was unsurprising since DED signs and symptoms are poorly correlated, compounded by variability between seasons, time of day, and findings among eye examinations, suggesting that symptoms may not truly reflect the whole dry eye state in patients [14, 15]. Though the cornea may be damaged, patients may still be asymptomatic. One possible explanation is that with damage to the ocular surface, the central cornea sensitivity decreases, making the patient less symptomatic [14, 16]. Similarly, the cornea may be healthy even as patients report multitude of symptoms. With fluorophotometry's capability to differentiate dry eyes from normal eyes, one possibility could be to use fluorophotometry as one of DED screening tools to detect subclinical DED in seemingly healthy patients. Earlier detection could lead to earlier treatment, or possible prevention of progression to severe DED when it may be more difficult to intervene. Higher values of fluorophotometry in DED patients correlate with increased permeability of the cornea, so fluorophotometry could be used to measure progression of corneal damage and assess whether current treatments for DED are sufficient, adjusting as needed depending on the results [17].

This study is not without limitations. Sample size was limited, and this factor most likely contributed to the relatively high variability in fluorescein concentrations with the fluorophotometer. More eyes may reduce this variability, but the biggest likely cause of this variation is the lumping of all DED eyes into one dry eye group. Mild DED was not differentiated from severe DED, as there was no clear way to do so without a gold standard or correlations with other exams. The next step would be to explore whether fluorophotometry correlates with DED severity, especially if it may be a tool that can grade DED severity on a sliding scale. Furthermore, we cannot eliminate some of the intrinsic problems associated with fluorescein, especially at higher concentrations, and the Fluorotron Master flurophotometer itself. For instance, because the machine cannot clearly distinguish the tear film from the cornea, we utilized a similar washing method from previous studies to eliminate any excess fluorescein remaining in the tear film and to standardize the technique [8, 12, 18, 19]. Although the process was controlled as much as possible, some patients may have more or less fluorescein left on the tear film, possibly due to mechanical issues such as excessive tearing or blinking. Finally, although we aimed to capture most factors that contribute to DED, not all possible diagnostic tests were done to reduce burden on the patients. In future studies, comparing fluorophotometry to more diagnostic tests such as tear osmolarity may be beneficial.

Conclusions

The degree of ocular surface disease as measured by fluorophotometry generally did not correlate with any other clinical DED tests. Given fluorophotometry's capability of differentiating between DED and normal eyes, there may be an aspect of DED that is missed in the current regimen of DED tests and only captured with fluorophotometry. Adding fluorophotometry as another diagnostic test for DED may be useful in screening, assessing, and monitoring patients with DED.

Ethics approval and consent to participate
Approval from Icahn School of Medicine at Mount Sinai's Institutional Review Board. Informed consent was obtained from all subjects.

Consent for publication
Not applicable.

Abbreviations
DED: dry eye disease; DIFF: increases in fluorescein concentration relative to its baseline; LOGDIFF: log values of DIFF; LOGPERC: log values of PERC; OSDI: ocular surface disease index; PERC: percent changes in fluorescein concentration relative to its baseline; TBUT: tear breakup time.

Competing interests
The authors declare that they have no competing interests.

Authors' contributions
KF performed data/statistical analysis, interpretation of data, and drafted the manuscript. NG and KL designed the study and acquired data. BB interpreted data and revised the manuscript. PA conceived the study, participated in the study design, and revised the manuscript. All authors read and approved the final manuscript.

Acknowledgements
Not applicable.

Funding
Financial support from these organizations is gratefully acknowledged: Martin and Toni Sosnoff Fund, Pfizer (unrestricted grant), Research to Prevent Blindness (unrestricted grant), and Fight for Sight. The funding organizations had no role in the design or conduct of this research.

References
1. Moss SE, Klein R, Klein BE. Prevalence of and risk factors for dry eye syndrome. Arch Ophthalmol. 2000;118:1264–8.
2. Yao W, Davidson RS, Durairaj VD, Gelston CD. Dry eye syndrome: an update in office management. Am J Med. 2011;124:1016–8.
3. Sullivan BD, Crews LA, Messmer EM, Foulks GN, Nichols KK, Baenninger P, et al. Correlations between commonly used objective signs and symptoms for the diagnosis of dry eye disease: clinical implications. Acta Ophthalmol. 2014;92:161–6.
4. Miyata K, Amano S, Sawa M, Nishida T. A novel grading method for superficial punctate keratopathy magnitude and its correlation with corneal epithelial permeability. Arch Ophthalmol. 2003;121:1537–9.
5. Yokoi K, Yokoi N, Kinoshita S. Impairment of ocular surface epithelium barrier function in patients with atopic dermatitis. Br J Ophthalmol. 1998;82:797–800.
6. Dundas M, Walker A, Woods RL. Clinical grading of corneal staining of non-contact lens wearers. Ophthalmic Physiol Opt. 2001;21:30–5.
7. Cui L, Huxlin KR, Xu L, MacRae S, Knox WH. High-resolution, noninvasive, two-photon fluorescence measurement of molecular concentrations in corneal tissue. Invest Ophthalmol Vis Sci. 2011;52:2556–64.
8. Fahim MM, Haji S, Koonapareddy CV, Fan VC, Asbell PA. Fluorophotometry as a diagnostic tool for the evaluation of dry eye disease. BMC Ophthalmol. 2006;6:20.
9. Gayton JL. Etiology, prevalence, and treatment of dry eye disease. Clin Ophthalmol. 2009;3:405–12.
10. Valim V, Trevisani VF, de Sousa JM, Vilela VS, Belfort R Jr. Current approach to dry eye disease. Clin Rev Allergy Immunol. 2015;49:288–97.

11. Kinoshita S, Adachi W, Sotozono C, Nishida K, Yokoi N, Quantock AJ, et al. Characteristics of the human ocular surface epithelium. Prog Retin Eye Res. 2001;20:639–73.
12. Yokoi N, Kinoshita S. Clinical evaluation of corneal epithelial barrier function with the slit-lamp fluorophotometer. Cornea. 1995;14:485–9.
13. Yokoi N, Komuro A, Nishida K, Kinoshita S. Effectiveness of hyaluronan on corneal epithelial barrier function in dry eye. Br J Ophthalmol. 1997;81:533–6.
14. Barboza MN, Barboza GN, de Melo GM, Sato E, Dantas MC, Dantas P, et al. Correlation between signals and symptoms of dry eye in Sjögren's syndrome patients. Arq Bras Oftalmol. 2008;71:547–52.
15. Zeev MS, Miller DD, Latkany R. Diagnosis of dry eye disease and emerging technologies. Clin Ophthalmol. 2014;8:581–90.
16. Bourcier T, Acosta MC, Borderie V, Borrás F, Gallar J, Bury T, et al. Decreased corneal sensitivity in patients with dry eye. Invest Ophthalmol Vis Sci. 2005;46:2341–5.
17. Nelson JD. Simultaneous evaluation of tear turnover and corneal epithelial permeability by fluorophotometry in normal subjects and patients with keratoconjunctivitis sicca (KCS). Trans Am Ophthalmol Soc. 1995;93:709–53.
18. Joshi A, Maurice D, Paugh JR. A new method for determining corneal epithelial barrier to fluorescein in humans. Invest Ophthalmol Vis Sci. 1996;37:1008–16.
19. McNamara NA, Fusaro RE, Brand RJ, Polse KA, Srinivas SP. Measurement of corneal epithelial permeability to fluorescein. A repeatability study. Invest Ophthalmol Vis Sci. 1997;38:1830–9.

24

Acute acquired comitant esotropia related to excessive Smartphone use

Hyo Seok Lee, Sang Woo Park and Hwan Heo[*]

Abstract

Background: To describe the clinical characteristics and outcomes of acute acquired comitant esotropia (AACE) related to excessive smartphone use in adolescents.

Methods: The medical records of 12 patients with AACE and a history of excessive smartphone use were retrospectively reviewed, and the duration of smartphone use, angle of deviation, refractive error, stereopsis, and treatment options were analyzed.

Results: All patients showed convergent and comitant esotropia ranging from 15 to 45 prism diopters (PD; average: 27.75 ± 11.47 PD) at far fixation. The angle of deviation was nearly equivalent for far and near fixation. Every patient used a smartphone for more than 4 h a day over a period of several months (minimum 4 months). Myopic refractive errors were detected in eight patients (average: -3.84 ± 1.68 diopters (D)), and the remaining four patients showed mild hyperopic refractive error (average: $+0.84 \pm 0.53$ D). Reductions in esodeviation were noted in all patients after refraining from smartphone use, and bilateral medial rectus recession was performed in three patients with considerable remnant esodeviation. Postoperative exams showed orthophoria with good stereoacuity in these patients.

Conclusion: Excessive smartphone use might influence AACE development in adolescents. Refraining from smartphone use can decrease the degree of esodeviation in these patients, and remnant deviation can be successfully managed with surgical correction.

Keyword: Esotropia, Medial rectus recession, Smartphone, Video display terminal

Background

Acute acquired comitant esotropia (AACE) is an unusual presentation of esotropia in older children and adults [1]. Its prevalence remains unknown, but it is generally considered rare [2]. Three main types have been defined and later modified by previous investigators: (1) Swan type: esotropia due to the disruption of fusion (precipitated by monocular occlusion or loss of vision in one eye); (2) Burian-Franceschetti type: esotropia characterized by minimal hypermetropia and diplopia, often associated with physical or psychological stress; and (3) Bielschowsky type: esotropia that occurs in adolescents and adults with varying degrees of myopia, and shows equal deviation at distance and near fixation [3, 4]. The mechanism of Bielschowsky type AACE is thought to be uncorrected myopia with excessive near work (holding printed materials or sewing excessively close to the eye), resulting in an inability to maintain balance between the converging and diverging forces of the eye, and the subsequent development of increased tonus of the medial rectus muscles, leading to esotropia [3]. Other rare types of AACE have also been reported, such as refractive-accommodative type AACE, and AACE associated with accommodative spasm or intracranial diseases [2, 5, 6].

The adoption of mobile technologies and wireless communication infrastructure is a global phenomenon [7, 8]. Among the existing technologies, smartphones have been one of the most prominent success stories of the last decade. In a relatively short period of time, smart mobile technology has significantly penetrated society in the Western world and globally, including South Korea. Since the introduction of the iPhone 3GS (Apple Inc., Cupertino, CA, USA) in South Korea in November

* Correspondence: opheye@hanmail.net
Department of Ophthalmology, Chonnam National University Medical School and Hospital, 42 Jebong-ro, Dong-Gu, Gwang-Ju 61469, South Korea

2009, smartphone distribution has dramatically increased and has become popular in a short period of time owing to South Korea's advanced information technology development. According to a report from the Korea Communications Commission, the number of smartphone users was estimated to be over 35 million in July, 2013 [9].

More specifically, smartphone possession has become surprisingly popular among adolescents and young adults. In 2010, only 5.8 % of adolescents in South Korea owned smartphones, but this number strikingly increased to 36.2 % in 2011, and exploded by nearly 15-fold to 81.5 % in 2013 [10]. However, the rapid spread of smartphones in today's society is associated with potentially serious social problems, such as smartphone addiction. According to a survey about smartphone addiction conducted by the National Information Society Agency in 2012, the incidence was 8.4 % in South Korea, which was higher than the average internet addiction rate of 7.7 % [9, 11]. Moreover, teenagers and individuals in their twenties showed higher addiction rates than those in their thirties and forties, thereby illustrating the vulnerability of adolescents to smartphone addiction [12]. Addictive tendencies toward smartphones in adolescence are not confined to South Korea alone, but have rapidly become a significant mental health problem in other nations [13]. Since smartphones are closely connected to most of our daily life activities—functioning as a mobile phone, portable computer with internet access, and mp3 or video player—and many people spend a considerable amount of time fumbling with their smartphones, smartphone use can be regarded as representative near work in today's contemporary era, replacing "classic" near work: reading or sewing. Thus, it is conceivable that smartphone addiction is a major contributor to excessive near work.

In this retrospective case series, we aimed to review our experience with AACE associated with excessive smartphone use, including its etiologies and outcomes.

Methods

The medical records of all adolescents with AACE who were examined at the Pediatric Ophthalmology and Strabismus Service of Chonnam National University Hospital, between January 2009 and June 2014 were reviewed. Patients who met the following criteria were included in this retrospective study: (1) age of onset after 1 year of age; (2) age ≤16 years; (3) acute onset of comitant strabismus (same deviation in all gaze directions); (4) photographic evidence of absence of strabismus before esotropia onset; (5) corrected visual acuity of 20/20 in both eyes; and (6) a minimum follow-up period of 3 months [14]. Patients with a history of eye problems, including strabismus and amblyopia, previous ocular

surgery, ophthalmic eye drop use, systemic diseases (including diabetes mellitus), or head trauma, were excluded. In total, 19 patients fulfilled the inclusion criteria. Among these, three patients were diagnosed with Burian-Franceschetti type AACE; one patient was diagnosed with Bielschowsky type AACE; and three patients were diagnosed with AACE related to neurologic disease. However, the other 12 patients did not meet the diagnostic characteristics for the three main types of AACE or AACE related to neurologic disease. Following extensive history taking and examination, the remaining 12 patients were identified as excessive smartphone users (smartphone use more than 4 h a day for more than four consecutive months, based on the statements of the patients and their parents) [9, 11]. This tendency was not found in the other seven patients, who either did not have a smartphone or used a smartphone for less than 2 h a day. Interestingly, the AACE patients presented to our clinic after the beginning of 2012, which corresponds with the period of rapid distribution of smartphones in South Korea. Therefore, we decided to analyze the clinical characteristics of the AACE patients who did not fit into the preexisting AACE classification. The following data were abstracted from the medical records: age, gender, presence of diplopia, visual acuity, duration of smartphone use, angle of deviation for near and distance fixation, manifest refractive error, cycloplegic refractive error, measurement of near stereoacuity with the Titmus test, Bagolini striated glasses test results, medical and surgical treatment, and recurrence. The alternate prism cover test was performed to measure the angle of deviation at 6 m and 33 cm fixation, as well as for all gaze directions with refractive correction. The manifest refractive error was measured with an automated refractometer (KR8900, Topcon Corp., Tokyo, Japan). Cycloplegic autorefraction was performed by a single investigator (HSL). To achieve adequate cycloplegia, 1 % atropine sulfate eye drop was instilled three times a day for 3 days by the parents or guardians at home, prior to visiting the clinic. On the 4th day, cycloplegia was assessed by pupil diameter ≥6 mm and no reaction to light or the accommodative target. Refractive error measurements were obtained by using an automated refractometer (KR8900, Topcon Corp.); five readings with a maximum 0.25 diopter (D) difference were recorded and averaged. The manifest and cycloplegic spherical equivalents of refractive error were calculated by using the algebraic sum of the dioptric powers of the sphere and half of the cylinder. All patients in this study underwent a complete neurological examination, including brain magnetic resonance imaging, conducted by a pediatric neurologist; the examinations revealed normal results in all patients except for the three who were diagnosed with AACE related to neurologic disease. Approval for this study was obtained from the Institutional Review Board of Chonnam National University Hospital (IRB No.: CNUH-2014-189), and the study adhered to the tenets of the Declaration of Helsinki. Written informed consent was given by the participants and their caregivers (legal guardian) for their clinical records to be used in this study. SPSS version 18.0 (SPSS Institute Inc., Chicago, IL, USA) was used for statistical analyses. The Wilcoxon signed rank test was used to compare the angle of deviation before and after smartphone restriction. P values < 0.05 were considered statistically significant.

Results

The mean age of the 12 patients was 13.33 ± 3.31 years (range, 7–16 years; Table 1A and B), seven of which were female. The onset of esotropia preceded presentation at our clinic by an average of 5.83 ± 2.89 months (range, 2–10 months). Results of neurological examination as well as brain magnetic resonance imaging were normal. The average duration of smartphone use per day was 6.08 ± 1.78 h. The average duration of smartphone use prior to the eye examination was 10.5 ± 5.13 months. All patients stated that they usually viewed smartphones at a close reading distance (<30 cm). Nine patients complained of horizontal diplopia, but five patients stated that diplopia happened only intermittently, usually at distance fixation. None of the patients complained that the diplopia severely interfered with their daily lives.

The mean manifest refractive errors were -2.81 ± 2.13 D in the right eyes and -2.88 ± 2.13 D in the left eyes. After cycloplegia, myopic refractive errors were detected in eight patients (average: -3.80 ± 1.74 D in the right eyes and -3.89 ± 1.73 D in the left eyes), and the remaining four patients showed mild hyperopic refractive error (average: $+0.81 \pm 0.55$ D in the right eyes and $+0.88 \pm 0.60$ D in the left eyes). Each patient presented with a visual acuity of 20/20 in both eyes on their first visit to our clinic (patients 1, 5, 9, and 10 had an uncorrected visual acuity of 20/20 in both eyes and all other patients showed visual acuity of 20/20 with their glasses). The esodeviations at initial presentation were comitant, ranging from 15 to 45 prism diopters (PD) at far (mean, 27.75 ± 11.47 PD) with full correction of refractive errors. In each patient, the angles of esodeviation were nearly equivalent for distance and for near fixation (differing by $\leq \pm 5$ PD; mean, 28.33 ± 11.15 PD). After refraining from smartphone use for 1 month, all patients noted esodeviation improvement (17.50 ± 6.45 PD at far fixation [$p = 0.003$]; 17.13 ± 6.24 PD at near fixation [$p = 0.002$]) Slit lamp and fundoscopic examination revealed normal results in all patients. There were no apparent gaze limitations in either eye of any patient.

Strabismus surgery was advised for five patients who showed a small decrease in esodeviation after smartphone restriction and/or considerable remnant esodeviation (>15 PD). Three of these patients underwent bilateral medial rectus recession appropriate for the degree of esotropia under general anesthesia, whereas the other patients (7 and 9) refused surgical treatment. Postoperatively, all patients achieved orthophoria. The initial and final stereoacuity test results, and surgical interventions used, along with other parameters are presented in Table 1A and B.

Discussion

Both similarities and differences exist between Bielschowsky type AACE (described originally by Bielschowsky and later modified by Hoyt and Good), and the patients described in our case series [3, 4]. Comitant esodeviation without evidence of paralysis of the extraocular muscles, similar deviation at distance and near fixation, as well as various degrees of myopia, are consistent with the definition suggested by Bielschowsky, Hoyt and Good. Further, we assumed that dynamic preponderance of the medial rectus muscles after sustained near work played a pivotal role in the development of esotropia in our patients. However, unlike Bielschowsky's postulation in which uncorrected myopia was the key etiology of this form of strabismus, eight of 12 patients with myopic refractive error in our study wore glasses, and none of these patients was reluctant to wear glasses before or after presentation to our clinic. In addition, the corrected visual acuity of the eight patients with myopia was 20/20 in both eyes, and the uncorrected visual acuity was 20/20 in both eyes in the other four patients with hyperopia,

The Bagolini striated glasses test was performed in all patients at initial presentation, and the results showed unsuppressed esotropia in all cases [15]. We repeated the Bagolini striated glasses test in patients who underwent strabismus surgery at 3 months after the operation, and the results revealed normal binocular single vision in all three patients. And all patients who received strabismus surgery regained normal stereopsis proved by Titmus test. Moreover, mere smartphone restriction for 1 month led to a significant decrease in esodeviation in all patients, which would not occur in decompensated monofixation syndrome. Based on these observations, we believe that monofixation syndrome can be excluded in our patients [16].

Myasthenia gravis may present with acute comitant strabismus. However, our patients did not show any sign of ptosis, change in strabismus pattern, or other signs of muscle weakness throughout the follow-up period; further, the angle of deviation did not vary on repeated testing from day to day throughout the follow-up period.

Table 1 Clinical characteristics of patients with acute acquired comitant esotropia

A

Patient Number	1	2	3	4	5	6
Age (years)/Sex	13/F	16/M	16/M	12/F	7/M	15/F
Wearing spectacles	−	+	+	+	−	+
Duration of esotropia (months)	3	8	8	10	10	5
Smartphone use per day (hours)	5	8	4	6	4	8
Duration of smartphone use (months)	6	12	10	12	12	8
Presence of diplopia	−	+	+	+	−	+
Presenting VA, Rt/Lt (logMAR)	0.0/0.0	0.0/0.0	0.0/0.0	0.0/0.0	0.0/0.0	0.0/0.0
UCVA, Rt/Lt (logMAR)	0.0/0.0	0.5/0.5	0.4/0.3	0.8/0.8	0.0/0.0	0.5/0.4
BCVA, Rt/Lt (logMAR)	0.0/0.0	0.0/0.0	0.0/0.0	0.0/0.0	0.0/0.0	0.0/0.0
Manifest refraction (SE), Rt/Lt (D)	+0.25/+0.25	−3.00/−3.50	−4.00/−3.75	−4.50/−4.50	−0.75/−0.5	−4.50/−4.25
Cycloplegic refraction (SE), Rt/Lt (D)	+1.50/+1.50	−2.00/−2.25	−3.50/−3.50	−4.00/−4.25	+0.25/+0.25	−4.50/−4.25
Spectacle glasses power (SE), Rt/Lt (D)	Nil	−3.00/−3.50	−3.75/−3.50	−4.00/−4.25	Nil	−4.25/−4.00
Sensory function (arc seconds) at initial presentation	Nil	Nil	Nil	Nil	Nil	Nil
Bagolini striated glasses test results	Unsuppressed esotropia	Unsuppressed esotropia	Unsuppressed esotropia	Unsuppressed esotropia	Unsuppressed esotropia	Unsuppressed esotropia
Esodeviation at initial presentation, distance/near (PD)	45/45	35/35	45/45	35/35	25/25	20/20
Esodeviation after restriction of smartphone use, distance/near (PD)	35/35	30/30	30/30	15/15	8/12	12/4
Operation	BMR	BMR	BMR	−	−	−
Esodeviation at last follow up visit, distance/near (PD)	Ortho/Ortho	Ortho/Ortho	Ortho/Ortho	15/15	8/12	12/6
Sensory function at last follow up visit (arc seconds)	40	40	100	100	100	40
Bagolini striated glasses tset results after operation	Normal binocular single vision	Normal binocular single vision	Normal binocular single vision	Nil	Nil	Nil
Recurrence	−	−	−	−	−	−
Follow-up period (months)	14	12	8	11	4	6

B

Patient Number	7	8	9	10	11	12
Age (years)/Sex	15/F	16/M	15/F	7/M	16/F	12/F
Wearing spectacles	+	+	−	−	+	+
Duration of esotropia (months)	4	8	2	3	6	3

Table 1 Clinical characteristics of patients with acute acquired comitant esotropia *(Continued)*

Smartphone use per day (hours)	8	5	5	4	8	8
Duration of smartphone use (months)	6	12	24	12	8	4
Presence of diplopia	+	+	+	–	+	+
Presenting VA, Rt/Lt (logMAR)	0.0/0.0	0.0/0.0	0.0/0.0	0.0/0.0	0.0/0.0	0.0/0.0
UCVA, Rt/Lt (logMAR)	1.0/1.0	1.0/1.0	0.0/0.0	0.0/0.0	0.8/0.8	0.4/0.4
BCVA, Rt/Lt (logMAR)	0.0	0.0/0.0	0.0/0.0	0.0/0.0	0.0/0.0	0.0/0.0
Manifest refraction (SE), Rt/Lt (D)	–4.25/–4.75	–4.50/–4.75	+0.50/+0.25	+0.75/+1.125	–7.5/–7.5	–1.625/–1.625
Cycloplegic refraction (SE), Rt/Lt (D)	–4.125/–4.25	–3.50/–4.00	+0.50/+0.50	+1.0/+1.25	–7.25/–7.25	–1.5/–1.375
Spectacle glasses power (SE), Rt/Lt (D)	–4.00/–4.50	–4.00/–4.375	Nil	Nil	–7.0/–7.0	–1.50/–1.375
Sensory function (arc seconds) at initial presentation	Nil	100	Nil	800	100	400
Bagolini striated glasses test results	Unsuppressed esotropia	Unsuppressed esotropia	Unsuppressed esotropia	Unsuppressed esotropia	Unsuppressed esotropia	Unsuppressed esotropia
Esodeviation at initial presentation, distance/near (PD)	25/30	15/15	35/35	20/20	8/10	25/25
Esodeviation after restriction of smartphone use, distance/near (PD)	20/20	15/12	25/25	10/10	6/0	15/15
Operation	–	–	–	–	–	–
Esodeviation at last follow up visit, distance/near (PD)	20/20	15/12	25/25	10/10	6/0	15/15
Sensory function at last follow up visit (arc seconds)	Nil	100	Nil	100	60	100
Recurrence	–	–	–	–	–	–
Follow up period (months)	3	3	3	3	6	6

Abbreviations: VA visual acuity, *UCVA* uncorrected visual acuity, *BCVA* best corrected visual acuity, *Rt* right, *Lt* left, *PD* prism diopter, *SE* spherical equivalent, *D* diopter, *BMR* bilateral medial rectus recession, *Ortho* Orthophoria

Although spasm of near reflex or accommodation is a possible differential diagnosis, this can be excluded based on the absence of episodic miosis, psychogenic or organic causes, consistency of eye deviation and refractive error in our patients after cycloplegia [17, 18]. Refractive esotropia is also a possible differential diagnosis, but all patients in our study were myopic or mildly hyperopic, and refractive correction did not show any change in the degree of esodeviation in patients with hyperopia. Bilateral sixth nerve paresis might evolve into comitant esodeviation without motility limitations in the future. However, the absence of trauma history, brain lesions, or vascular disorder, the similarity in esodeviation at near and far fixation, and the reduction in esodeviation after smartphone restriction could be discriminating factors between bilateral sixth nerve paresis and comitant esodeviation in our patients.

As proposed in previous articles, many authors have emphasized that a high index of clinical suspicion should be maintained for intracranial lesions as a cause of AACE, because AACE can be the sole sign of intracranial disease [19–21]. However, all patients in our case series had undergone neurologic examination, including neuroimaging, and no abnormalities were detected.

Burian-Franceschetti type AACE can also be a possible diagnosis. Comitant convergent strabismus without a definitive underlying cause, the presence of diplopia, the moderate degree of the angle of deviation, and good functional outcome after strabismus surgery meets the diagnostic criteria. However, most of our patients were myopic and none of our patients had experienced recent physical or psychological stress due to exhaustion that might have caused acute onset of eyeball deviation in the aforementioned type of esotropia.

The type of esotropia observed in our case series most closely resembles "acute concomitant esotropia of adulthood" described by Spierer [22]. They share common characteristics, such as the development of comitant esotropia with normal corrected visual acuity in both eyes, regaining of normal stereopsis after surgical correction of esotropia, as well as similar angle of deviation at distance and near fixation, absence of neurologic disease, and mainly myopic refraction error. The mechanism by which patients with myopia and good stereopsis develop comitant esotropia is still not clear.

Video display terminal (VDT) work itself was shown to induce abnormalities in accommodation and vergence compared with ordinary hard copy work (non-VDT work) [23, 24]. Thus, it is conceivable that excessive smartphone use at a close reading distance and the resultant abnormalities in accommodation and vergence in adolescents with low fusional divergence capacity or previous latent esophoria (inherently susceptible to the development of esotropia) can lead to dynamic preponderance of the medial rectus muscles, resulting in the development of manifest esotropia; the mechanism of which was initially proposed by Bielschowsky [3, 4, 25].

The absence of diplopia in some patients and the presence of only intermittent diplopia at distance fixation in others might indicate that dynamic hypertonus of the medial rectus muscles and the resultant development of esotropia progress slowly [26]. Refraining from smartphone use caused a decrease in the degree of esodeviation, which partially supports this mechanism. However, evidence is insufficient to supportthis proposal. The exact mechanism by which comitant esotropia develops in myopic or slightly hyperopic patients without previous manifest deviation remains unclear and has yet to be determined.

The orthophoric position and normal fusional capacity were re-established postoperatively in three patients who received bilateral medial rectus recession. As Spierer [22] proposed, normally developed binocular vision is disrupted after the onset of strabismus; therefore, the binocular capacity is potentially preserved and is later regained after the strabismus is surgically corrected.

The limitations of this case series include small sample size and the fact that we studied only patients with AACE who used smartphones excessively. AACE is a disease entity with undefined prevalence, but it is certainly considered rare. Therefore, although medical chart review was performed for patients who had visited the tertiary pediatric ophthalmology and strabismus service during a period of several years, the sample size was small [14]. In addition, we could not perform a comparative analysis between AACE patients with and without history of excessive smartphone use because of the paucity of AACE patients.

A distinct causal relationship between AACE and excessive smartphone use was not proven in our patients. However, other types of AACE, such as Bielschowsky type, Burian-Franceschetti type, AACE caused by intracranial tumor, and other causes of esotropia in adolescences, can be excluded in our case series. Further, extensive and comprehensive questioning and history taking revealed that only excessive smartphone use (more than 4 h per day) for a long period of time was common in all patients with AACE who were not diagnosed with Bielschowsky type, Burian-Franceschetti type, and AACE related to neurologic disease. In addition, smartphone restriction led to a significant decrease in esodeviation in all patients. Therefore, we speculate that excessive smartphone use could lead to the development of AACE.

Further, it is unclear whether other confounding factors (e.g., other forms of near work such as reading or sewing) may have influenced the clinical results. However, according to questioning and history taking, a gross difference did not exist in hours spent studying, reading, or other possible near-visual activities in AACE patients with a history of excessive smartphone use, when compared with AACE patients due to other causes. Further case-controlled studies with larger study populations are warranted. Moreover, we did not obtain an accommodation measurement by using dynamic retinoscopy or other devices that would give a more objective measure of accommodative power.

Conclusion

In conclusion, excessive smartphone use at a close reading distance might influence the development of rarely occurring AACE in patients with myopia or mild hyperopia, good corrected visual acuity, and binocularity. AACE can potentially be induced by increased tonus of the medial rectus muscles resulting from the sustained near work itself, and disrupted accommodation and vergence by VDT work. In these cases, refraining from smartphone use can decrease the amount of esodeviation, and successful management of residual esotropia and restoration of binocularity can be achieved with bilateral medial rectus recession. Further studies with larger sample sizes and long-term follow-up periods are warranted.

Abbreviations
AACE: acute acquired comitant esotropia; D: diopters; PD: prism diopters; VDT: video display terminal.

Competing interests
The authors declare that they have no competing interests.

Authors' contributions
All authors (HSL, SWP, and HH) conceived of and designed the study protocol. HSL collected the data. HSL and HH were involved in the analysis. HSL wrote the first draft of the manuscript. SWP and HH reviewed and revised the manuscript and produced the final version. All authors read and approved the final manuscript.

Authors' information
Not applicable.

Acknowledgements
The study was supported by the CNUH Biomedical Research Institute (CRI 15014-1). The funders had no role in study design, data collection and analysis, decision to publish or preparation of the m anuscript. None of authors have any financial interest in any of the material described herein.

References
1. Clark AC, Nelson LB, Simon JW, Wagner R, Rubin SE. Acute acquired comitant esotropia. Br J Ophthalmol. 1989;73:636–8.
2. Legmann Simon A, Borchert M. Etiology and prognosis of acute, late-onset esotropia. Ophthalmology. 1997;104:1348–52.
3. Burian HM, Miller JE. Comitant convergent strabismus with acute onset. Am J Ophthalmol. 1958;45:55–64.
4. Hoyt CS, Good WV. Acute onset concomitant esotropia: when is it a sign of serious neurological disease? Br J Ophthalmol. 1995;79:498–501.
5. Kemmanu V, Hegde K, Seetharam R, Shetty BK. Varied aetiology of acute acquired comitant esotropia: a case series. Oman J Ophthalmol. 2012;5:103–5.
6. Hussaindeen JR, Mani R, Agarkar S, Ramani KK, Surendran TS. Acute adult onset comitant esotropia associated with accommodative spasm. Optom Vis Sci. 2014;91:S46–51.
7. Boulos MNK, Wheeler S, Tavares C, Jones R. How smartphones are changing the face of mobile and participatory healthcare: an overview, with example from eCAALYX. Biomed Eng Online. 2011;10:24.
8. Brian RM, Ben-Zeev D. Mobile health (mHealth) for mental health in Asia objectives, strategies, and limitations. Asian J Psychiatry. 2014;10:96–100.
9. Kwon M, Kim DJ, Cho H, Yang S. The Smartphone addiction scale: development and validation of a short version for adolescents. PLoS One. 2013;8, e83558.
10. Lee CH, Kim KH, Jang SA. A study on policy measures to protect youths with the spread of Smartphone. National Youth Policy Institute Research. 2013;12:1–311.
11. Kwon M, Lee JY, Won WY, Park JW, Min JA, Hahn C, et al. Development and validation of a Smartphone addiction scale (SAS). PLoS One. 2013;8, e56936.
12. Bernheim A, Halfon O, Boutrel B. Controversies about the enhanced vulnerability of the adolescent brain to develop addiction. Front Pharmacol. 2013;4:118.
13. Wang H, Zhou X, Lu C, Wu J, Deng X, Hong L. Problematic internet use in high school students in Guangdong province china. PloS One. 2011;6, e19660.
14. Kothari M. Clinical characteristics of spontaneous late-onset comitant acute nonaccommodative esotropia in children. Indian J Ophthalmol. 2007;55:117–20.
15. Ing MR, Roberts KM, Lin A, Chen JJ. The stability of the monofixation syndrome. Am J Ophthalmol. 2014;157:248–53. e1.
16. Buch H, Vinding T. Acute acquired comitant esotropia of childhood: a classification based on 48 children. Acta Ophthalmol. 2015;93:568–74.
17. Chan RVP, Trobe JD. Spasm of accommodation associated with closed head trauma. J Neuro Ophthalmol. 2002;22:15–7.
18. Knapp C, Sachdev A, Gottlob I. Spasm of the near reflex associated with head injury. Strabismus. 2002;10:1–4.
19. Musazadeh M, Hartmann K, Simon F. Late onset esotropia as first symptom of a cerebellar tumor. Strabismus. 2004;12:119–23.
20. Lee JM, Kim SH, Lee JI, Ryou JY, Kim SY. Acute comitant esotropia in a child with a cerebellar tumor. Korean J Ophthalmol. 2009;23:228–31.
21. Schreuders J, Thoe Schwartzenberg GWS, Bos E, Versteegh FGA. Acute-onset esotropia: should we look inside? J Pediatr Ophthalmol Strabismus. 2012;49:e70–2.
22. Spierer A. Acute concomitant esotropia of adulthood. Ophthalmology. 2003;110:1053–6.
23. Ishikawa S. Examination of the near triad in VDU operators. Ergonomics. 1990;33:787–98.
24. Mutti DO, Zadnik K. Is computer use a risk factor for myopia? J Am Optom Assoc. 1996;67:521–30.
25. Campos EC. Why do the eyes cross? a review and discussion of the nature and origin of essential infantile esotropia, microstrabismus, accommodative esotropia, and acute comitant esotropia. J AAPOS. 2008;12:326–31.
26. Godts D, Mathysen DGP. Distance esotropia in the elderly. Br J Ophthalmol. 2013;97:1415–9.

25

Biometry and visual function of a healthy cohort in Leipzig, Germany

Maria Teresa Zocher[1], Jos J. Rozema[2,3], Nicole Oertel[1], Jens Dawczynski[1], Peter Wiedemann[1], Franziska G. Rauscher[1*] and For the EVICR.net

Abstract

Background: Cross-sectional survey of ocular biometry and visual function in healthy eyes across the life span of a German population aged 20 to 69 years ($n = 218$). Subject number in percent per age category reflected the percentage within the respective age band of the population of Leipzig, Germany.

Methods: Measurements obtained: subjective and objective refraction, best-corrected visual acuity, accommodation, contrast sensitivity, topography and pachymetry with Scheimpflug camera, axial length with non-contact partial coherence interferometry, and spectral-domain optical coherence tomography of the retina. Pearson correlation coefficients with corresponding p-values were given to present interrelationships between stature, biometric and refractive parameters or their associations with age. Two-sample T-tests were used to calculate gender differences. The area under the logarithmic contrast sensitivity function (AULCSF) was calculated for the analysis of contrast sensitivity as a single figure across a range of spatial frequencies.

Results: The results of axial length (AL), anterior chamber depth (ACD) and anterior chamber volume (ACV) differed as a function of the age of the participants (rho (p value): AL −0.19 (0.006), ACD −0.56 (< 0.001), ACV-0.52 (< 0.001)). Longer eyes had deeper ACD (AL:ACD 0.62 (< 0.001), greater ACV (AL:ACV 0.65 (< 0.001) and steeper corneal radii (AL:R1ant; R2ant; R1post; R2post 0.40; 0.35; 0.36; 0.36 (all with (< 0.001)). Spherical equivalent was associated with age (towards hyperopia: 0.34 (< 0.001)), AL (−0.66 (< 0.001)), ACD (−0.52 (< 0.001)) and ACV (−0.46 (< 0.001)). Accommodation was found lower for older subjects (negative association with age, $r = -0.82$ (< 0.001)) and contrast sensitivity presented with smaller values for older ages (AULCSF −0.38, (< 0.001)), no change of retinal thickness with age. 58 % of the study cohort presented with a change of refractive correction above ±0.50 D in one or both eyes (64 % of these were habitual spectacle wearers), need for improvement was present in the young age-group and for older subjects with increasing age.

Conclusion: Biometrical data of healthy German eyes, stratified by age, gender and refractive status, enabled cross-comparison of all parameters, providing an important reference database for future patient-based research and specific in-depth investigations of biometric data in epidemiological research.

Trial registration: ClinicalTrials.gov # NCT01173614 July 28, 2010

Keywords: Ocular biometry, Visual function, Gullstrand, Cross section, Dioptric distance

* Correspondence: franziska.rauscher@medizin.uni-leipzig.de
[1]Department of Ophthalmology, Leipzig University Hospital, Liebigstrasse 10-14, 04103 Leipzig, Germany
Full list of author information is available at the end of the article

Background

The optics of the human eye is based on the refractive parameters of the individual ocular structures, each of which is affected differently by age. Well known examples of this are the thickening of the crystalline lens with aging and the gradual flattening of the anterior chamber [1]. Although normal aging has been studied extensively in the literature, some studies limit themselves to subsections of the population, such as subjects over 40 years, children, certain nationalities or ethnicities, or emmetropes [2–4]. Other studies presented only certain parameters of ocular biometry, or concentrated on prevalence of specific eye conditions (e.g., cataract, AMD) [5, 6]. This study concentrates on various biometric parameters in connection with refraction and retinal measurements with optical coherence tomography (OCT) in a healthy population. Although measurements in healthy eyes across the life span could provide an invaluable reference in the form of a normative database for a multitude of ocular biometric factors, few studies have presented recent data for a European population since many of the population – based studies have been conducted in developing countries [7–9]. In Europe, three larger population-based studies have focused on the aspects of biometric data to determine the prevalence, incidence and major risk-factors of age-related macular degeneration, glaucoma and diabetic retinopathy in adults over 35 years [10–14]. Results on refractive error and related ocular biometry were presented for British adults over 48 years of age [15].

As those previous eye studies in Europe concentrated on older eyes and on the prevalence of ocular pathologies, the current study aimed to obtain a full cross-section of a healthy population using modern measuring devices to establish reliable reference values for future work. A specific strength of this study is the investigation of many different biometric values together with detailed information on refraction and retinal properties. OCT was implemented to eliminate subjects with retinal changes or pathologies from the sample. Based on these data differences in parameters across the different age groups can be determined, and it provides reference values stratified by age range, gender and refractive status. This may help to find inter – correlations of optical parameters in the human eye.

Methods

Study population

The cohort presented in this work was measured under the framework of "Project Gullstrand" (Ethics Committee of the Antwerp University Hospital (No. B30020072406)), a multi-centred cross – sectional study performed at different European clinical sites [16, 17]. The Leipzig dataset, for the first time, presents various biometric measures

in a group of healthy German subjects with strictly examined absence of degenerative changes of the retina. This cohort was recruited to mirror the distribution of age and gender of the population of Leipzig (Saxony, Germany) [18]. The data presented here were obtained between July and December 2011. The study adhered to the Tenets of the Declaration of Helsinki and approval for the study was obtained from the Ethics Committee of the Medical Faculty of the University of Leipzig (No. 162/11) and is registered as ClinicalTrials.gov # NCT01173614.

Subjects were recruited through public announcements and press releases. However, in a first telephone interview the interested subjects were asked a series of health related questions in order to exclude subjects based on the inclusion criteria (age 20–69 years old, ametropia between −10 D and +10 D) before examinations, and the exclusion criteria, which were prior ocular surgery, amblyopia, refraction larger than ± 10 D, corneal or retinal pathologies in either eye, systemic diseases (e.g., diabetes mellitus, hypertension, multiple sclerosis, Grave's disease, …), pregnancy of more than 5 months at the moment of testing, as well as recent wear of hard contact lenses. Likewise, a 2-day break prior to testing was required with soft contact lens use.

Examination procedures

After informed consent was obtained, an interview was conducted to determine ocular and medical history, level of education and height and weight as self – reported by the subject. Then subjects were asked to fill out the 25 item National Eye Institute visual functioning questionnaire (NEI – VFQ – 25), developed at RAND under the sponsorship of the National Eye Institute [19, 20].

The following refraction parameters were used following the uniform method for visual acuity notation in scientific publication [21]. Refraction was estimated with an autorefractometer (Automatic Refractor/Keratometer Model 599, Humphrey Instruments, Carl Zeiss Meditec AG, Jena, Germany). A single operator then performed a non – cycloplegic subjective refinement of the refractive correction until the best corrected visual acuity (BCVA) was obtained. Uncorrected and corrected distance visual acuity (UDVA, CDVA) were measured monocularly and binocularly with a trial frame at 4 m, using an ETDRS chart [22], which was housed in a light box. Participants who failed to read the largest letter unaided at 4 m were retested at 2 m then at 1 m. Testing began with the first letter on the top row. When having difficulty reading a letter, the subject was encouraged to guess. Visual acuity was scored as the total number of letters read correctly in logMAR units (logarithm of the minimum angle of resolution). The full refraction was noted and for further analysis the spherical equivalent (SE) or the dioptric distance (described below, [23]) were used as measures of refractive error.

After determining the best CDVA, accommodation was tested for each eye separately and binocularly using the negative lens test with an ETDRS chart at 4 m distance, while wearing the distance correction [24]. The subject was asked to focus two lines above the lowest line still readable with best correction. A lens of −10 D was placed in front of the eye and the subject was asked if he or she could still read the line. If this was not the case, the same was repeated with a lens of 0.5 D lower power until the subject was able to see the line clearly again.

Contrast sensitivity was measured with the Visual Contrast Test System (VCTS; Vistech Consultants, Dayton, USA) panel in a room with 80–100 lux illuminance. Before, the pupil size was determined with a pupil size gauge. This contrast sensitivity panel uses a grid of contrast levels for a range of spatial frequencies, which allows a rough reconstruction of the entire contrast sensitivity curve. With the VCTS panel the contrast increases from left to right and the spatial frequency from top to bottom. Each column contains gratings with spatial frequencies of 1.5, 3, 6, 12 and 18 cycles per degree (cpd). Each line contains 8 grids with progressively decreasing levels of contrast and a uniform grey field at the end of each line. The subject was seated at a distance of 2 m from the panel and had the task of describing the orientation of the lines of the respective grating being either vertical or 15° to the right or to the left. When the contrast of a grid has fallen below the threshold value, only a single grey field is perceived. The last grating of each row that was identified correctly was noted. The testing was carried out monocularly and binocularly with optical correction, if applicable.

Topography and pachymetry were measured with a Pentacam Scheimpflug camera (Oculus Optikgeräte GmbH, Wetzlar, Germany). Using non – contact partial coherence laser interferometry (IOL Master; Carl Zeiss Meditec AG, Jena, Germany), five measurements for axial length (AL) were obtained and the mean of these measurements as calculated by the IOL Master was noted in the datasheet. AL was measured as the distance from the anterior corneal vertex to the retinal pigment epithelium along fixation, automatically adjusted to the distance to the internal limiting membrane as used as a reference plane in ultrasound techniques [25]. The displayed results of the axial length measurements are therefore compatible with immersion ultrasound measurements through the use of an internal, statistically verified calculation algorithm [26, 27].

Further measurements were carried out employing optical coherence tomography (OCT) (Spectralis OCT, Heidelberg Engineering) to measure retinal thickness in the foveal region. The OCT was also useful in detecting diseases of the retina or pre – clinical abnormalities. OCT instrumentation and imaging technique have been described in detail elsewhere [28–31]. The central retinal thickness was defined as the distance between the internal limiting membrane to the outer border of the retinal pigment epithelium via the automatic segmentation algorithms of the Spectralis software by which the macular region is sectioned into three circular rings (1 mm, 3 mm and 6 mm diameter) which are subdivided into four quadrants to form nine regions of analysis. An average retinal thickness and retinal volume can be reported for central, superior inner, inferior inner, temporal inner, nasal inner, superior outer, inferior outer, temporal outer, nasal outer regions. The average of all points within the inner circle of 1-mm diameter is defined as central foveal subfield thickness (CFST). With accurate centration, the central foveal subfield (1 mm) includes the foveal minimum. The minimum retinal thickness is defined as minimal central retinal thickness (CRTmin).

Calculations and statistical analysis

Statistical analysis was performed using Minitab 14 (Minitab Inc., State College, Pennsylvania, USA). Due to the high degree of correlation between the eyes of a subject, only data of the right eye are presented in this study. All variables were first analysed by calculating the mean, standard deviation (SD) and 95 % confidence interval (95 % CI) after tests for normality using Q-Q-plots [32]. Further, mean and SD of the variables was calculated for age decades. Pearson correlation coefficient rho (r) and its corresponding p-value was calculated to present the interrelationships between stature and biometric and refractive parameters. Labeling systems exist to roughly categorize r values where correlation coefficients (in absolute value) of ≤ 0.35 are generally considered to represent low or weak correlations, 0.36 to 0.67 reflect modest or moderate correlations, and 0.68 to 1.0 identify strong or high correlations, and r coefficients of ≥ 0.90 represent very high correlations [33]. This notation was used throughout the manuscript. Meaningful clinical relevance of such associations should be established by calculating the coefficient of determination. It is obtained by simply squaring the correlation coefficient rho. R^2 is defined as the percent of the variation in the values of the dependent variable (y) that can be explained by variations in the values of the independent variable (x). This presents an index for the strength of an association, a value of $R2 \geq 50$ % (rho > 0.7) can be considered a relevant correlation [34]. Two-sample T-tests were used to calculate gender differences (p-values stated without Bonferoni correction, based on the planned outline of the procedure). ANOVA analysis with post-hoc t-tests were not carried out to investigate possible differences for individual parameters between age-categories (20–29, 30–39, 40–49, 50–59, 60–69 years of age) stated in Table 1, as a correlation with age itself is given for each biometric parameter measured as part of the result section.

The mean and SD of contrast sensitivity values in log units by age and gender are provided. To obtain log units from the contrast sensitivity level, a value key for the Vistech VCTS 6500 contrast sensitivity test system was used and log units of these values were calculated [35]. For further analysis of the contrast sensitivity as a single figure across a range of spatial frequencies, the area under the logarithmic contrast sensitivity function (AULCSF) was calculated according to the method of Applegate and colleagues [36]. In brief, the AULCSF was calculated by integrating a third order polynomial fitted to the log contrast sensitivity data between the fixed limits of 0.18 (corresponding to 1.5 cpd) and 1.26 (18 cpd) on the log spatial frequency scale; based on the raw data supplied by the test employed. It is, however, also possible to employ linear interpolation and integration between 1.5 and 18 cpd to compute an area under the contrast sensitivity curve [37]. Such a single-index criterion represents contrast sensitivity data as one number and therefore facilitates comparison and statistical analysis.

For further analysis, data were analysed by refractive status categorised by spherical equivalent (SE; sphere plus half cylinder based on sphere (S) and cylinder (C)) or categorised by dioptric distance (described below). Separation by SE was done by division into three groups (myopia (M), emmetropia (E) and hyperopia (H)).

Myopia was defined as a SE less than −0.5 D and hyperopia as a SE greater than +0.5 D. For facilitation of subanalysis of future publications, the data are also given as five subcategories, to indicate that there is a considerable functional difference between uncorrected eyes with a refraction smaller than ±2D and eyes with refractive error larger that ±2D. ±2D also roughly corresponds to the emmetropic peak of the refraction distribution. Tables 5, 6 and 7, as a reference: manifest myopia (< −2D), low myopia (−2D ≤ −0.5D), emmetropia (−0.5D ≥ ≤ +0.5D), low hypermetropia(+0.5D ≥ +2D) and manifest hypermetropia (> +2D).

Where possible, the mean difference between subpopulations was given (e.g., difference between men and women for various age groups amounting to an overall mean difference for men and women). However, other publications provide only the overall mean (e.g., mean of all women irrespective of age), therefore some cross – referencing in our study was only possible by computation based on values given in another investigation. This comparison (i.e., men and women) of averaged data, is referred to as difference of the mean(s) to distinguish the difference.

Description of refractive error by means of spherical equivalent is widely employed by ophthalmologists and optometrists. However, in a mathematical description of ophthalmic lenses, it is more suitable to employ matrix formalism [23, 38], which enables an accurate derived measure of every full refraction as a single term, making it independent of unit conversion problems otherwise present. While sphere and cylinder refer to power along principal directions, power components refer to fixed

Table 1 "Subjective refraction data stratified by gender and age"

	Women					Men				
	n	Sphere [D]	Spherical equivalent [D]	Dioptric Distance to habitual correction [D]	Dioptric Distance to a 0.00D lens [D]	n	Sphere [D]	Spherical equivalent [D]	Dioptric Distance to habitual correction [D]	Dioptric Distance to a 0.00D lens [D]
20–29 years	24	−0.85 ± 1.64	−0.99 ± 1.64	0.45 ± 0.27	1.23 ± 1.48	26	−1.07 ± 1.39	−1.46 ± 1.46	0.43 ± 0.26	1.78 ± 1.16
30–39 years	19	−1.34 ± 2.06	−1.63 ± 2.17	0.32 ± 0.29	2.06 ± 1.79	20	−1.62 ± 2.29	−2.00 ± 2.35	0.46 ± 0.36	2.07 ± 2.31
40–49 years	32	−0.86 ± 1.93	−1.13 ± 2.00	0.50 ± 0.35	1.33 ± 1.90	29	−0.24 ± 2.13	−0.56 ± 2.11	0.41 ± 0.33	1.39 ± 1.75
50–59 years	19	+0.91 ± 1.22	+0.74 ± 1.17	0.52 ± 0.43	1.15 ± 0.79	19	0.16 ± 2.36	−0.13 ± 2.41	0.70 ± 0.50	1.64 ± 1.76
60–69 years	16	+0.63 ± 1.94	+0.24 ± 2.18	0.73 ± 0.36	1.68 ± 1.47	14	+1.07 ± 1.66	+0.68 ± 1.76	0.55 ± 0.17	1.27 ± 1.06
All	110	−0.42 ± 1.95	−0.66 ± 2.02	0.49 ± 0.35	1.45 ± 1.56	108	−0.47 ± 2.15	−0.81 ± 2.18	0.49 ± 0.35	1.64 ± 1.67

Caption: Mean (± standard deviation) of sphere, spherical equivalent (SE) and dioptric distance (DD) to a 0.00D lens and dioptric distance of habitual spectacle correction to new subjective refraction, determined by best corrected visual acuity per age decade for women and men. SE (subjective) for the right eyes of 20–29 year olds was found to be −1.24 ± 1.55 D; 30–39: −1.82 ± 2.24 D; 40–49: −0.86 ± 2.06 D; 50–59: +0.31 ± 1.92 D; 60–69: +0.45 ± 1.97 D, see also Fig. 1. The hyperopic shift resulted in more emmetropic eyes in the 40–49 years decade, followed by a higher percentage of hyperopic eyes from 50 years onwards: 20–29: H = 4 %, E = 34 %, M = 62 %; 30–39: H = 8 %, E = 31 %, M = 62 %; 40–49: H = 8 %, E = 52 %, M = 39 %; 50–59: H = 45 %, E = 26 %, M = 29 %; 60–69: H = 50 %, E = 30 %, M = 20 % (% rounded to present full numbers). It is possible that some of the differences found between younger and older age groups may reflect other factors (e.g., changes in prevalence of refractive error) and therefore differences in refractive error observed may not properly account for changes in refractive error over time
The dioptric distance to habitual correction specifies the average deviation of the subject's habitual corrective lens (or no correction in-situ) to the optimum spectacle correction. The deviation of the habitual corrective state to its optimal corrective state, identified as part of the study, increased with increasing age and was greatest for older subjects. A second at-risk group for malcorrection was identified in the 20–29 age bracket, where about half a dioptre blur was measured

coordinate axes and are grouped into a matrix. The dioptric power matrix, F, is defined as

$$F = \begin{pmatrix} S + C \sin^2 \alpha & -C \cos\alpha \sin\alpha \\ -C \cos\alpha \sin\alpha & S + C \cos^2\alpha \end{pmatrix}$$, and it accounts

for all paraxial properties of the ophthalmic lens (prismatic effects are not considered here). In order to determine the mean refractive status for the study population, data for sphere, cylinder, and axis (α) measured by subjective refraction were transformed into a dioptric power matrix. In order to compare measures of refraction (e.g., old and new refraction), the dioptric distance (DD) was used. The dioptric distance DD is defined as the distance in the power domain between lenses with different astigmatic effects. This distance between two points based on the Frobenius norm, is

$$DD = \sqrt{0.5 \left((Fxx1-Fxx2)^2 + (Fyy1-Fyy2)^2 + 2(Fxy1-Fxy2)^2 \right)}$$

with Fxx, Fyy, Fxy as the elements of the matrix. The factor of 2 results from the equal diagonal elements of the matrix as depicted above. The prefactor 0.5 is conveniently employed in order to scale the dioptric distance to compare data logically (i.e., the dioptric distance of two spherical refractions equates to the distance between spheres).

Furthermore, the overall refractive error of the study population was provided by calculating the mean dioptric distance to a 0.00 D lens, as this transfers each measured refraction into a single number which allows such averaging. Additionally, the mean dioptric matrix and the mean dioptric distance were determined for different age decades. The dioptric distance to a 0.00 D lens results in a simplification of the above formula, as the second terms are replaced by zero.

$$DD = \sqrt{\left(S + \frac{C}{2}\right)^2 + \frac{C^2}{4}}$$

In order to establish how many subjects were in need of a new correction, a change in SE of 0.50 or a visual acuity improvement of one line of the ETDRS chart (equal to 0.1 logMAR) is commonly used [29, 39–41]. A change of 0.50 D for SE was employed to calculate differences between habitual correction and best corrected refraction. Differences are given as percentages above this criterion to indicate potential need of improved correction. For dioptric distance such a cut – off criterion for when a new correction would be required, needed to be similarly established. Here, for practical reasons, a dioptric distance between old corrective state and new best corrected refraction of 0.35 D was chosen for previous spectacle wearers and a dioptric distance of 0.50 D was chosen for non-spectacle wearers. This threshold of change of 0.35 D (and 0.50 D) is above the

known diurnal fluctuation [42] in refractive status and therefore underlining a true change in refraction. A dioptric distance of 0.35 D is equivalent to a change in sphere of 0.35 D or equivalent to a change in cylinder of 0.50 D, both of which constitute a similar influence on visual acuity. The dioptric distance of 0.50 D is equivalent to a change in sphere of 0.50 D or a change in cylinder of 0.71 D, again both affecting visual acuity to the same extent. The effect on visual acuity is based on previous research showing that the influence on vision is the same for refractions resulting in the same dioptric distance [43].

Results

Of the 245 participants eligible for participation based on the telephone interview, 27 subjects had to be excluded because it was established during examination that they did not fulfil the inclusion criteria (amblyopia (7), previously unknown health problems (4, diabetes mellitus, arterial hypertension, multiple sclerosis and glaucoma), rigid gas permeable lens wear (3) and pathologies of the cornea or retina as established by eye examination and OCT (13)), leaving 218 Caucasian subjects for the analysis. The data presented are based on 108 men and 110 women aged 21–69 years with mean ± SD age of 42 ± 13 years and 43 ± 13 years, respectively. See Fig. 1 for distribution of age across the sample.

The aim of this investigation is to establish normal sample data of biometric measurements based on strict inclusion criteria. The study cohort was specifically recruited to reflect the age and gender distribution of the population of Leipzig and is therefore unbiased by a specific selection [18]. In order to mirror this distribution for the final sample, (i) age and gender brackets were formed by referring to population data of Leipzig and then (ii) those bins were filled in sequence by subjects who fulfilled the strict exclusion criteria based on the telephone interview. Therefore many subjects, especially in the older age groups were not allowed to participate and it took longer to fill those bins with adequate subjects in order to have true normal data. (iii) Some subjects had to be excluded again based on OCT or other measures when abnormalities or degenerations were found. This procedure (i) to (iii) resulted in a match of the bins with the age and gender distribution of the population of Leipzig at the time stamp of analysis.

Biometric measurements
Height and weight
The mean height of the study population was 173 ± 10 cm (range 151 to 198 cm). The mean weight was 75 ± 17 kg (range 43 to 155 kg). Mean height and weight for women were 166 ± 6 cm and 66 ± 13 kg. Mean height and weight for men were 180 ± 8 cm and 84 ± 16 kg. As

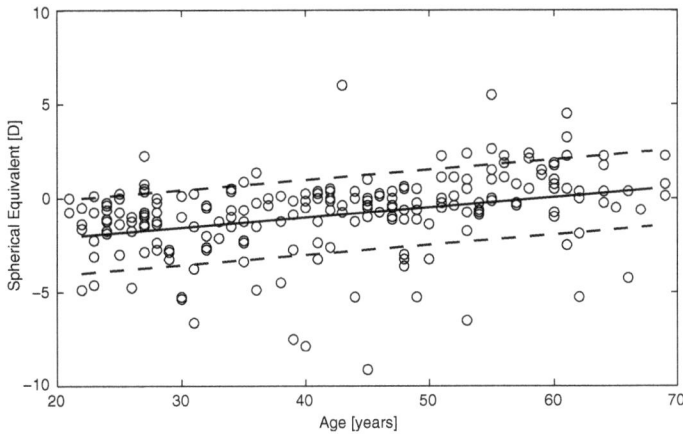

Fig. 1 "Spherical equivalent by age of subject ($n = 218$)". Caption: Scatterplot of age and spherical equivalent for subjective refraction. In the study population there was weak association between age and subjective refractive error ($r = 0.335$, $p < 0.001$). Regression equation: Spherical equivalent = $-3.03 + 0.054$ Age; 50 % confidence interval: 1.96 D

this data is self-reported, the data can only serve as an indicator. The body mass index (BMI) was then calculated, resulting in a mean of 25.0 ± 4.6 kg/m^2 (normal weight) (range 16.8 severe underweight to 46.8 kg/m^2 adipositas III). Women had a calculated BMI of 24.0 ± 4.2 kg/m^2 and men had a calculated BMI of 25.9 ± 4.5 kg/m^2. Taller people had longer eyes ($r = 0.374$, $p < 0.001$), deeper anterior chamber depths ($r = 0.240$, $p < 0.001$) and greater radii of corneal curvature ($r = 0.325$, $p < 0.001$). For regression equations, see Table 8. Body height was associated with several biometric parameters reported; height-adjusted variables are presented in Table 8.

Corneal curvature
The mean horizontal radius of curvature of the anterior cornela surface was 7.91 ± 0.26 mm (range 6.92 to 8.74 mm) with its corresponding refracting power being 47.62 ± 1.59 D (range 43.00–54.37 D). The radius was correlated significantly only with AL ($r = 0.398$, $p < 0.001$), but only with modest effect. The mean vertical radius of curvature of the anterior corneal surface was 7.73 ± 0.28 mm (range 6.45–8.59 mm) and the corresponding refracting power was 48.68 ± 1.78 D (range 43.78–58.27 D). The mean radius of curvature of the anterior corneal surface was 7.82 ± 0.26 mm (range 6.81–8.66 mm). The mean horizontal radius of curvature of the posterior corneal surface was 6.65 ± 0.27 mm (range 5.88–8.00 mm) and the corresponding refracting power was -6.03 ± 0.24 D (range -6.80 to -5.00 D). The mean vertical radius of curvature of the posterior corneal surface was 6.29 ± 0.26 mm (range 5.41–6.90 mm) with its corresponding refracting power being -6.37 ± 0.26 D (range -7.40 to -5.80 D). The mean radius of curvature

of the posterior corneal surface was 6.47 ± 0.25 mm (range 5.68–7.09 mm). See Table 4 for stratification by gender and age.

Corneal eccentricity (e) as the measure of corneal asphericity was assessed [44]. Mean eccentricity of the anterior corneal surface (e ant) was 0.38 ± 0.19 (range -0.12 to 0.72) and mean eccentricity of the posterior corneal surface (e post) was 0.16 ± 0.36 (range -0.48 to 0.90). Eccentricities for both the anterior and posterior surfaces were mildly associated with age (e ant = $0.56 - 0.004$ Age, $r = 0.340$, $p < 0.001$; e post = $-0.41 + 0.013$ Age, $r = 0.439$, $p < 0.001$). The eccentricity of anterior and posterior corneal surface was each associated differently with anterior chamber depth. The anterior eccentricity was independent of ACD ($r = 0.046$, $p = 0.496$), i.e., the shape of the surface of the front of the cornea is not associated with ACD. The posterior eccentricity was moderately negatively correlated with ACD ($r = -0.430$, $p < 0.001$): a shallower ACD resulted in eccentricities closer to 1 reflecting an ellipse (e between 0 and 1) or even a parabola(e =1), whereas deeper ACD were associated with a more spherical shape (if e =0 the curve is a circle) [44].

Central corneal thickness
Mean central corneal thickness (CCT) was 554 ± 32 μm (range 454–666 μm). CCT was not associated with age ($r = 0.026$, $p = 0.701$), refractive error SE ($r = 0.039$, $p = 0.568$), AL ($r = 0.116$, $p = 0.087$) nor ACD ($r = -0.018$, $p = 0.793$).

Axial length
Mean axial length was 23.80 ± 1.05 mm (range 20.89–27.42 mm). Women had shorter ALs ($p < 0.001$) and axial length differed as a function of age (AL = 24.4 –

0.0141 Age), although, the correlation was very weak ($r = -0.184$, $p < 0.001$). Myopic eyes were longer than hyperopic eyes ($r = -0.674$, $p < 0.001$). Longer eyes had a deeper ACD ($r = 0.623$, $p < 0.001$) and a greater ACV ($r = 0.652$, $p < 0.001$). There was an increase in corneal curvature radii with increasing axial length ($r = 0.398$, $p < 0.001$). AL moderately correlated with UDVA ($r = 0.431$, $p < 0.001$). Stratification by age and gender is displayed in Table 4, stratification by refractive category is depicted in Tables 5, 6 and 7.

Anterior chamber depth
Mean anterior chamber depth (ACD) was 2.83 ± 0.37 mm (range 1.84–3.74 mm). Men (2.92 mm) had deeper mean ACD than women (2.74 mm) ($p < 0.001$) and in general older people had shallower anterior chamber depths than younger people as a modest negative correlation was found with age (ACD = 3.50 – 0.0155 Age; $r = -0.555$, $p < 0.001$). ACD was moderately associated with refractive error based on SE of subjective refraction (ACD = 2.76 – 0.0938 SE; $r = -0.519$, $p < 0.001$), showing myopic subjects had a greater ACD than hyperopic subjects.

Anterior chamber volume
Mean anterior chamber volume (ACV) was 160.1 ± 39.5 mm^3 (range 71.00–283.00 mm^3). Men had greater ACVs ($p < 0.001$). Age and ACV were moderately correlated ($r = -0.519$, $p < 0.001$, ACV = 225 – 1.52 Age). The association between ACV and ACD ($r = 0.900$, $p < 0.001$) and the association between ACV and AL ($r = 0.652$, $p < 0.001$) can be described further: subjects with greater ACD (ACV = –108 + 94.7 ACD) and longer eyes (ACV = –420 + 24.3 AL) had greater ACV. ACV was associated with refractive error ($r = -0.468$, $p < 0.001$). Myopic subjects, when stratified by subjected best corrected SE, had the greatest ACV (H < E < M: 125 < 157 < 178 mm^3). See also stratification by five refractive state in Tables 5, 6 and 7.

Retinal thickness
Measurements of retinal thickness were available for 206 subjects. Each OCT scan was manually centred to optimize grid location according to foveal centre, correcting for any possible decentration due to fixation errors. Central retinal thickness, defined here as central foveal subfield thickness (CFST, i.e., mean thickness within the circular central subfield (1 mm diameter, [22])) for the subject group was normally distributed. Minimal central retinal thickness (CRTmin) defined as the thinnest value was not normally distributed. The average across subjects for the CFST was 279 ± 21 μm (range: 227–337 μm). For CRTmin the mean was 232 ± 20 μm (range: 191–317 μm), the median was 230 μm. The mean

± SD of CRTmin and CFST thicknesses in men were 233 ± 20 μm (median 232 μm) and 285 ± 20 μm, respectively. CFST was statistical significantly different for men compared to women ($p < 0.001$). The mean ± SD of CRTmin and CFST thickness in women were 230 ± 20 μm (median 228 μm), and 274 ± 19 μm, respectively. No relationship of CRTmin with gender (Mann-Whitney U test (MW-U); $p = 0.162$,) or age (rank correlation; $r = 0.13$, $p = 0.06$) was found. Although the younger age categories presented with thinner retinas, this comparison was not statistically significant, $p = 0.403$. CRTmin presented with the following median thicknesses separated by gender for the decades investigated, 20–29: male (m):225 μm, female (f):218 μm; 30–39: m: 233 μm, f: 225 μm; 40–49: m: 234 μm, f:232 μm; 50–59: m: 234 μm, f: 228 μm; 60–69: m: 235 μm, f: 231 μm.

When CFST and CRTmin were stratified based on three groups of SE (subjective best corrected), there was no statistically significant difference between CRTmin or CFST between the investigated refractive categories. However the trend presented with slightly smaller CFST and CRTmin values for myopic eyes compared to emmetropes or hyperopic eyes, i.e., longer eyes presented with thinner retinal thickness (CFST = 295– 0.65 AL, $r = -0.033$, $p = 0.634$).

Optics and visual function
Refractive error
The mean of the subjective refractive error across the sample was calculated by employing the dioptric distance (DD) to a 0.00 D lens per subject, allowing averaging across the sample. Based on that, the mean refractive error was DD: 1.55 ± 1.63 D (range 0.00–8.38 D); women 1.45 ± 1.59 D; men 1.64 ± 1.67 D.

Mean sphere (based on subjective, right eye) was -0.45 ± 2.05 D (range –8.00 to +6.50 D). Mean cylinder (subjective, right eye) was -0.58 ± 0.61 D (range 0.00 to –4.00 D). Mean SE (objective, right eye) was -0.75 ± 2.06 D (range –9.125 to +6.00 D), see also Fig. 1. The spherical equivalent of the best corrected subjective refraction resulted in -0.69 ± 2.13 D for the right eye (81 emmetropic eyes) and in -0.66 ± 2.09 D for the left eye with a mean best corrected visual acuity of -0.12 ± 0.08 logMAR for either eye respectively.

A weak correlation of sphere (subjective) and age ($r = 0.356$, $p < 0.001$) and spherical equivalent (subjective) and age ($r = 0.335$, $p < 0.001$) suggests a hyperopization for older ages (Table 1). SE was additionally weakly to moderately associated with UDVA ($r = -0.544$, $p < 0.001$), ACD ($r = -0.519$, $p < 0.001$), ACV ($r = -0.468$, $p < 0.001$) and AL ($r = -0.661$, $p < 0.001$). For stratification by gender and age see Table 4, for stratification by refractive state see Tables 5, 6 and 7.

There was a strong correlation between sphere ($r = 0.978$, $p < 0.001$) and spherical equivalent ($r = 0.979$, $p < 0.001$) from respectively subjective and objective refraction. Therefore the values of the subjective refraction were chosen for analysis in the present paper because BCVA was taken as the gold standard.

Inclusion criteria restricted large refractive error, and therefore the reported data are truncated deliberately. 44 % of the study population were myopic (M), 37 % emmetropic (E) and 19 % hyperopic (H). The average uncorrected and corrected visual acuity were +0.25 ± 0.42 logMAR (range –0.26 to +1.50 logMAR) and –0.12 ± 0.08 logMAR (range –0.30 to +0.20 logMAR), respectively.

Spherical equivalent and dioptric distance
Additionally to the refractive error summarized above, the difference between the subjective refraction and the existing spectacle lens of a subject was calculated by employing the dioptric distance [23]. For the 218 subjects, the mean dioptric distance found between best visual acuity based refractive correction and habitual correction was 0.50 ± 0.35 D ranging from 0.00 to 1.63 D; women 0.50 ± 0.36 D; men 0.50 ± 0.35 D. There was an increase of need for optimised correction with age, for stratification by age, see Tables 1 and 2.

In comparison to other studies and with respect to the clinical routine, the SE measure is more commonly used.

Using spherical equivalent as a marker, it was investigated how the refractive status was distributed across the study cohort and if improvement of vision by new subjective refraction resulted in changed correction. Interestingly, 118 (54 %) were habitual spectacle wearers, of those 81 (69 %) presented with a change of refraction of over ±0.50 D in one or both eyse established by subjective best corrected refraction in comparison to habitual correction. 100 (46 %) wore no glasses prior to the study and for 46 (46 %) of those a change of refraction of over ±0.75 D in one or both eyes was found. This resulted in 58 % of the study cohort with a change of refraction which might require a need of new or updated spectacle correction (64 % of those already habitual spectacle wearers).

To allow cross-comparison with previous work where the more time-consuming measure of subjective refraction had not been carried out [45, 46], the change of refraction was additionally assessed based on the objective refraction. In order to investigate if a subject required a new refractive correction in comparison to such studies, the change in refractive error is additionally presented here based on the objective refraction measurements carried out. Based on this, the change in objective refraction resulted in 76 (64 %) of 118 spectacle wearers (i.e., 54 % of the study population) with a change of refraction of over ±0.50 D in one or both eyes. 100 (46 %) wore no glasses prior to the study, 16 (16 %) of those were found to be require a

Table 2 "Visual acuity and refractive data stratified by refractive error"

	Myopes	Emmetropes	Hyperopes
UDVA [logMAR]	+0.52 ± 0.43	–0.09 ± 0.09	+0.32 ± 0.32
CDVA [logMAR]	–0.10 ± 0.08	–0.15 ± 0.07	–0.10 ± 0.09
Sphere [D]	–2.01 ± 1.81	0.11 ± 0.34	2.05 ± 1.30
SE [D]	–2.40 ± 1.83	–0.06 ± 0.31	+1.79 ± 1.23
DD to habitual correction [D]	0.52 ± 0.35	0.34 ± 0.26	0.73 ± 0.38
DD to a 0.00D lens [D]	2.47 ± 1.82	0.34 ± 0.19	1.74 ± 1.21
AL [mm]	24.38 ± 1.06	23.54 ± 0.73	22.98 ± 0.79
CRTmin [µm]	231.08 ± 20.07	231.76 ± 20.50	232.51 ± 18.75
CFST [µm]	279.01 ± 20.58	279.49 ± 20.70	279.28 ± 20.67
height adjusted data (for procedure see Table 8)			
AL_adj [mm]	24.32 ± 1.01	23.57 ± 0.65	23.03 ± 0.74
CRTmin_adj [µm]	230.96 ± 19.76	232.03 ± 20.47	233.17 ± 18.89
CFST_adj [µm]	278.10 ± 19.66	279.61 ± 20.18	280.41 ± 19.60

Caption: Data stratified by refractive state based on spherical equivalent (SE) of subjective refraction (mean ± standard deviation) determined by best corrected visual acuity. Data grouped into three refractive states by SE based on the following criteria: hyperopia > +0.50 and myopia < –0.50. Uncorrected distance visual acuity (UDVA) was best for emmetropes, corrected distance visual acuity (CDVA) was relatively equal between groups, mean SE identified that myopia was the highest absolute refractive error of the sample. Dioptric distance (DD) was employed to present the change of the best corrected subjective refraction to the previous corrective state (e.g., spectacle correction if present). Here a value of zero would indicate that former correction and current refraction matched. Based on this, the mean DD between best corrected refraction and current spectacle correction was 0.52D (SD ±0.35) for myopes, 0.34D (±0.26) for emmetropes and 0.73D (±0.38) for hyperopes. To summarise the refractive error present in the sample (218 subjects) by dioptric distance to a 0.00D lens, the group presented with 1.55 ± 1.63 D (range 0.00 to 8.38 D); women 1.45 ± 1.59 D; men 1.64 ± 1.67 D. Stratified by SE, these values for DD were 2.47D (±1.82) for myopic subjects, 0.24D (±0.19) for emmetropes and 1.74D (±1.21) for hyperopes, which is supplied here for comparison with the routinely used measure of SE when stratified into the three groups change of refraction of over ±0.75 D in one or both eyes; i.e., change to a value of zero, representing no previous habitual correction). Here, 42 % of the study cohort presented a deviation of objective refraction to habitual spectacle correction (83 % of those already previous spectacle wearers). Using dioptric distance as a marker, it was investigated how the refractive status was distributed across the study cohort and if improvement of vision by new subjective refraction resulted in changed correction. Here, 71 (60 %) of 118 (54 %) habitual spectacle presented with a change of refraction of over ±0.35 D in one or both eyes. 101 (46 %) wore no glasses previous to the study, 47 (47 %) of those had a change of refraction of over ±0.50 D in one or both eyes. This resulted in 54 % of the study cohort with a change of refraction which might require a need of new or updated spectacle correction (60 % already habitual spectacle wearers). As can be seen from Table 1, older subjects presented with poorer accuracy of current spectacle lens correction. The deviation of the habitual corrective state to its optimum increased with increasing age. A second group identified with need for improvement of refractive correction was 20–29 years old, where about half a dioptre blur was measured.

Accommodation

Mean binocular amplitude of accommodation was 2.65 ± 1.92 D, 2.67 ± 2.07 D in women and 2.63 ± 1.77 D in men. Accommodation was found to differ between age groups and the amplitude of accommodation was progressively less for older ages (Accommodation = 10.2 − 0.158 Age, $r = -0.826$, $p < 0.001$). Detailed binocular amplitudes of accommodation for age groups were 20–29 years 4.32 ± 2.13 D, 30–39 years 3.92 ± 1.86 D, 40–49 years 2.12 ± 0.96 D, 50–59 years 1.07 ± 0.50 D and 60–69 years 1.29 ± 0.67 D. Accommodation had moderate correlations

with ACD ($r = 0.498$, $p < 0.001$) and ACV ($r = 0.484$, $p < 0.001$).

Contrast sensitivity

Mean contrast sensitivity (log units) in spatial frequencies of 1.5, 3, 6, 12 and 18 cpd was 1.70 ± 0.18, 1.99 ± 0.18, 2.04 ± 0.20, 1.90 ± 0.26 and 1.58 ± 0.27, respectively. For comparison of levels of spatial frequency data, women seemed to have a better contrast sensitivity than men. As can be seen from Fig. 2, contrast sensitivity differed amongst the stratified age groups and was lower at each spatial frequency for older subjects. This association with age was confirmed by the analysis on the basis of the area under the log contrast sensitivity function (AULCSF) curve (AULCSF = 2.29 - 0.005 Age, r = −0.379, p < 0.001). As shown in Fig. 3, hyperopic subjects seemed to have reduced contrast sensitivity. The AULCSF curve was 2.08 ± 0.19 and 31.16 ± 3.19 with linear integration if spatial frequencies were not logarithmic. AULCSF data for women was 2.04 ± 0.18 and for men was 2.09 ± 0.18, this difference was statistically significantly different from zero ($p = 0.038$). Separated by refractive category, myopes presented with an AULCSF of 2.04 ± 0.19, emmetropes with an AULCSF of 2.07 ± 0.17 and hyperopes with an AULCSF of 2.11 ± 0.18, respectively, however there was no significant difference between them. There was no clinical relevant association with AULCSF and best corrected SE (AULCSF = 2.07 + 0.012 SE, $r = 0.136$, $p = 0.045$).

NEI − VFQ − 25

The composite score of the NEI − VFQ − 25 can range between 0 and 100, depending on the answers of the subject. Our sample presented with scores ranging from 74 to 100. Most subjects (72 %) had scores over 90. The

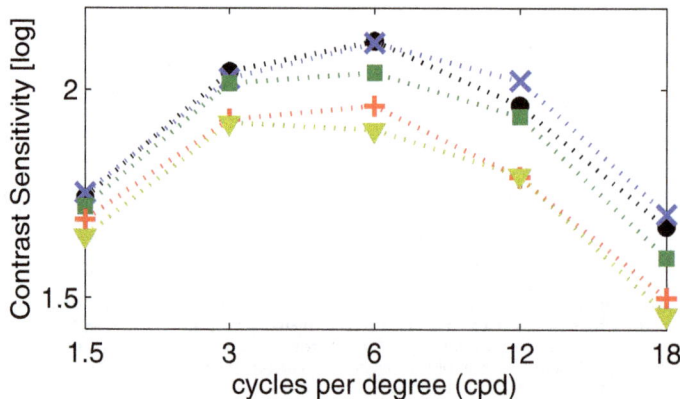

Fig. 2 "Contrast sensitivity measured with the Visual Contrast Test System chart and its association with age". Caption: Contrast sensitivity for all age groups: ● 20–29 years; x 30–39 years; □ 40–49 years; + 50–50 years; Δ 60–69 years. Gratings examined consisted of spatial frequencies of 1.5, 3, 6, 12 and 18 cycles per degree

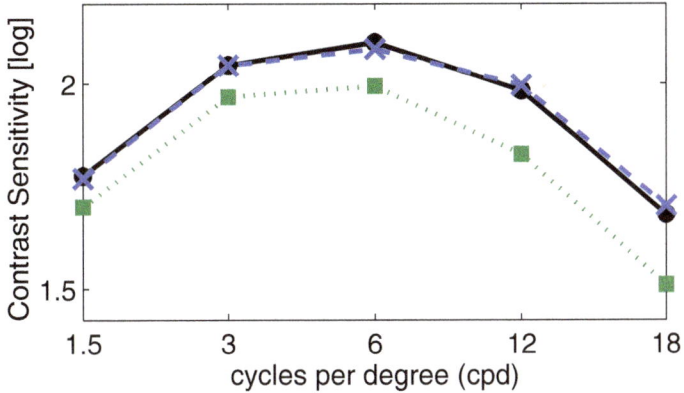

Fig. 3 "Contrast sensitivity results for different spatial frequencies stratefied by refractive status". Caption: Contrast sensitivity for the three refractive states, stratified by spherical equivalent of subjective refraction determined by best corrected visual acuity: ● myopia; x emmetropia; □hyperopia. Gratings examined consisted of spatial frequencies of 1.5, 3, 6, 12 and 18 cycles per degree

subscale "General Health" had a mean score of 70. All subscales had a score over 80.

Discussion

The data presented are part of a multicentre European study on ocular biometric values and visual functions in healthy eyes across the life span. The main purpose of the study is to create a large reference catalogue. This study provides normative data on ocular biometry in a Caucasian adult population of the clinical centre in Leipzig (n = 218) aged 21–69 years. In addition to ocular biometric data, we present data on refraction and stature.

Biometric measurements

Height and weight

As expected, taller people had longer eyes, deeper anterior chamber depths and greater corneal curvature radii. This is in agreement with findings of previous studies [4, 7, 45]. Based on previous reports difference

in stature was shown to be partially responsible for gender differences found in ocular biometry [7, 47–49]. The current study investigated the effect of body height in association with statistical significant gender differences found for corneal radii, CCT, ACD, ACV, AL and CFST. After adjustment for body height on the basis of a regression model, parameters shown in Table 8 no longer exhibited such gender difference.

Corneal findings

Front surface and back surface corneal curvature measured with Pentacam presented four values per subject. The averages are presented in Table 3. Pentacam studies have to take into consideration that corneal power (CP) as given by the built in software employs a refractive index of 1.3375 in order to present a comparable measure to Placido disc systems and allowing for the CP value to be used directly in standard intraocular lens calculations. Instead of the historically used refractive index

Table 3 "Axial length in the literature"

	Year	Method	Axial Length [mm]
Gullstrand		Biometry of enucleated eyes and calculations	24.387
Leipzig	2011	IOLMaster	23.80 ± 1.10
Leipzig_height adjusted data	2011	IOL Master	23.80 ± 0.98
Statistical eye model for normal eyes	2011	IOLMaster	23.67 ± 1.12
The Singapore Malay Eye Study	2010	IOLMaster	23.55 ± 0.05
The Liwan Eye Study	2009	A-mode ultrasound	23.11 ± 0.63
The Meiktila Eye Study	2007	A-mode ultrasound	22.74 ± 0.93
Optical components interactions in emmetropes	2007	A-mode ultrasound	23.34 ± 0.71
The Reykjavik Eye Study	2005	A-mode ultrasound	23.89 ± 1.09
The Los Angeles Latino Eye Study	2005	A-mode ultrasound	23.38 ± 1.01
The Tanjong Pagar Survey	2003	A-mode ultrasound	23.24 ± 0.05

Caption: Axial length values (mean ± standard deviation) for several studies with IOLMaster or ultrasound [2, 4, 7, 47, 50, 51, 55, 56, 89]

Table 4 "Corneal biometry, anterior chamber and axial length stratified by gender and age"

	CC R1 ant [mm]	CC R2 ant [mm]	CC R1 post [mm]	CC R2 post [mm]	CCT [µm]	ACD [mm]	ACV [mm³]	AL [mm]	CRTmin [µm] n=206	CFST [µm] n=206	CRTmin_adj [µm] n=206	CFST_adj [µm] n=206
All (218)	7.91±0.26	7.73±0.28	6.65±0.27	6.29±0.26	554±32	2.81±0.38	160±40	23.8±1.1	231±20	279±21	231±20	279±20
Women (110)	7.85±0.27	7.68±0.27	6.60±0.26	6.26±0.25	549±32	2.74±0.38	149±37	23.4±1.0	230±20	273±19	231±20	278±19
20–29 (24)	7.85±0.30	7.69±0.32	6.62±0.27	6.27±0.28	547±35	3.01±0.34	174±31	23.4±1.0	222±17	271±20	224±16	274±19
30–39 (19)	7.93±0.24	7.73±0.26	6.72±0.24	6.32±0.26	541±41	2.91±0.32	168±33	24.0±0.9	228±22	273±19	229±21	275±17
40–49 (32)	7.78±0.26	7.62±0.23	6.52±0.25	6.17±0.19	554±31	2.76±0.30	144±26	23.5±1.0	233±14	278±17	235±14	282±18
50–59 (19)	7.89±0.31	7.72±0.30	6.59±0.29	6.28±0.29	549±27	2.42±0.22	122±38	23.0±0.8	234±27	274±19	235±26	278±19
60–69 (16)	7.87±0.23	7.72±0.20	6.61±0.24	6.30±0.21	551±21	2.50±0.37	130±32	23.3±0.9	233±20	274±25	236±20	279±24
Men (108)	7.96±0.24	7.78±0.28	6.69±0.28	6.33±0.26	559±32	2.92±0.35	172±39	24.2±1.0	233±20	285±20	232±20	280±20
20–29 (26)	7.94±0.21	7.74±0.22	6.67±0.24	6.27±0.26	559±39	3.18±0.19	196±21	24.4±0.8	231±20	283±21	229±20	278±22
30–39 (20)	7.94±0.30	7.78±0.31	6.65±0.27	6.34±0.34	557±28	3.05±0.19	187±23	24.5±1.1	237±23	289±23	235±23	284±24
40–49 (29)	8.01±0.28	7.83±0.28	6.72±0.28	6.35±0.27	559±31	2.85±0.31	167±41	24.2±1.1	233±19	284±17	232±19	281±17
50–59 (19)	7.95±0.20	7.80±0.21	6.68±0.22	6.35±0.19	560±38	2.81±0.44	160±45	23.9±1.2	233±17	285±20	231±17	280±20
60–69 (14)	7.97±0.19	7.76±0.42	6.78±0.39	6.35±0.19	558±22	2.55±0.30	128±26	23.7±0.7	234±23	280±23	234±23	279±22
Statistical comparison women to men (all)	p=0.001	p=0.008	p=0.015	p=0.028	p=0.025	p<0.001	p<0.001	p<0.001	p=0.162	p<0.001	p=0.903	p=0.324

Caption: Data stratified by gender and age (mean ± standard deviation). Additionally the statistical comparison of each parameter analysed by two sample t-test stratified by gender is given in the lower portion of the table in keratometry (1.3375), the Pentacam gives more detailed information on the radii and enables CP calculation employing the corneal refractive index of 1.376. Therefore, this study relied on corneal radii when interpreting the curvature data. Front surface corneal radius is an important measure for many clinical investigations, for example fitting of contact lenses. In this study, no age effect on corneal radius was found. A relationship with age was also not found for CP in this study, which is in line with literature. However, former research suggested an association with gender: It has been suggested that women have greater CP (mean difference 0.72 D [50]; mean difference: 0.74 D [40, 51] difference of the means 0.32 D [52]). In terms of radii, the same applied, women were found to have smaller radii than men (mean difference of 0.14 mm [2], 0.11 mm [4] and 0.12 mm (difference of the means, [52]). The results of this study are in line with this, with a mean difference of 0.09 mm and difference of the mean of 0.13 mm. Statistical analysis presented with a gender effect for anterior and posterior corneal radii, see Tables 4 and 8. Height-adjusted mean anterior and posterior corneal radii presented with no further gender effect, see Table 8.

There was a trend in that men had thicker central corneas than women (mean difference 10 μm and difference of the means 10 μm) see Tables 4 and 8, partially this gender effect might be explained by differences in height, see Table 8. There was no effect of age on CCT. This confirms the findings of the Reykjavik Eye Study who found no significant changes in CCT with age, nor any difference between the eyes of men and women. A

recent investigation found that men had thicker central corneas than women (difference of the means 5 μm), and suggested that younger subjects had thicker corneas [13].

The eccentricities of the anterior and posterior corneal surface found in this study were in agreement with the findings of an Iran population, where the mean corneal eccentricity was +0.27 ± 0.63 measured with the Pentacam HR [53]. Asgari et al. further discussed a great variety of the normal range of eccentricity between studies, which might be due to different corneal topography devices used. For example, Sicam et al. [54] found mean eccentricities for the anterior and posterior corneal surface of 0.87 ± 0.11 and 0.77 ± 0.17 measured with the Topcon SL-45 Scheimpflug camera.

Axial length, anterior chamber depth and anterior chamber volume

Axial length was statistically significantly larger in men compared to women ($p < 0.001$), this had been shown before [47–49]. Height-adjusted axial length presented with no further gender effects, see Tables 8. Stratified into five refractive categories, men presented with statistically significantly larger axial lengths compared to women in all but the low hyperopia category ($p = 0.160$), see also Tables 5, 6 and 7.

In the present study, axial length was slightly larger (men: 24.18 ± 1.01 mm; women: 23.41 ± 0.98 mm) than reported in previous work, e.g., the Reykjavik study [47, 52] (men: 23.74 ± 1.0 mm; women: 23.20 ± 0.98 mm), the Zagreb study (men: 23.49 ± 0.75 mm; women: 23.18 ±

Table 5 "Corneal biometry, anterior chamber and axial length stratified by refractive error-all subjects"

		CC R1 ant	CC R2 ant	CC R1 post	CC R2 post	CCT	ACD	ACV	AL
Manifest myopia (< −2D)	mean	7.77	7.55	6.57	6.16	552.81	3.11	185.59	25.07
	SD	0.26	0.33	0.36	0.25	34.05	0.24	27.69	1.12
Low myopia (−2D ≤ −0.5D)	mean	7.89	7.73	6.65	6.33	549.02	3.04	179.31	24.20
	SD	0.23	0.25	0.24	0.26	31.35	0.33	35.30	0.90
Emmetropia (−0.5D ≤ ≥ +0.5D)	mean	7.91	7.74	6.64	6.27	554.13	2.83	159.18	23.54
	SD	0.26	0.25	0.25	0.24	34.07	0.32	35.05	0.72
Low hypermetropia (+0.5D ≥ +2D)	mean	8.01	7.84	6.71	6.38	556.86	2.54	135.06	23.41
	SD	0.28	0.28	0.27	0.28	32.38	0.28	35.11	0.79
Manifest hypermetropia (> +2D)	mean	7.90	7.74	6.71	6.32	559.94	2.34	109.76	22.51
	SD	0.30	0.28	0.29	0.27	29.54	0.29	24.78	0.74

Caption: Data stratified by refractive state based on sphere of subjective best corrected vision (mean ± standard deviation). Anterior radii of the cornea (flat: R1 ant, steep: R2 ant) and posterior radii of the cornea (flat: R1 post, steep:R2 post) presented with the following relationship compared for myopic and hyperopic groups: for manifest myopia, the flattest anterior radius (R1) was steeper compared to manifest hypermetropia, the steep counterpart (R2 ant) again was steepest for the myopic group. The corresponding posterior radius presented with a similar change in steepness (again R1 post and R2 post being steepest for myopes). The difference for all four radius parameters was ~0.2 from manifest myopia to manifest hyperopia, reflecting the appearance of a minus lens of the cornea within the optics of the eye. The difference between R1 ant and R2 ant was about 0.2 mm within each refractive category, i.e. for manifest myopia to manifest hyperopia, between R1 post and R2 post this difference for each refractive category was ~ 0.4 mm. Central corneal thickness (CCT) was similar for manifest myopia and manifest hyperopia groups. Anterior chamber depth (ACD) and – volume (ACV) was smaller in hypermetropic subjects. Axial length (AL) was shortest for subjects with manifest hypermetropia. See Tables 6 and 7 for stratification based on gender

Table 6 "Corneal biometry, anterior chamber and axial length stratified by refractive error - women"

		CC R1 ant	CC R2 ant	CC R1 post	CC R2 post	CCT	ACD	ACV	AL
Manifest myopia (< −2D)	Mean	7.72	7.50	6.48	6.13	542.81	3.09	180.38	24.64
	SD	0.30	0.28	0.26	0.26	36.93	0.27	29.88	1.07
Low myopia (−2D ≤ −0.5D)	Mean	7.86	7.72	6.65	6.34	551.11	2.87	160.53	23.73
	SD	0.22	0.24	0.22	0.20	33.83	0.38	36.71	0.83
Emmetropia (−0.5D ≤ ≥ +0.5D)	Mean	7.84	7.69	6.59	6.22	551.34	2.76	147.52	23.21
	SD	0.25	0.23	0.25	0.21	33.37	0.32	28.72	0.66
Low hypermetropia (+0.5D ≥ +2D)	Mean	8.01	7.82	6.72	6.38	546.50	2.46	131.70	23.21
	SD	0.25	0.23	0.25	0.21	33.37	0.32	28.72	0.66
Manifest hypermetropia (> +2D)	Mean	7.67	7.53	6.50	6.18	557.13	2.20	96.13	21.98
	SD	0.19	0.15	0.20	0.23	33.88	0.15	9.08	0.59

Caption Data stratified by gender (female) and refractive state based on sphere of subjective best corrected vision (mean ± standard deviation). Women presented with steeper anterior radii of the cornea (flat: R1 ant, steep:R2 ant) and steeper posterior radii of the cornea (flat: R1 post, steep:R2 post) compared to men (see Table 7)

0.67 mm) [55] and the EPIC-Norfolk Eye Study (men: 23.80 ± 1.16 mm; women: 23.39 ± 1.15 mm) [15]. However, the Zagreb study measured only emmetropic subjects and Foster et al. included 52 % hyperopic subjects. A Belgian dataset measured 23.67 ± 1.12 mm [56]. Eysteinsson et al. [47] although men in our study were taller, the main difference in AL observed in Table 3 may be related to the fact that our subjects were measured with the IOL Master. See Table 3 for comparison of different studies, where IOL Master values for AL were higher on average than ultrasound measurements.

Studies by Lam et al., Santodomingo – Rubido et al. and Sheng et al. have shown the IOL Master to be more repeatable than ultrasound for axial length measurement [57–59]. Sheng et al. showed that the repeatability of the IOL Master was excellent regardless of the experience of the observer. Therefore, we chose to measure the axial length with the IOL Master. Table 2 shows that the axial length measured with the IOL Master is slightly longer than the A – scan ultrasound axial length. (This was also shown by Sheng et al.) The differences in axial length between the listed studies may be due to differences in races in population based samples of biometrical data.

Considering different races, AL of Caucasian eyes in this study were longer than East Asian eyes (AL 23.55 mm) measured with IOL Master [4]. In general, AL was associated with ACD and ACV, with an increase in ACD resulting in an increase in ACV. AL decreased with increasing age and women had smaller values, which was in agreement with other findings [2, 4, 47, 50]. However, the current findings established only a low association of age or gender with AL. The decrease of ACD and ACV with age resulted mainly from an increase in lens thickness [60]. In this sample, some association of SE was established with ACD ($r = -0.519$), ACV ($r = -0.468$) and AL ($r = -0.661$). This is contradictory to previous findings where no correlation was found between SE and ACD ($r = -0.13$, $p = 0.42$) [61]. The previous results were based on myopic subjects (0.00 to −14.88 D), whereas the current investigation included a range of

Table 7 "Corneal biometry, anterior chamber and axial length stratified by refractive error - men"

		CC R1 ant	CC R2 ant	CC R1 post	CC R2 post	CCT	ACD	ACV	AL
manifest myopia (< −2D)	Mean	7.82	7.60	6.67	6.20	562.81	3.12	190.81	25.51
	SD	0.20	0.37	0.42	0.22	28.62	0.21	25.17	1.01
low myopia (−2D ≤ −0.5D)	Mean	7.92	7.74	6.65	6.33	547.50	3.16	193.04	24.55
	SD	0.23	0.26	0.25	0.31	30.00	0.22	27.54	0.79
emmetropia (−0.5D ≤ ≥ +0.5D)	Mean	7.99	7.81	6.69	6.33	557.30	2.90	172.43	23.90
	SD	0.24	0.25	0.25	0.26	34.96	0.30	37.13	0.62
low hypermetropia (+0.5D ≥ +2D)	Mean	8.02	7.87	6.69	6.38	569.81	2.63	139.25	23.66
	SD	0.27	0.28	0.25	0.23	37.76	0.29	31.91	0.85
manifest hypermetropia (> +2D)	Mean	8.11	7.94	6.89	6.44	562.44	2.45	121.89	22.99
	SD	0.23	0.23	0.23	0.26	26.94	0.33	28.36	0.49

Caption: Data stratified by gender (male) and refractive state based on sphere of subjective best corrected vision (mean ± standard deviation). Men presented with flatter anterior radii of the cornea (flat: R1 ant, steep:R2 ant) and flatter posterior radii of the cornea (flat: R1 post, steep:R2 post) compared to women (see Table 6)

hyperopic to myopic subjects (+6.00 to −9.13 D). Gender differences in the current study observed for ACD and ACV were accounted for by body height adjustment, see Tables 4 and 8.

Retinal thickness

Retinal thickness was investigated using CFST and CRTmin. Measured within the central 1 mm diameter area of the retina, statistically significant smaller CFST was found for women compared to men, see Table 8. This confirmed previous findings for CFST on the same OCT device [62, 63] by Wagner-Schuman et al. who established 265 ± 23 μm for men and 254 ± 19 μm for women; $p = 0.0086$ [64]. In cross-reference, Wagner-Schuman and colleagues reviewed several other studies on various OCT devices which also found sex-related differences in retinal thickness with smaller thicknesses for women [64]. In the past, healthy subjects have been investigated on the OCT device of the current study [54, 62]. Wolf-Schnurrbusch et al. [65] in a comparative

study with Spectralis SD-OCT Grover et al. found a mean CFST of 271 ± 20 μm [63]. In an earlier study mean CFST was 270 ± 23 μm (men 274 ± 23 μm; women 266 ± 22 μm) based on the small sample size the gender effect had not been found significant ($p = 0.1$) [62]. The CFST data for Caucasians ($n = 28$) in the Grover sample of 50 healthy subjects (273 ± 21 μm) was slightly smaller than the findings of the current investigation [62]. Wolf-Schnurrbusch on the other hand established a CFST of 289 ± 16 μm (right eye) across their sample of 20 subjects [65]. The current study presents normative retinal thickness data on 206 Caucasian subjects and it can therefore be assumed that 279 ± 21 μm is more representative of the population.

One could expect that myopic eyes, which are longer, to have thinner retinal thickness, but this trend apparent in the data was not confirmed statistically. Whereas other studies based on larger subject numbers found in fact that central macular thickness is greater in myopic eyes. The work of Choovuthayakorn et al. demonstrated

Table 8 "Selected gender effects adjusted for by body height"

Variable under investigation men: $n = 108$ women: $n = 110$	Statistical significant difference male (m) versus female (f)	Regression analysis	Variable after adjustment for body height based on regression model
Mean anterior corneal radius (CCRant)	m: 7.87 (SD 0.25); f: 7.77 (SD 0.26); $p = 0.003$	CCRant = 6.37 + 0,00837 Height	m: 7.82 (SD 0.24); f: 7.83 (SD 0.26); $p = 0.701$
Mean posterior corneal radius (CCRpost)	m: 6.51 (SD 0.24); f: 6.43 (SD 0.25); $p = 0.014$	CCRpost = 5.26 + 0,00699 Height	m: 6.46 (SD 0.23); f: 6.48 (SD 0.24); $p = 0.591$
Central corneal thickness (CCT)	m: 558.7 (SD 32.3); f: 548.7 (SD 32.0); $p = 0.023$	CCT = 532 + 0.128 Height	m: 557.3 (SD 32.3); f: 549.2 (SD 32.2); $p = 0.064$
Anterior chamber depth (ACD)	m: 2.92 (SD 0.35); f: 2.74 (SD 0.38); $p < 0.001$	ACD = 1.25 + 0,00912 Height	m: 2.86 (SD 0.35); f: 2.81 (SD 0.38); $p = 0.314$
Anterior chamber volume (ACV)	m: 171.6 (SD 39.2); f: 148.9 (SD 36.7); $p < 0.001$	ACV = − 43.0 + 1,17 Height	m: 163.9 (SD 38.6); f: 157.8 (SD 36.8); 0.235
Axial length (AL)	m: 24.16 (SD 1.01); f: 23.44 (SD 0.97); $p < 0.001$	Axial length = 17.0 + 0.0393 Height	m: 23.88 (SD 0.97); f: 23.72 (SD 0.98); $p = 0.219$
Central foveal subfield thickness (CFST) Men: $n = 103$ Women: $n = 103$	m: 284.6 (SD 20.3); f: 273.9 (SD 19.4); $p < 0.001$	CFST = 182 + 0.562 Height	m: 280.4 (SD 20.3); f: 277.7 (SD 19.2); $p = 0.324$
Minimal retinal thickness (CRTmin) Men: $n = 103$ Women: $n = 103$	m: 233.4 (SD 20.1) median 232.0; f: 229.8 (SD 19.7) median 228.0; p(MW-U) = 0.162	CRTmin = 194 + 0,216 Height	m: 232.1 (SD 20.1) median: 230.6; f: 231.4 (SD 19.5) median 229.4; p (MW-U) = 0.903

Caption: Mean data stratified by gender for men ($n = 108$) and women ($n = 110$) for corneal radii, CCT, ACD, ACV, AL and retinal thickness measured as CFST and CRTmin. All but CRTmin presented with statistically significant gender effects
Association of respective variables with body height was investigated and adjusted based on a regression model where variable_new = variable_old −regression function + mean (variable_old). After adjustment for body height, all investigated variables presented with no gender effects, therefore differences in stature between men and women may explain some of the differences in the biometric data reported

an increasing CFST and decreasing inner and outer sub-field thicknesses with greater axial length [66]. The UK Biobank Study found a mean CFST of 265 ± 23 μm and showed that CFST was positively correlated with greater myopia ($p < 0.001$) [67].

Optics and visual function
Refractive error
In the present study, subjects tended to be more hyper-opic in older age groups (SE (subjective) in right eyes of 40–49 year olds: -0.86 ± 2.06 D; 50–59: $+0.31 \pm 1.92$ D; 60–69: $+0.45 \pm 1.97$ D), see also Fig. 1 and caption of Table 1. Nevertheless, the differences in refractive error amongst the sample age groups do not necessarily sug-gest a change as a function of age. The hyperopic shift resulted in more emmetropic eyes in the 40–49 years decade, followed by a higher percentage of hyperopic eyes from 50 years onwards. This is in line with previous findings. In the Gutenberg Health Study (GHS) myopia was present in 35 % of the study sample and hyperopia in 32 %, with refractive errors ranging from -21.50 to $+13.88$ D [46]. Wolfram et al. found a higher prevalence of myopia in younger age groups, with a hyperopic shift up to the age of 69 years for their population of 35 to 74 years of age. In a Spanish study population aged 40 to 79 years the prevalences of myopia and hyperopia were 25 % and 44 %, respectively. Myopia did not change significantly with age but hyperopia increased with age [68]. This trend towards hyperopia by increas-ing age was confirmed by a Norwegian study, whose study population was between 38 and 87 years old [12]. British adults aged 48 to 88 years presented with refract-ive errors of 27 % myopia and 52 % hyperopia [15]. In a recent meta-analysis of European refractive error studies, the prevalence of myopia and hyperopia was 30.6 % and 25.2 %, respectively [69]. They also reported a hyperopic shift in the older age groups. Several studies with East Asian subjects reported more myopic cohorts compared to the present study, but the general trend also was a hyperopic shift towards old age [2]. High myopia in young Chinese reported recently [70, 71] is not yet part of those subjects; this may influence this observation in future. The present data included age groups from 20–69 years and may have examined more subjects with a higher level of education, which has been associated with a more myopic refraction [72], and thus the preva-lence of myopia may be higher in the current investiga-tion ((M) 44 %, (E) 37 %, (H) 19 %). However, the association of the level of education and myopic refrac-tion could not be confirmed in our study sample. Fur-thermore, Williams et al. used refractive error categories, where emmetropia ranges from -0.74 to 0.99 D, which differed from ours as defined in the methods section. This resulted in a higher prevalence of

emmetropia of 43.5 % in the meta-analysis and the re-sults are not useful for direct comparison.

Grouped by gender and age, the spherical equivalent for the cohort in this study is presented in Table 1. A higher prevalence of hyperopia was seen in older com-pared to younger persons also when separated by gen-der. Similarly to the presented findings, older women were more hyperopic than men of the same age in American Latino [50], Northern European [13, 47] and Singaporian Chinese subjects [2].

Table 4 shows subjects separated by gender and age decade. This allowed interpretation of ocular biomet-ric values (ACD, ACV, AL, CC and CCT) in separate categories and therefore enabled direct comparison. Tables 5, 6, and 7 presents the same data stratified by refractive state (based on sphere of best corrected sub-jective refraction), here it is clearly visible that param-eters are dependent on refractive status. Myopic subjects compared to manifest hypermetropic subjects presented with steeper anterior and posterior corneal radii, had slightly thinner corneas (CCT) on average and presented with much longer mean anterior cham-ber depths (ACD), as well as bigger anterior chamber volume (ACV), and their axial length (AL) was longer, see Tables 5, 6 and 7 for additional stratification based on gender.

Spherical equivalent and dioptric distance
This study was able to perform an accurate comparison between best – corrected subjective refraction and ha-bitual corrective status, e.g., old glasses. Commonly, the spherical equivalent (SE, sphere plus half of cylinder) is used to compare measures of refraction. However, this is unsuitable when comparing the change in power of two spherocylindrical lenses accurately, as SE does not take the axis into account. Therefore, to display the dif-ference between new refraction to previous correction of a subject, the dioptric distance between both lenses was calculated [23]. The dioptric distance is a helpful tool, especially as it allows accurate grouping of such changes across the population. Future observations may therefore benefit from accurate calculations using dioptric distance.

There was a difference between the state of undercor-rection depending on reporting objective (42 %, 83 % of which were previous spectacle wearers) or subjective best corrected data (58 %, 64 % of which were previous spectacle wearers), specifically for the lower refractive errors of non-spectacle wearers (16 % objective versus 46 % subjective). This might be due to the repeatability and validity of the autorefractor used (Humphrey Au-tomated refractor/Keratometer (HARK) 599), this has to be investigated separately. The objective data (S: $-0.51D \pm 2.02$; SE: $-0.75D \pm 2.1$) and subjective data

(S: −0.44D ± 2.04; SE = −0.73D ± 2.1) across the whole subject group presented with similar refractive error and SD over all. Previously it was shown that the between-visits-repeatability for all refractive error measurements were <0.75 D and the mean difference between the subjective refraction and the HARK autorefraction for spherical equivalent was statistically significant under non-cycloplegic conditions (−0.90 D, $P < .0001$) and cycloplegic conditions (−2.05 D, $P < .0001$) [73]. Thus, this may have affected specifically the reporting of low refractive errors of previous non-spectacle wearers. Therefore it can be concluded that the subjective best corrected results of the current study represent the true state of the sample investigated. The Gutenberg Health Study presented autorefraction data (HARK) and compared this to self-reported information on the current spectacle or contact lens correction worn and found that 3.5 % of subjects who were in need of refractive correction did not previously possess one based on the criteria of binocular myopia or hyperopia [46]. This is much lower than the state of undercorrection in non-spectacle wearers (16 % based on autorefraction; 46 % based on subjective refraction) in the current investigation even though the present study included a higher percentage of emmetropic subjects (37 vs. 33 % GHS). Additionally, the current study is able to report on the clinical significant change in refraction of spectacle wearers (based on autorefraction: 64 %, based on subjective refraction: 69 %). The Blue Mountains Eye Study stated that undercorrected refractive error was present in 10.2 % of the study population [45]. But they investigated initial visual acuity in comparison with the subject's habitual correction and defined undercorrection as an improvement of ≥ 10 letters (two lines on the log-MAR chart), after refraction in subjects with a presenting visual acuity <45 letters. The high percentages for improvement of correction of refractive error found in this healthy cross-section might have implications on visual acuity for driving, quality of visual performance for the work force and quality of life parameters based on vision. This suggests that the population might benefit from regular eye examinations and vision testing.

Visual acuity

Uncorrected and corrected visual acuity were +0.25 ± 0.42 logMAR (−0.26 to +1.50 logMAR) and −0.12 ± 0.08 logMAR (−0.30 to 0.20 logMAR), respectively. Divided into age and gender no differences were found. Visual acuity is therefore only weakly correlated with age ($r = 0.202$). A weak association with age was found in an older Chinese population (40 to over 75 years) ($r = 0.390$) [74], which might be due to older age and larger percentage of vision problems which specifically had been excluded from the present study. No association

was found between visual acuity and education in line with findings by Xu et al. [74].

Accommodation

Cause for the reduced ability to accommodate with increasing age is a progressive age – related loss of elasticity of the lens capsule, nuclear sclerosis or a lens thickening by lifelong growth of the lens [75], [1]. For this reason accommodation presented with moderate correlations with ACD ($r = 0.498$, $p < 0.001$) and ACV ($r = 0.484$, $p < 0.001$) as a thicker lens influences ACD and ACV, i.e., they are reduced, and in turn this is associated with a decreased ability to accommodate. Yuan et al. [76] reported that ACD decreased significantly with accommodation compared to the non-accommodative condition.

Contrast sensitivity

Mean contrast sensitivity (log units) for different spatial frequencies was in line with other studies.

With an increase in spatial frequencies employed (1.5 to 18 cpd, see above) contrast sensitivity increased to its peak at 6 cpd followed by a decrease to its lowest value at 18 cpd [77], [78]. This was expected as contrast sensitivity in the normal human eye peaks at a level of 6 cpd.

The present study was able to establish that contrast sensitivity decreased with age at each spatial frequency based on a larger number of subjects across the life span (20–69 years of age), see Fig. 2. Additionally, pupil diameter in the given population decreased with age ($r = -0.388$, $p < 0.001$), which may in turn have an influence on contrast sensitivity [79]. In comparison with data obtained using the Optec 6500 Functional Acuity Contrast Test (Stereo Optical Company, Chicago, IL), the present study found lower contrast sensitivity measures for lower spatial frequencies (1.5, 3, 6 cpd) whereas for higher spatial frequencies higher contrast values were found [77]. In a different study, the contrast sensitivity function of an older population (40–64 years) was generally lower [80]. However, Hashemi et al. employed the CSV – 1000 (VectorVision, Greenville, OH) and it can generally be noted that the VCTS – 6500 (Vistech, Dayton, OH) produces higher scores than the former apparatus [81]. Note that the younger population tested there also presented lower scores in comparison to the present findings. Contrast sensitivity has been shown to be influenced by refractive error, with myopes showing lower contrast sensitivity values than hyperopes [80]. The present investigation, however, found hyperopic eyes with lower contrast sensitivity than myopic eyes, but this is due to increasing hyperopia with age in the population and therefore age is the predominant factor and not hyperopia, see Figs. 2 and 3 for cross-reference.

The concept of computing the area under the log contrast sensitivity function (AULCSF) provided the advantage of giving one number per subject containing information from all spatial frequencies [82, 83]. This enabled comparison with other measures, additionally serving as a baseline for future studies. Another German study using the functional acuity and contrast chart (FACT) as part of the Contrast Sensitivity Tester 1800 (CST 1800; Vision Science Research Corp.; San Ramon, CA), which is comparable to the VCTS chart, found a decrease in contrast sensitivity (AULCSF) in the older age group (50–69 years) compared to the younger age group (21–47 years) [84]. With the OPTEC 6500 device the relationship of the AULCSF with age has been shown to be $r = 0.57$ (photopic) and $r = 0.54$ (mesopic) where a reduction of contrast sensitivity is associated with increasing age [85].

NEI VFQ – 25
Most subjects (72 %) had composite scores over 90. It can be concluded that subjects interviewed in our study are content with their vision and therefore think of their vision as "good". The subscale "General Health" presented with a mean score of only 70, although the subjects had no chronic disease or any health problems. The questionnaire can be considered a subjective tool and therefore subjects may underestimate their health. All subscales have a score over 80. In comparison, overall lower scores were found for both the English and Spanish speaking groups in a healthy and visually normal subsample of the Latino Eye study [87]. Data on visually impaired Chinese subjects showed a clear association of lower scores with severity of impairment [86]. Another German study examined 511 subjects with good eye health and found a similar composite score of 91.6 ± 7.1 and a higher score for general health (79.9 ± 17.4), and based on their subscales they were able to establish that the subjects had good eye health. They concluded that as a screening tool the VFQ – 25 was not specific or sensitive enough to detect subjects with eye conditions from a random population [88].

Possible shortcomings of our study were the relatively small sample size, limited by the various measurements carried out, the non-randomized study population and - although intended - the missing ethnic diversity, as the study presented results for an exclusive German cohort without other Caucasian subgroups.

The study recruited subjects of all levels of education. In the analysis there was no correlation of the level of education with any result of the examinations found. This may have been due to small numbers per education level, as previous research showed a link between education and refractive status, i.e., myopia was linked to higher education levels [72].

Conclusion
The data obtained present an overview of the average ocular biometry within the population of Leipzig, Germany. The large subset of parameters established for each subject allows comparison between datasets providing the background for creation of a database. This enables cross-referencing to determine associations between parameters for healthy eyes. The reference values established therefore permit multiple comparisons with patient data for further investigations, especially in view of the correlations established as part of this study.

In this paper, biometrical data based on in – vivo measurements of healthy German eyes are presented and compared stratified by age, gender and refractive status. This resulted in the following conclusions: a decrease with age was found for anterior corneal curvature, anterior chamber depth, and anterior chamber volume. The spherical equivalent was more hyperopic with age. A decrease with age was found for accommodation and contrast sensitivity. Greater anterior corneal curvature, greater anterior chamber depth and greater anterior chamber volume were established for hyperopic subjects than for myopic subjects.

We verified relationships or differences between those parameters based on our data and in reference to the current literature. Our dataset is useful for future work on either a smaller number of subjects or a selected patient group, as data can be directly compared with each aspect given in our study, allowing other research to extract answers for their data without having to establish an age correlated normal sample themselves. In future, with aid of this data existing statistical eye models can be updated [56]. This data of strictly controlled eyes on a multitude of biometric reference parameters in the same eye based on gold-standard techniques, serves as starting points for disease prevention as well as a reference for health policy and practice. Together with detailed information on current habitual correction versus new corrective lenses based on best corrected visual acuity, it provides background to the goal of extending good functional vision into old age.

Abbreviations
ACD, anterior chamber depth; ACV, anterior chamber volume; AL, axial length; AULCSF, area under the logarithmic contrast sensitivity function; BCVA, best corrected visual acuity; BMI, body mass index; C, cylinder; CC, corneal curvature; CC R ant, mean anterior corneal radius; CC R post, mean posterior corneal radius; CC R1 ant, flat anterior corneal radius; CC R1 post, flat posterior corneal radius; CC R2 ant, steep anterior corneal radius; CC R2 post, steep posterior corneal radius; CCT, central corneal thickness; CDVA, corrected distance visual acuity; CFST, central foveal subfield thickness; CP, corneal power; cpd, cycles per degree; CRTmin, minimal central retinal thickness; DD, Dioptric distance; E, Emmetropia; e, Corneal eccentricity; e ant, eccentricity of anterior corneal surface; e post, eccentricity of posterior corneal surface; f, female; H, hyperopia; logMAR, logarithm of the minimum angle of resolution; M, myopia; M, male; NEI-VFQ-25, National Eye Institute visual functioning questionnaire 25; OCT, optical coherence tomography; S, sphere; SD, standard deviation; SE, spherical equivalent; UDVA, uncorrected distance visual acuity; VCTS, visual contrast test system

Acknowledgements
We would like to thank Dr. Bernd Klaus (Centre for Statistical Data Analysis, European Molecular Biology Laboratory (EMBL), Heidelberg) for help with the statistics, Dr. Björn Zocher (Institute for Theoretical Physics, University of Leipzig) for the design of the graphs and Carolin Blankenburg, Marlen Kendziora (both Beuth University of Applied Science, Berlin) and Silvana Hermsdorf (Ernst Abbe University of Applied Sciences, Jena) for assistance with examining study subjects. Furthermore we would like to thank Professor Ralf Blendowske (Department of Optical Technologies and Image Processing, University of Applied Sciences, Darmstadt, Germany) for discussions and help on the concept of dioptric power matrix and dioptric distance.
European Vision Institute Clinical Research Network, AIBILI, Azinhaga de Santa Comba, Celas, 3000-548 Coimbra, Portugal.

Authors' contributions
MTZ: recruitment of subjects; telephone interview; acquisition of data; analysis and interpretation of data; statistical analysis; drafting of the manuscript; drafting of figures and tables; JJR: conception and design of the study; guidance of analysis; involved in revising the manuscript; NO: acquisition, analysis and interpretation of Pentacam Scheimpflug camera data; JD: participated in set-up and coordination of the study in Leipzig; helped to revise the manuscript. PW: helped to revise manuscript critically for important intellectual content. FGR: substantial contributions to set-up of the study in Leipzig; training of MTZ to carry out measurements; analysis and interpretation of data; statistical analysis; helped with drafting of the manuscript; drafting and finalising of tables; revised manuscript critically for important intellectual content. All authors read and approved the final manuscript.

Competing interests
The authors declare that they have no competing interests.

Consent for publication
Written informed consent to publish the obtained anonymized data was obtained for each subject prior to the study.

Ethics approval and consent to participate
The study adhered to the Tenets of the Declaration of Helsinki and approval for the study was obtained from theEthics Committee of the Medical Faculty of the University of Leipzig (No. 162/11) and is registered asClinicalTrials.gov # NCT01173614. Written informed consent to participate was obtained for each subject prior to the study.

Author details
[1]Department of Ophthalmology, Leipzig University Hospital, Liebigstrasse 10-14, 04103 Leipzig, Germany. [2]Department of Ophthalmology, Antwerp University Hospital, Wilrijkstraat 10, 2650 Edegem, Belgium. [3]Department of Medicine and Health Science, University of Antwerp, Universiteitsplein 1, 2610 Wilrijk, Belgium.

References
1. Fisher RF. Presbyopia and the changes with age in the human crystalline lens. J Physiol. 1973;228:765–79.
2. Wong TY, Foster PJ, Ng TP, Tielsch JM, Johnson GJ, Seah SKL. Variations in ocular biometry in an adult Chinese population in Singapore: The Tanjong Pagar Survey. Invest Ophthalmol Vis Sci. 2001;42:73–80.
3. Atchison DA, Markwell EL, Kasthurirangan S, Pope JM, Smith G, Swann PG. Age-related changes in optical and biometric characteristics of emmetropic eyes. J Vision. 2008;8:1–20.
4. Lim LS, Saw SM, Jeganathan VSE, Tay WT, Aung T, Tong L, Mitchell P, Wong TY. Distribution and determinants of ocular biometric parameters in an Asian population: The Singapore Malay eye study. Invest Ophthalmol Vis Sci. 2010;51:103–9.
5. Dandona R, Dandona L, Srinivas M, Giridhar P, McCarty CA, Rao GN. Population-based assessment of refractive error in India: The Andhra Pradesh eye disease study. Clin Exp Ophthalmol. 2002;30:84–93.
6. Nirmalan PK, Tielsch JM, Katz J, Thulasiraj RD, Krishnadas R, Ramakrishnan R, Robin AL. Relationship between vision impairment and eye disease to vision – specific quality of life and function in rural India: The Aravind comprehensive eye survey. Invest Ophthalmol Vis Sci. 2005;46:2308–12.
7. Wu HM, Gupta A, Newland HS, Selva D, Aung T, Casson RJ. Association between stature, ocular biometry and refraction in an adult population in rural Myanmar: The Meiktila eye study. Clin Experiment Ophthalmol. 2007;35:834–9.
8. Shah SP, Jadoon MZ, Dineen B, Bourne RRA, Johnson GJ, Gilbert CE, Khan MD. Refractive errors in the Pakistani population: The National blindness and visual impairment survey. Ophthalmic Epidemiol. 2008;15:183–90.
9. Jonas JB, Xu L, Wang YX. The Beijing eye study. Acta Ophthalmol. 2009;87:247–61.
10. Vingerling JR, Dielemans I, Hofman A, Grobbee DE, Hijmering M, Kramer CFL, de Jong PTVM. The prevalence of age-related maculopathy in the Rotterdam Study. Ophthalmology. 1995;102:205–10.
11. Wolfs RCV, Klaver CC, Vingerling JR, Grobbee DE, Hofman A, de Jong PTVM. Distribution of central corneal thickness and its association with intraocular pressure: The Rotterdam Study. Am J Ophthalmol. 1997;123:767–72.
12. Bertelsen G, Erke MG, von Hanno T, Mathiesen EB, Peto T, Sjolie AK, Njolstad I. The Tromso Eye Study. Study design, methodolgy and results on visual acuity and refractive errors. Acta Ophthalmol. 2013;91:635–42.
13. Mirshahi A, Ponto KA, Hoehn R, Wild PS, Pfeiffer N. Ophthalmological aspects of the Gutenberg Health Study (GHS): an interdisciplinary prospective population-based cohort study. Ophthalmologe. 2013;110:210–7.
14. Korb CA, Kottler UB, Wolfram C, Hoehn R, Schulz A, Zwiener I, Wild PS, Pfeiffer N, Mirshahi A. Prevalence of age-related macular degeneration in a large European cohort: Results from the population-based Gutenberg Health Study. Graefes Arch Clin Exp Ophthalmol. 2014;252:1403–11.
15. Foster PJ, Broadway DC, Hayat S, Luben R, Dalzell N, Bingham S, Wareham NJ, Khaw KT. Refractive error, axial length and anterior chamber depth of the eye in British adults: the EPIC-Norfolk Eye Study. Br J Ophthalmol. 2010;94:827–30.
16. Jongenelen S, Rozema JJ, Tassignon MJ, EVICR.net & Project Gullstrand Study Group. Distribution of the crystalline lens power in vivo as a function of age. Invest Ophthalmol Vis Sci. 2015;56:7029–35.
17. Rozema JJ, Tassignon MJ, EVICR.net & Project Gullstrand Study Group. The Bigaussian nature of ocular biometry. Optom Vis Sci. 2014;91:713–22.
18. Stadt Leipzig, Amt für Statistik und Wahlen. Statistisches Jahrbuch 2011. Stadt Leipzig, Amt für Statistik und Wahlen. 2011;Band 42: 24 (Table 208).
19. Mangione CM, Berry S, Spritzer K, Janz NK, Klein R, Owsley C, Lee PP. Identifying the content area for the 51-item national eye institute visual function questionnaire: results from focus groups with visually impaired persons. Arch Ophthalmol. 1998;116:227–33.
20. Mangione CM, Lee PP, Gutierrez PP, Spritzer K, Hays RD. Development of the 25-item national eye institute visual function questionnaire. Arch Ophthalmol. 2001;119:1050–8.
21. Williams MA, Moutray TN, Jackson AJ. Uniformity of visual acuity measures in published studies. Invest Ophthalmol Vis Sci. 2008;49:4321–7.
22. Early Treatment Diabetic Retinopathy Study Research Group. Classification of diabetic retinopathy from fluorescein angiograms. ETDRS report number 11. Ophthalmology. 1991;98(5 Suppl):807–22.
23. Diepes H, Blendowske R. Optik und Technik der Brille. Druckhaus Beltz, Hemsbach. Chapter. 2005;21:473–510.
24. Wold JE, Hu A, Chen S, Glasser A. Subjective and objective measurement of human accomodative amplitude. J Cataract Refract Surg. 2003;29:1878–88.
25. Ip JM, Huynh SC, Kifley A, Rose KA, Morgan IG, Varma R, Mitchell P. Variation of the contribution from axial length and other oculometric parameters to refraction by age and ethnicity. Invest Ophthalmol Vis Sci. 2007;48:4846–53.
26. Haigis W, Lege B, Miller N, Schneider B. Comparison of immersion ultrasound biometry and partial coherence interferometry for intraocular lens calculation according to Haigis. Graefes Arch Clin Exp Ophthalmol. 2000;238:765–73.
27. He M, Wang D, Zheng Y, Zhang J, Yin Q, Huang W, Mackey DA, Foster PJ. Heritability of anterior chamber depth as an intermediate phenotype of angle-closure in Chinese: The Guangzhou Twin Eye Study. Invest Ophthalmol Vis Sci. 2008;49:81–6.

28. Huang D, Swanson EA, Lin CP, Schuman JS, Stinson WG, Chang W, Hee MR, Flotte T, Gregory K, Puliafito CA. Optical coherence tomography. Science. 1991;254:1178–81.
29. Hee MR, Izatt JA, Swanson EA, Huang D, Schuman JS, Lin CP, Puliafito CA, Fujimoto JG. Optical coherence tomography of the human retina. Arch Ophthalmol. 1995;113:325–32.
30. Fercher AF, Drexler W, Hitzenberger CK, Lasse T. Optical coherence tomography-principles and applications. Rep Prog Phys. 2003;66:239–303.
31. Williams DR. Imaging single cells in the living retina. Vision Res. 2011;51:1379–96.
32. Gilchrist WG. Validation, Chapter 10. In: Statistical modelling with quantile functions. London: Chapman Hall/CRC; 2000. p. 224.
33. Taylor R. Interpretation of the correlation coefficient: a basic review. J Diagn Med Sonogr. 1990;1:35–9.
34. Bühl Achim. SPSS 22: Einführung in die moderne Datenanalyse. Berlin: Pearson Deutschland GmbH; 2014.
35. Kim EA, Koo YJ, Han YB. Contrast sensitivity changes in patients with diabetic retinopathy. J Korean Ophthalmol Soc. 1995;36:1523–8.
36. Applegate RA, Howland HC, Sharp RP, Cottingham AJ, Yee RW. Corneal aberrations and visual performance after radial keratotomy. J Refract Surg. 1998;14:397–407.
37. Marcos S. Aberration and visual performance following standard laser vision correction. J Refract Surg. 2001;17:596–601.
38. Harris WF. Power vectors versus power matrices, and the mathematical nature of dioptric power. Optom Vis Sci. 2007;84:1060–3.
39. Arditi A, Cagenello R. On the statistical reliability of letter-chart visual acuity measurements. Invest Ophthalmol Vis Sci. 1993;34:120–9.
40. Bailey IL, Bullimore MA, Raasch TW, Taylor HR. Clinical grading and the effects of scaling. Invest Ophthalmol Vis Sci. 1991;32:422–32.
41. Rosser DA, Cousens SN, Murdoch IE, Fitzke FW, Laidlaw DAH. How Sensitive to Clinical Change are ETDRS logMAR Visual Acuity Measurements? Invest Ophthalmol Vis Sci. 2003;44:3278–81. doi:10.1167/iovs.02-1100.
42. Chakraborty R, Read SA, Collins MJ. Diurnal variations in ocular aberrations of human eyes. Curr Eye Res. 2014;39:271–81.
43. Raasch TW. Spherocylindrical refractive errors and visual acuity. Optom Vis Sci. 1995;72:272–5.
44. Calossi A. Corneal asphericity and spherical aberration. J Refract Surg. 2007;23:505–14.
45. Thiagalingam S, Cumming RG, Mitchell P. Factors associated with undercorrected refractive errors in an older population: the Blue Mountains Eye Study. Br J Ophthalmol. 2002;86:1041–5.
46. Wolfram C, Hoehn R, Kottler U, Wild P, Blettner M, Buehren J, Pfeiffer N, Mirshahi A. Prevalence of refractive errors in the European adult population: the Gutenberg Health Study (GHS). Br J Ophthalmol. 2014;98:857–61.
47. Eysteinsson T, Jonasson F, Arnarsson A, Sasaki H, Sasaki K. Relationships between ocular dimensions and adult stature among participants in the Reykjavik Eye Study. Acta Ophthalmol Scand. 2005;83:734–8.
48. Lee KE, Klein BEK, Klein R, Quandt Z, Wong TY. Age stature and education associations with ocular dimensions in an older white population. Arch Ophthalmol. 2009;127:88–93.
49. Roy A, Kar M, Mandal D, Ray RS, Kar C. Variation of axial ocular dimensions with age, sex, height, BMI- and their relation to refractive status. J Clin Diagn Res. 2015;9:AC01–4.
50. Shufelt C, Fraser-Bell S, Ying-Lai M, Torres M, Varma R, The Los Angeles Latino Eye Study. . Refractive error, ocular biometry, and lens opalescence in an adult population: The Los Angeles Latino Eye Study. Invest Ophthalmol Vis Sci. 2005;46:4450–60.
51. He M, Huang W, Li Y, Zheng Y, Yin Q, Foster PJ. Refractive error and biometry in older Chinese adults: The Liwan Eye Study. Invest Ophthalmol Vis Sci. 2009;50:5130–6.
52. Olsen T, Arnarsson A, Sasaki H, Jonasson F. On the ocular refractive components: The Reykjavik Study. Acta Ophthalmol. 2007;85:361–6.
53. Asgari S, Hashemi H, Mehravaran S, Khabazkhoob M, Emamian MH, Jafarzadehpur E, Shariati M, Fotouhi A. Corneal refractive power and eccentricity in the 40- to 64-year-old population of Shahroud, Iran. Cornea. 2013;32:25–9.
54. Sicam VADP, Dubbelman M, van der Heijde RGL. Spherical aberration of the anterior and posterior surfaces of the human cornea. J Opt Soc Am A. 2006;23:544–9.
55. Kuzmanovic Elabjer B, Petrinovic-Doresic J, Duric M, Busic M, Elabjer E. Cross-sectional Study of ocular optical components interactions in emmetropes. Coll Antropol. 2007;31:743–9.
56. Rozema JJ, Atchison DA, Tassignon MJ. Statistical eye model for normal eyes. Invest Ophthalmol Vis Sci. 2011;52:4525–33.
57. Lam AK, Chan R, Pang PC. The repeatability and accuracy of axial length and anterior chamber depth measurements from the IOLMaster. Ophthalmic Physiol Opt. 2001;21:477–83.
58. Santodomingo-Rubido J, Mallen EAH, Gilmartin B, Wolffsohn JS. A new non-contact optical device for ocular biometry. Br J Ophthalmol. 2002;86:458–62.
59. Sheng H, Bottjer CA, Bullimore MA. Ocular componenet measurement using the Zeiss IOLMaster. Optom Vis Sci. 2004;81:27–34.
60. Klein BE, Klein R, Moss SE. Correlates of lens thickness: The Beaver Dam Eye Study. Invest Ophthalmol Vis Sci. 1998;39:1507–10.
61. Utine CA, Altin F, Cakir H, Perente I. Comparison of anterior chamber depth measurements taken with the Pentacam, Orbscan IIz and IOLMaster in myopic and emmetropic eyes. Acta Ophthalmol. 2009;87:386–91.
62. Grover S, Murthy RK, Brar VS, Chalam KV. Normative data for macular thickness by high-definition spectral-domain optical coherence tomography (Spectralis). Am J Ophthalmol. 2009;148:266–71.
63. Grover S, Murthy RK, Brar VS, Chalam KV. Comparison of retinal thickness in normal eyes using Stratus and Spectralis optical coherence tomography. Invest Ophthalmol Vis Sci. 2010;51:2644–7.
64. Wagner-Schuman M, Dubis AM, Nordgren RN, Lei Y, Odell D, Chiao H, Weh E, Fischer W, Sulai Y, Dubra A, Carroll J. Race- and sex-related differences in retinal thickness and Foveal pit morphology. Invest Ophthalmol Vis Sci. 2011;52:625–34.
65. Wolf-Schnurrbusch UEK, Ceklic L, Brinkmann CK, Iliev ME, Frey M, Rothenbuehler SP, Enzmann V, Wolf S. Macular thickness measurements in healthy eyes using six different optical coherence tomography instruments. Invest Ophthalmol Vis Sci. 2009;50:3432–7.
66. Choovuthayakorn J, Laowong T, Watanachai N, Patikulsila D, Chaikitmongkol V. Spectral-domain optical coherence tomography of macula in myopia. Int Ophthalmol. 2015. doi:10.1007/s10792-015-0119-x.
67. Patel PJ, Foster PJ, Grossi CM, Keane PA, Ko F, Lotery A, Peto T, Reisman CA, Strouthidis NG, Yang Q, on behalf of the UK Biobank Eyes and Vision Consortium. Spectral-domain optical coherence tomography imaging in 67312 adults: associations with macular thickness in the UK Biobank Study. Ophthalmology. 2016;123:829–40.
68. Anton A, Andrada MT, Mayo A, Portela J, Merayo J. Epidemiology of refractive errors in an adult European population: The Segovia study. Ophthal Epidemiol. 2009;16:231–7.
69. Williams KM, Verhoeven VJM, Cumberland P, Bertelsen G, Wolfram C, Buitendijk GHS, Hofman A, Duijn CM, Vingerling JR, Kuijpers RWAM, Hoehn R, Mirshahi A, Khawaja AP, Luben RN, Erke MG, von Hanno T, Mahroo O, Hogg R, Gieger C, Cougnard-Grégoire A, Anastasopoulos E, Bron A, Dartigues J, Korobelnik J, Creuzot-Garcher C, Topouzis F, Delcourt C, Rahi J, Meitinger T, Fletcher A, Foster, Pfeiffer N, Klaver CCW, Hammond CJ. Prevalence of refractive error in Europe: the European eye epidemiology (E3) Consortium. Eur J Epidemiol. 2015;30:305–15.
70. Saw SM, Tong L, Chua WH, Chia KS, Koh D, Tan DTH, Katz J. Incidence and progression of myopia in Singaporean school children. Invest Ophthalmol Vis Sci. 2005;46:51–7.
71. Sun J, Zhou J, Zhao D, Lian J, Zhu H, Zhou Y, Sun Y, Wang Y, Zhao L, Wei Y, Wang L, Cun B, Ge S, Fan X. High prevelance of myopia and high myopia in 5060 Chinese university students in Shanghai. Invest Ophthalmol Vis Sci. 2012;53:7504–9.
72. Mirshahi A, Ponto KA, Hoehn R, Zwiener I, Zeller T, Lackner K, Beutel ME, Pfeiffer N. Myopia and level of education. Ophthalmology. 2014;121:2047–52.
73. Bailey MD, Twa MD, Mitchell GL, Dhaliwal DK, Jones LA, McMahon TT. Repeatability of autorefraction and axial length measurements after laser in situ keratomileusis. J Refract Surg. 2005;31:1025–34.
74. Xu L, Li J, Cui T, Hu A, Zheng Y, Li Y, Sun B, Ma B, Jonas JB. Visual acuity in Northern China in an urban and rural population: The Beijing Eye Study. Br J Ophthalmol. 2005;89:1089–93.
75. Helmholtz. Über die Akkommodation des Auges. Graefes Arch Ophthalmol. 1859;2:1–74.
76. Yuan Y, Shao Y, Tao A, Shen M, Wang J, Shi G, Chen Q, Zhu D, Lian Y, Qu J, Zhang Y, Lu F. Ocular anterior segment biometry and high-order wavefront aberrations during accommodation. Invest Ophthalmol Vis Sci. 2013;54:7028–37.
77. Haughom B, Strand TE. Sine wave mesopic contrast – defining the normal range in a young population. Acta Ophthalmol. 2013;91:176–82.

78. Wachler BS, Krueger RR. Normalized contrast sensitivity values. J Refract Surg. 1998;14:463–6.
79. Alfonso JF, Fernandez-Vega L, Baamonde MB, Montes-Mico R. Correlation of pupil size with visual acuity and contrast sensitivity after implantation of an apodized diffractive intraocular lens. J Refract Surg. 2007;33:430–8.
80. Hashemi H, Khabazkhoob M, Jafarzadehpur E, Emamian MH, Shariati M, Fotouhi A. Contrast sensitivity evaluation in a population-based study in Shahroud. Iran Ophthalmology. 2012;119:541–6.
81. Franco S, Silva AC, Carvalho AS, Macedo AS, Lira M. Comparison of the VCTS-6500 and the CSV-1000 tests for visual contrast sensitivity testing. Neurotoxicology. 2010;31:758–61.
82. Hiraoka T, Okamoto C, Ishii Y, Kakita T, Oshika T. Contrast sensitivity function and ocular higher-order aberrations following overnight orthokeratology. Invest Ophthalmol Vis Sci. 2007;48:550–6.
83. Eppig T, Filser E, Goeppert H, Schroeder AC, Seitz B, Langenbucher A. Index of contrast sensitivity (ICS) in pseudophakic eyes with different intraocular lens designs. Acta Ophthalmol. 2015;93(3):e181–7. doi:10.1111/aos.12538. Epub 2014 Aug 27.
84. Buehren J, Terzi E, Bach M, Wesemann W, Kohnen T. Measuring contrast sensitivity under different lighting conditions: comparison of three tests. Optom Vis Sci. 2006;83:290–8.
85. Hohberger B, Laemmer R, Adler W, Juenemann AG, Horn FK. Measuring contrast sensitivity in normal subjects with OPTEC® 6500: influence of age and glare. Graefes Arch Clin Exp Ophthalmol. 2007;245:1805–14.
86. Wang CW, Chan CL, Jin HY. Psychometric properties of the Chinese version of the 25-item National Eye Institute Visual Function Questionnaire. Optom Vis Sci. 2008;85:1091–9.
87. Globe D, Varma R, Azen SP, Paz S, Yu E, Preston-Martin S & Los Angeles Latino Eye Study Group. Psychometric performance of the NEI VFQ-25 in visually normal latinos: The Los Angeles Latino Eye Study. Invest Ophthalmol Vis Sci. 2003;44:1470–8.
88. Hirneiss C, Schmid-Tannwald C, Kernt M, Kampik A, Neubauer AS. The NEI VFQ-25 vision – related quality of life and prevalence of eye disease in a working population. Graefes ArchClin Exp Ophthalmol. 2010;248:85–92.
89. Le Grand Y. Optiques physiologique – La dioptrique de l'optique de ceil et sa correction. Editions de la revue d'optique, Paris. 1952; 29–31.

26

Tarsoaponeurectomy as an alternative in difficult blepharoptosis cases

Selam Yekta Sendul[1*], Burcu Dirim[1], Mehmet Demir[1], Zeynep Acar[1], Atilla Gokce Demir[1], Ali Olgun[1], Semra Tiryaki[1], Cemile Ucgul[2] and Dilek Guven[1]

Abstract

Background: The purpose of this study was to evaluate the results of tarsoaponeurectomy in patients with unsuccessful results after repetitive surgery or who developed post-traumatic blepharoptosis.

Methods: The files of 107 patients (136 eyes) on whom surgery was performed between January 2010 and December 2014 due to blepharoptosis were scanned retrospectively. Among these patients, the files and operational notes of eight patients who underwent surgery through the method of tarsoaponeurectomy were examined in detail. The epidemiological data, indication for surgery, previous ptosis and/or eyelid surgeries and trauma histories, preoperative and postoperative measurement data (palpebral space (PS), margin reflex distance (MRD1, MRD2), levator muscle function (LMF)) of the patients were recorded. The follow-up time of the patients was 7 to 34 months with an average of 16 months.

Results: A total of eight patients consisting of three females and five males were included in the study. The age range was 19 to 63 years with an average of 39 ± 16.2 years. Four patients had traumatic ptosis history whereas four patients had previous multiple levator procedure surgery history. Those patients with a history of ptosis had undergone surgery with levator procedure at least two times. Additionally, one patient had upper eyelid entropion, one had anophthalmic socket syndrome, and one had exposure keratopathy and traumatic dilated pupil. Seven patients had ptosis in the left eye whereas one patient had ptosis in the right eye. All patients were given a tarsoaponeurectomy as the basic surgical procedure while the patient with entropion was given a tarsal fracture and ear cartilage grafting as additional surgery. Two patients with vertical notching were also given a vertical blepharotomy through which a strip of tarsus was removed.

Conclusions: Tarsoaponeurectomy is an alternative method for oculoplastic surgeons used to deal with patients on whom sufficient and desired results have not been achieved despite repetitive surgery and in post-traumatic cases where levator muscle and aponeurosis cannot be dissociated peroperatively.

Background

Blepharoptosis can be conventionally classified as congenital or acquired. Acquired blepharoptosis can be sub-classified as myogenic, neurogenic, aponeurotic and mechanical or traumatic [1]. In the treatment of blepharoptosis, while the surgical treatment alternatives essentially vary on the basis of levator muscle function, many surgical intervention methods have been defined and discussed [1–4]. While there are several fundamental success criteria, the most important success criterion is

postoperative patient satisfaction [4]. Some blepharoptosis cases constitute a difficult patient group in oculoplastic practice in terms of the results obtained. Particularly those patients who had previously undergone eyelid surgery due to various reasons, those whose initial surgical treatment had not been conducted by experienced oculoplastic surgeons and those cases with no success despite repetitive surgeries as well as those patients with eyelid anatomy disorders such as levator, tarsal and septum disorders as a result of multiple traumas may be included in this patient group.

In this study, we shall discuss the results achieved through the tarsoaponeurectomy technique in acquired ptosis cases with whom the desired results could not be

---

* Correspondence: sysendul@hotmail.com
[1]Department of Ophthalmology, Sisli Hamidiye Etfal Training and Research Hospital, Etfal Street 34280, Sisli, Istanbul, Turkey
Full list of author information is available at the end of the article

achieved despite repetitive surgeries and in post-traumatic ptosis cases.

Methods

In our clinic, the files of 107 patients (136 eyes) who underwent surgery due to blepharoptosis between January 2010 and December 2014 were scanned retrospectively. Forty five patients (58 eyes) out of 107 had been given frontalis sling surgery due to congenital or levator muscle function weakness. The remaining 62 patients (78 eyes) had been operated on using a levator procedure with different methods. Out of the latter, the files and operational notes of eight patients who had undergone a tarsoaponeurectomy operation were examined in detail. The epidemiological data, indication for surgery, previous ptosis and/or eyelid surgeries, trauma histories, preoperative and postoperative measurement data (palpebral space (PS), margin reflex distance (MRD1, MRD2), levator muscle function (LMF)) of the patients were recorded. The tarsoaponeurectomy indication was made preoperatively taking into consideration the previous multiple ptosis surgeries the patient had undergone, traumatic eyelid deformities, level of preoperative levator muscle function and damages on the tarsus in the upper eyelid. Upon reaching the levator aponeurosis and muscle peroperatively, a further evaluation was made and the decision to perform a tarsoaponeurectomy on patients who were considered as showing a low chance of success through the levator procedure was finalized.

The measured palpebral space (PS), levator muscle function (LMF) and MRD1 values and the postoperative complications of all patients were recorded preoperatively and postoperatively. Again, the recorded preoperative and postoperative eyelid deformations and eyelid contour disorders were examined and photographed (Fig. 1a, b, c). All patients were contacted and final follow-up examinations were made. The follow-up time of the patients was 7 to 34 months with an average of 16 months. The study was conducted in accordance with the tenets of the Declaration of Helsinki by obtaining written consent from all patients, with the approval of the local ethical committee.

Surgical technique

The incision line was marked with a pen preoperatively based on the eyelid sulcus line of the healthy eye. Jetokain (Lidocaine HCL 20 mm/ml+Epinephrine HCL 0.0125 mg/ml) was injected into the eyelid locally in order to reduce peroperative bleeding and all patients were operated under local anesthesia. Then, the marked section was incised and the cutaneous and subcutaneous tissues were passed. The upper eyelid tarsal tissue was reached through vertical dissection. The adhesions due to previous trauma and/or surgery were released through blunt and sharp

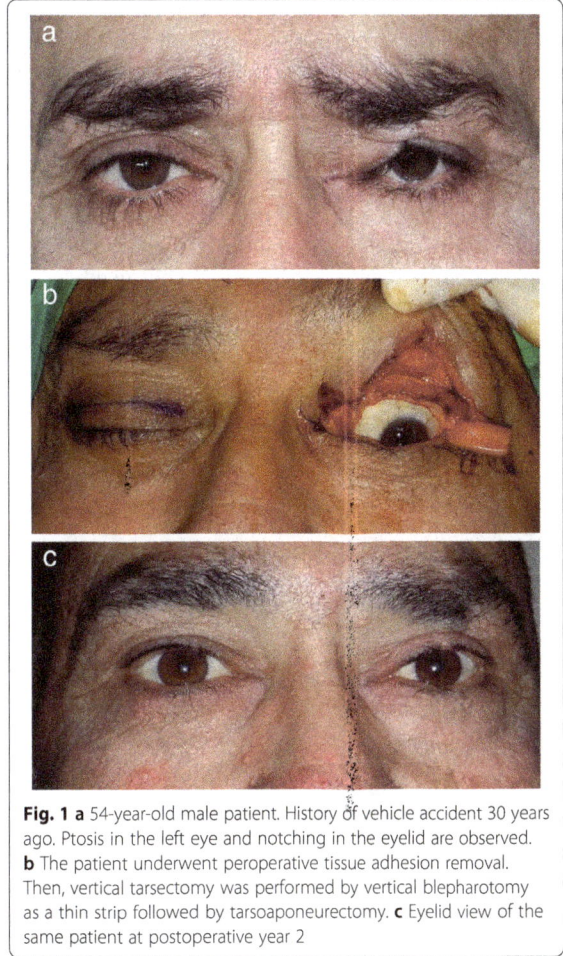

Fig. 1 a 54-year-old male patient. History of vehicle accident 30 years ago. Ptosis in the left eye and notching in the eyelid are observed. **b** The patient underwent peroperative tissue adhesion removal. Then, vertical tarsectomy was performed by vertical blepharotomy as a thin strip followed by tarsoaponeurectomy. **c** Eyelid view of the same patient at postoperative year 2

dissection. As the septum was in a damaged state due to previous surgical treatments and/or trauma, the levator aponeurosis and muscle were reached using the preaponeurotic fat tissue as an indicator. At this stage, those patients with intact levator muscles and aponeurosis were given conventional aponeurosis surgery whereas it was decided to perform tarsoaponeurectomy to those patients who did not have their muscles, aponeurosis or tarsus intact. At this stage, the amount of tarsus and aponeurosis complex (aponeurosis, Müller muscle, conjunctiva) to be excised was determined on the basis of preoperative measurements and in comparison with the peroperative eyelid level of the other eye. An average of 1–3 mm tarsal tissue and 1–5 mm aponeurosis complex were excised. Afterwards, the aponeurosis complex was sutured to the upper edge of the tarsus with three 6/0 vicryl sutures as central, nasal and temporal. At this stage, the eyelid contour and level were compared to the healthy eyelid of the patient as a preoperative check upon which middle sutures were made. Then, three sutures forming the upper eyelid crease were located in a way as to pass through the aponeurosis complex and the skin was closed with 6/0 prolene (polyproylene) suture. After surgery contact lenses were applied to all patients for 1 week in order to prevent postoperative corneal erosion (Fig. 2a, b, c, d).

Statistical analysis

In the descriptive statistics of the data, mean and standard deviations, median and min-max values were used. The distribution of the variables was controlled by the

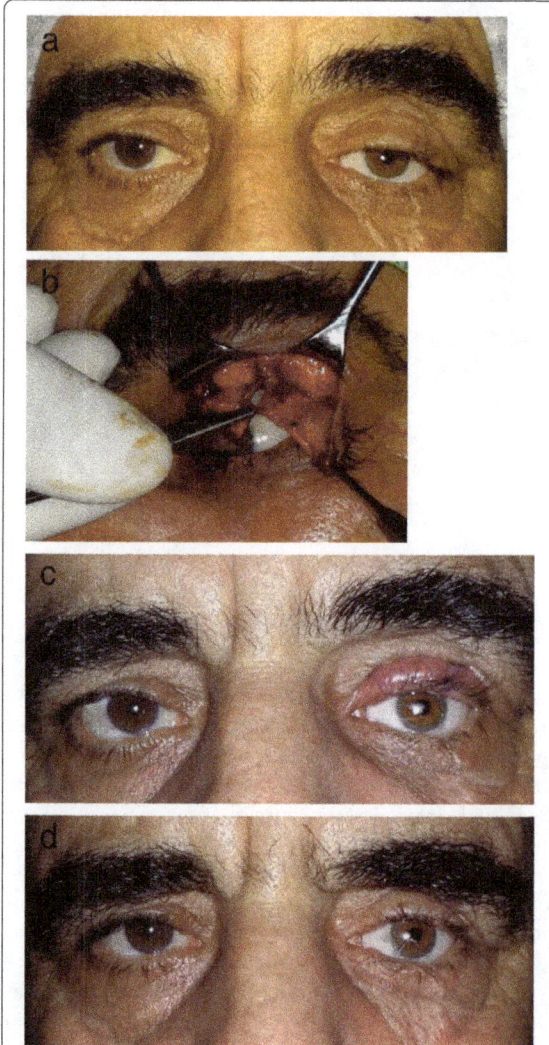

Fig. 2 a 63-year-old male patient. History of sharp object injury 10 years ago. Prosthesis in the left eye due to anophthalmic socket. Distinct ptosis and notching at the temporal are observed. Even more distinct ptosis in the nasal region of the right eye is apparent. **b** Peroperative view of the same patient. Vertical tarsectomy was performed by vertical blepharotomy as a thin strip followed by horizontal tarsoaponeurectomy. **c** View at postoperative week 1. Ptosis in the right eye continues. **d** View at postoperative year 1.5 following right levator advancement

Kolmogorov Smirnov test. In the analysis of the quantitative data, the Wilcoxon test and the matched sample t test were used. In the analyses, the SPSS 22.0 program was used.

Results

A total of eight patients consisting of three females and five males were included in the study. The age range was 19 to 63 years with an average of 39 ± 16.2 years. Four patients had a traumatic ptosis history whereas four patients had a previous multiple levator procedure surgery history. Each patient who had had previous multiple surgeries under a levator procedure had a history of at least two and at most four operations. Additionally, one patient had upper eyelid entropion, one had anophthalmic socket syndrome, and one had exposure keratopathy and traumatic fix dilated pupil. Seven patients had ptosis in the left eye whereas one patient had ptosis in the right eye (Table 1). All patients were given tarsoaponeurectomy as the basic surgical procedure while the patient with entropion was given tarsal fracture and ear cartilage grafting as additional surgery. Two patients with traumatic vertical notching were also given vertical blepharotomy through which tarsus in the shape of a tarsal strip was removed.

The basic success criterion was taken as a quantitative ptosis measurement (Table 2). All measurements were made during clinical examination. Preoperatively, the PS value was significantly lower in the eye with ptosis compared to the normal eye ($p < 0.05$) whereas postoperatively no significant difference was detected between the two eyes ($p > 0.05$) and again postoperatively a significant increase was detected in the eye with ptosis compared to the preoperative values ($p < 0.05$) (Fig. 3). With respect to levator muscle function, it was significantly reduced in the eye with ptosis both preoperatively and postoperatively compared to the healthy eyelid ($p < 0.05$) whereas no significant difference was detected in the postoperative levator function of the unhealthy eye compared to the preoperative value ($p < 0.05$) (Fig. 4). In terms of MRD1 value, the preoperative MRD1 value in the eye with ptosis was significantly lower than that of the healthy eye ($p < 0.05$) while there was no significant difference between the two postoperative values ($p > 0.05$). Again, in the eye with ptosis, the postoperative MRD1 value showed a significant increase compared to the preoperative value ($p < 0.05$) (Fig. 5). We did not observe any serious complications such as eyelid instability, ectropion or entropion in any of our cases. However, all cases showed temporary lagophthalmos of 1–3 mm continuing until postoperative month 1. Within this period, all patients were given intense eye-drop and gel therapy thereby preventing any ocular surface damage that might have developed due to lagophthalmos.

Table 1 Epidemiologic data, preopeartive and postoperative histories and complications of the patients.(*M* male, *F* female)

Patient	Age/Type	History	Additional disease	Additional surgery	Complications
1	27/m	ptosis - 3 times	entropion	-tarsal fracture -ear cartilage graft	corneal irritation in the early term
2	42/f	ptosis - 2 times	none	Revision surgery due to postoperative temporal drooping	corneal irritation in the early term
3	51/f	extravehicular traffic accident	-notching in the lid -exposure keratopathy -lower eyelid laxity -traumatic fix dilated pupil	lateral canthal sling (in a separate session)	- corneal irritation in the early term -continuous light sensitivity
4	63/m	sharp trauma 10 years ago	- notching in the lid -anophthalmic socket syndrome	Removal of vertical tarsal strip by vertical blepharotomy	none
5	54/m	traffic accident 30 years ago	notching in the lid	Removal of vertical tarsal strip by vertical blepharotomy	corneal irritation in the early term
6	19/m	-motorcycle accident -bilateral canalicular repair and lid reconstruction	multiple former wound scars in the facial area	none	none
7	21/m	ptosis - 2 times	none	none	none
8	35/f	ptosis - 4 times	none	none	none

Discussion

In the correction of blepharoptosis, three primary surgical methods exist. In congenital ptosis cases and/or in ptosis cases with poor levator function, frontalis sling techniques may be used whereas in acquired ptosis cases, levator resection or levator aponeurisis advancement techniques may be used depending on the strength of the levator muscle. It is possible to choose one of these methods on patients who apply for primary surgery [5–8]. However, there is a group of patients who are very difficult. This group includes those ptosis cases on whom no successful results are obtained despite repetitive surgery and also those ptosis cases that develop due to eyelid tissue damage following orbital or eyelid traumas. In this study, we evaluated the tarsoaponeurectomy method which we performed on this group of

patients, the indications for the procedure, the results thereof and postoperative complications.

Tarsal resection has a long history in blepharoptosis surgery. In his presentation, Reifler [9] detailed the basic points whereas Anatole Pierre Louis Gillet de Grandmont [10] reported that correction in ptosis was obtained through partial tarsal resection. Hervoue¨t and Tessier [11] published a study in 1956 and Mustarde [12] published another in 1975 where they defined tarsectomy combined with plication of the levator aponeurosis-Müller muscle complex, i.e. "split-level" operation.

Patel SM et al. [13] reported that they received excellent results in congenital ptosis cases with poor levator muscle functions through the levator aponeurosis-Müller-conjunctiva complex surgery combined with tarsus, and regarding

Table 2 Preoperative and postoperative statistical data

	Healthy eye			ptotic eye			*p*
	Avg. ± s.d.	Med(Min-Max)		Avg. ± s.d.	Med(Min-Max)		
Vision	1.8 ± 2.3	1.0	1-7	0.7 ± 0.4	0.7	0.0-1.0	0.068
Preop PS	8.8 ± 0.7	9.0	8-10	7.0 ± 1.4	7.0	5.0-10.0	0.004
Postop PS	8.8 ± 0.7	9.0	8-10	8.5 ± 0.5	8.5	7.5-9.0	0.305
Preop/Postop Change	1.000			0.030			
Preop LMF	16.1 ± 1.9	16.0	13-18	7.9 ± 4.0	7.0	2.0-15.0	0.012
Postop LMF	16.3 ± 2.0	16.5	13-18	11.0 ± 2.9	10.5	6.0-16.0	0.012
Preop/Postop Change	0.317			0.121			
Preop MRD1	3.4 ± 0.4	3.5	3-4	1.7 ± 1.2	1.0	1.0-4.5	0.016
Postop MRD 1	3.4 ± 0.4	3.5	3-4	3.1 ± 0.4	3.0	2.5-3.5	0.096
Preop/Postop Change	1.000			0.029			

Wilcoxon test/Matched sample *t* test

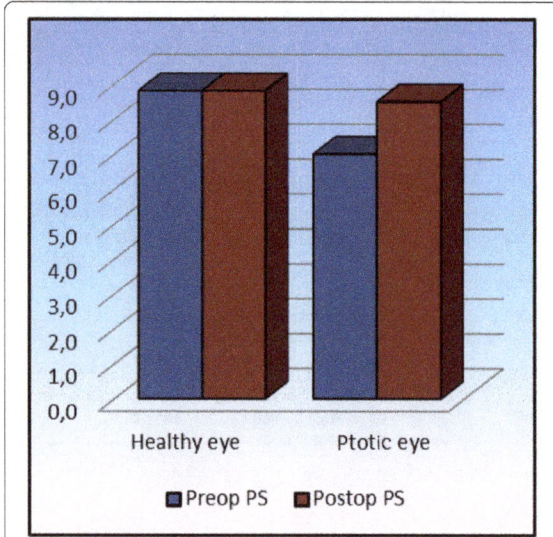

Fig. 3 Significant increase in palpebral space is observed postoperatively in ptotic eyes

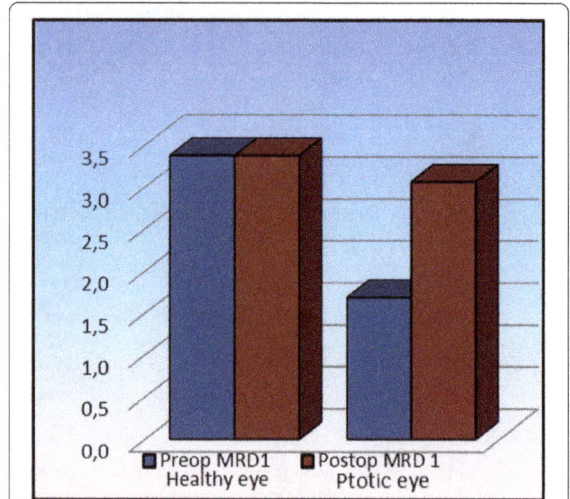

Fig. 5 Increase in MRD1 values is observed postoperatively in ptotic eyes

complications, they only detected temporary lagophthalmos and exposure keratopathy that both recover over time, however they further stated that they did not have sufficient long term information. On the other hand, Park J et al. [14], in their comparative study in which they performed super-maximum levator resection surgery alone or in combination with superior tarsectomy again in patients with poor levator muscle function, reported that the eyelid was

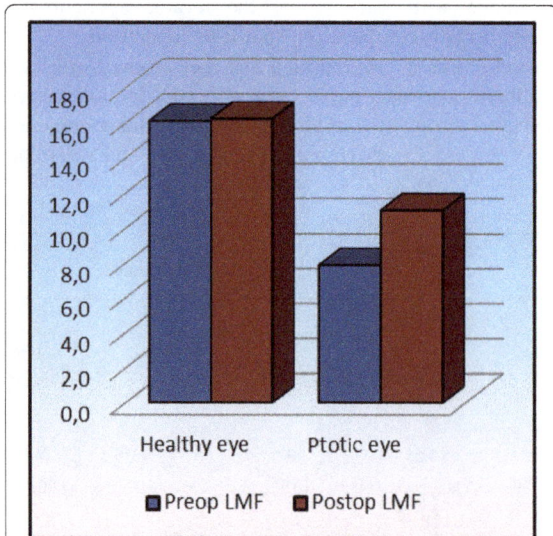

Fig. 4 Increase in LMF is observed postoperatively in ptotic eyes, although not at statistically significant rates. (It probably occurred due to the enlargement of the movement range of the muscle following the recovery of adhesions)

lifted more in the latter group. They also reported that they did not identify any possible complications that may have occurred in the resection of the tarsus such as eyelid instability, ectropion, entropion, etc. In our study, all patients consisted of cases with fair or good levator muscle function, and we obtained successful results on them. Again, similar to the above mentioned studies, although temporary lagophthalmos was detected in the early postoperative term, it recovered completely by the end of month 1. Again, although we detected discomfort due to suture irritation in our patients, we overcame this problem in the early postoperative term through the use of contact lenses and also intensive use of eye drops and gels. None of the cases showed eyelid instability.

The question that comes to mind in this matter is the amount of tarsus-aponeurosis-Müller-conjunctiva complex to be resected. Of course, in this regard, the amount and degree of ptosis come into play. [13–15] Beard [15] defines eyelid drooping up to 2 mm as mild, 3 mm as moderate and 4 mm and above as severe ptosis. In this matter, Patel et al. [13] reported that they made their decisions on the basis of the level of ptosis and that they performed the Müller-conjunctiva resection about twice as many times as the tarsal resection and that in mild ptosis cases with poor levator muscle function, they performed 2–3 mm tarsus and 4–6 mm Müller-conjunctiva, in moderate ptosis cases 3–4 mm tarsus, 6–8 mm Müller-conjunctiva, and in severe ptosis cases 4–5 mm tarsus and 8–10 mm Müller-conjunctiva resection. We conducted surgery under local anesthesia and therefore we made our decisions by taking into consideration the preoperative measurement data and comparing it with the peroperative healthy eyelid level. After we performed the first resection and made the first sutures, just like the case in the levator advancement technique, we compared it with the other eyelid by giving the patient instructions and making the patient sit when necessary. At this stage, we made additional resections when insufficient corrections or contour disorders were in question. Due to the fact that the muscle function levels of our patients were fair to good, the tarsus-aponeurosis-Müller-conjunctiva complex reduced the resection amount.

Another question was as to what can be done in the case of insufficient correction or overcorrection. Park et al. [16] reported that two patients in group 2 were detected with insufficient correction, they performed the frontalis sling on one and the levator resection on the other and they performed a combined treatment on their patients who had unsuccessful results from group 1. As a matter of fact, this was the question that worried us most during surgery in that we had little chance as to what we could do in the case of overcorrection. Therefore, we performed the surgery by keeping the resection amount at low levels peroperatively and constantly comparing it with the other eyelid. In our study, only one patient developed temporal eyelid drooping and we corrected this case through a second surgery by simply removing some conjunctiva-müller-aponeurosis complex from the temporal area. According to us, the major disadvantage of this surgery is that there are no alternatives other than placing graft to the posterior lamellar area when overcorrection happens. Thankfully, we did not come across any postoperative overcorrections in any of our patients.

Another question to be examined is what are the long term results of this surgery. Unfortunately, there is no sufficient study or data in the literature in this regard. According to our experience of about 3 years of follow-ups, insufficient corrections are revealed at the end of postoperative month 1. We did not detect any changes in our patients in the subsequent follow-ups. However, it is not proper to reach a final judgment in this regard due to the low number of patients.

Conclusions
In conclusion, with regard to the tarsoaponeurectomy method, we submit the following points: 1. Tarsoaponeurectomy should never be the initial choice in patients with good levator muscle function; 2. The tissue to be resected should be kept minimal during peroperative resection because, in case of overcorrection, there is no other alternative but placing a new graft; and 3. Tarsoaponeurectomy is an alternative method for oculoplastic surgeons to be used only for those patients in whom sufficient and desired results are not obtained despite repetitive surgery and in post traumatic cases where levator muscle and aponeurosis cannot be dissociated peroperatively.

Ethics approval and consent
This study was approved by Sisli Hamidiye Etfal Training and Research Hospital Local Ethical Committee. Further, written consent was obtained from the patients shown in the figures. (Approval date:01.09.2015, Approval number:1063).

Abbreviations
PS: palpebral space; MRD1: margin reflex distance1; MRD2: margin reflex distance2; LMF: levator muscle function.

Competing interest
All authors declare that they have no competing interests.

Authors' contributions
SYS performed examination, surgery and follow-up of the patients and contributed in drafting the manuscript; BD contributed in study design and drafting; AGD collected and examined retrospective patient files; MD contributed in study design and drafting; ZA examined patient files and contributed in drafting the manuscript; AO performed statistical analysis; ST contributed in study design and obtaining the ethical committee approval; CU contributed in drafting and editing the manuscript; DG carried out the study and performed final editing of the manuscript. All authors read and approved the final manuscript.

Acknowledgments
We thank Ayse Unal and Mark Scott for editing the paper in terms of English.

Funding
No financial support was received for this study.

Author details
[1]Department of Ophthalmology, Sisli Hamidiye Etfal Training and Research Hospital, Etfal Street 34280, Sisli, Istanbul, Turkey. [2]Department of Ophthalmology, Ulucanlar Eye Training and Research Hospital, Ulucanlar street, 06030, Altındag, Ankara, Turkey.

References
1. Waqar S, McMurray C, Madge SN. Transcutaneous blepharoptosis surgery - advancement of levator aponeurosis. Open Ophthalmol J. 2010;4:76–80.
2. Lee EI, Ahn TJ. Mild ptosis correction with the stitch method during incisional double fold formation. Arch Plast Surg. 2014;41:71–6.
3. Buttanri IB, Serin D. Levator resection in the management of myopathic ptosis. Korean J Ophthalmol. 2014;28(6):431–5.
4. Scoppettulol E, Chadha V, Bunce C, Olver JM, Wright M. British Oculoplastic Surgery Society (BOPSS) national ptosis survery. Br J Ophthalmol. 2008;92: 1134–8.
5. Nemet AY. The effect of Hering's law on different ptosis repair methods. Aesthet Surg J. 2015;35(7):774–81.
6. Frueh BR, Musch DC, McDonald H. Efficacy and efficiency of a new involutional ptosis correction procedure compared to a traditional aponeuroticapproach. Trans Am Ophthalmol Soc. 2004;102:199–206.
7. Ichinose A, Leibovitch I. Transconjunctival levator aponeurosis advancement without resection of Müller's muscle in aponeuroticptosis repair. Open Ophthalmol J. 2010;4:85–90.
8. McDonald H. Minimally invasive levator advancement: a practical approach to eyelid ptosis repair. Semin Plast Surg. 2007;21(1):41–6.
9. Reifler DM. The tarsectomy operation of A.P.L. Gillet de Grandmont (1837–1894) and its periodic rediscovery. Doc Ophthalmol. 1995;89:153–62.
10. de Grandmont G. Nouvelle operation du ptosis congenital. Recueil d'Ophthalmologie. 1891;13:267–70.
11. Hervouët F, Tessier P. Nouvelle technique ope'ratoire du ptosis. Bull Mem Soc Fr Ophthlmol. 1956;69:239–42.
12. Mustarde JC. Problems and possibilities in ptosis surgery. Plast Reconstr Surg. 1975;56:381–8.

13. Patel SM, Linberg JV, Sivak-Callcott JA, Gunel E. Modified tarsal resection operation for congenital ptosis with fair levator function. Ophthal Plast Reconstr Surg. 2008;24(1):1–6.
14. Perry JD, Kadakia A, Foster JA. A new algorithm for ptosis repair using conjunctival Müllerectomy with or without tarsectomy. Ophthal Plast Reconstr Surg. 2002;18(6):426–9.
15. Beard C. Ptosis. 2nd ed. St. Louis: CV Mosby Co.; 1976.
16. Pak J, Shields M, Putterman AM. Superior tarsectomy augments süper-maximum levator resection in correction of severe blepharoptosis with poor levator function. Ophthalmology. 2006;113(7):1201–8.

27

Bimatoprost, latanoprost, and tafluprost induce differential expression of matrix metalloproteinases and tissue inhibitor of metalloproteinases

Hiroshi Yamada[1], Masahiko Yoneda[2], Masahiko Gosho[3], Tomohiro Kato[1] and Masahiro Zako[1*]

Abstract

Background: Differences in the increase in matrix metalloproteinase (MMP) and decrease in tissue inhibitor of metalloproteinase (TIMP) activity may contribute to the different characteristics observed clinically on decreased intraocular pressure in patients with glaucoma or ocular hypertension. The purpose of this study was to investigate differences in the expression profiles of MMPs and TIMPs induced by the prostaglandin analogs bimatoprost, latanoprost, and tafluprost in human non-pigmented ciliary epithelial cells (HNPCECs).

Methods: HNPCECs were cultured for 24 h with 0, 10, 100, or 1000 μM of the free acid forms of bimatoprost, latanoprost, and tafluprost. We measured the expression levels of MMPs and TIMPs using real-time polymerase chain reaction, and compared the results. Enzyme activities of MMP-2 and −9 in conditioned media were measured by gelatin zymography.

Results: All prostaglandin analogs we examined dose-dependently increased expression levels of MMP-1, −2, −3, −9, and −17, whereas expression levels of TIMP-1 and −2 decreased with increasing concentrations of each analog. Each prostaglandin analog induced different levels of increases in MMPs and decreases in TIMPs.

Conclusions: Unique expression profiles of MMPs and TIMPs induced by bimatoprost, latanoprost, and tafluprost, as shown in HNPCECs, may contribute to clinically different effects on intraocular pressure decreases in patients with glaucoma or ocular hypertension.

Keywords: Human non-pigmented ciliary epithelial cells, Matrix metalloproteinases, Prostaglandin analog, Tissue inhibitor of metalloproteinases

Background

Bimatoprost (amide prodrug of 17-phenyl-$PGF_{2\alpha}$), latanoprost (ester prodrug of $PGF_{2\alpha}$), and tafluprost (difluoroprostaglandin derivative of $PGF_{2\alpha}$) are prostaglandin analogs (PGAs) available for clinical use to lower patients' intraocular pressure (IOP). Recently, PGAs were approved as a first-line treatment for glaucoma based on their efficacy in lowering IOP, lack of relevant systemic side effects, and requirement for once-daily dosing [1].

The mechanism by which PGAs reduce IOP has been well-studied and is believed to occur by enhancement of uveoscleral outflow due to the regulation of matrix metalloproteinases (MMPs) and resulting remodeling of the extracellular matrix [2–4]. Clinically, we often experience different effects from the different PGAs. Different receptor subtypes for PGAs were proposed, and different PGAs may lower IOP by different mechanisms of action through these different receptor subtypes [5, 6]. However, the precise mechanism through which these PGAs exhibit different effects in individual patients is still unclear. Previous studies reported differential expression of MMPs in the ciliary body or ciliary muscle after bimatoprost, latanoprost, or tafluprost treatment [2–4, 7]. The

* Correspondence: zako@aichi-med-u.ac.jp
[1]Department of Opthalmology, Aichi Medical University, Nagakute, Aichi 480-1195, Japan
Full list of author information is available at the end of the article

activity of these endopeptidases is inhibited by endogenous tissue inhibitor of metalloproteinases (TIMPs); thus, the balanced expression of MMPs and TIMPs is important for maintaining homeostasis of the extracellular matrix and for reducing IOP by these PGAs.

Human non-pigmented ciliary epithelial cells (HNPCECs), which comprise the blood-aqueous barrier (BAB), are involved in controlling IOP. HNPCECs secrete aqueous humor. A decrease in aqueous humor secretion occurs in association with uveitis, especially uveitis involving the ciliary body epithelium (iridocyclitis) [8]. We previously showed that TNF-α (tumor necrosis factor-α) promotes the induction of MMPs in HNPCECs, which degrade claudin-1 and occludin, major constituents of tight-junctions between HNPCECs [9]. We found significantly increased permeability of a monolayer of HNPCECs after MMP treatment. We hypothesized that the balance of MMPs and TIMPs that degrade the components of tight junctions in the BAB in HNPCECs modifies the production of aqueous humor, which consequently decreases aqueous secretion and IOP.

In the present study, we measured and compared the expression levels of MMPs and TIMPs in HNPCECs cultured with various concentrations of bimatoprost, latanoprost, or tafluprost. Differences in the increase in MMP and decrease in TIMP activity may contribute to the different characteristics observed clinically on decreased IOP in patients with glaucoma or ocular hypertension.

Methods

Cell culture
HNPCECs were prepared as described previously [9].

Cell treatment
Free-acid forms of bimatoprost, latanoprost, or tafluprost (Cayman Chemical Ann Arbor, MI, USA) were prepared in dimethyl sulfoxide (DMSO) and diluted to experimental concentrations (10, 100, and 1000 μM) with serum-free medium and added to the HNPCECs. The cells were then incubated for 24 h.

RNA isolation and cDNA synthesis
Total cellular RNA was isolated from the HNPCECs, and total RNA was used as a template for cDNA synthesis with random primers as described previously [9].

qPCR
cDNA was synthesized from total RNA (50 ng) for each treatment group. The cDNA served as the template for the real-time quantitative polymerase chain reaction (qPCR) assays. The primer sequences for human MMP-1, –2, –3, and –9 were described previously [9]. The primer sequences were human MMP-17 forward (5′-CACCAAGTGGAACAAGAGGAACCT-

3′) and reverse (5′-TGGTAGTACGGCCGCATGATG-GAGTGTGCA-3′). The primer sequences for human TIMP-1, and –2 were described previously [9]. The qPCR gene expression results were normalized as described previously [9]. The qPCR reaction was carried out as described previously [9].

Gelatin zymography
Gelatin zymography was performed and gelatinolytic band densities were quantified as described previously [9].

Statistical analysis
Experiments were repeated four times. The results are presented as the mean ± standard deviation (SD). Statistical analyses were performed using an analysis of variance model with Bonferroni's post hoc test for multiple comparisons. The value measured without PAGs was defined as a control. We used the SAS 9.4 software (SAS Institute, Cary, NC, USA) for all statistical analyses. Differences with P-values < 0.05 were considered significant.

Results
We examined the expression levels of MMPs and TIMPs in cellular extracts from HNPCECs treated with 10, 100, or 1000 μM of bimatoprost, latanoprost, or tafluprost. The qPCR results demonstrated that MMP-1, MMP-2, MMP-3, MMP-9, and MMP-17 mRNA expression levels were dose dependently increased with increasing bimatoprost, latanoprost, or tafluprost concentrations (Fig. 1, Table 1). When the concentrations of the PGAs were 1000 μM, the MMP-1, MMP-2, MMP-3, MMP-9, and MMP-17 expression levels significantly increased compared to the control levels. When the PGA concentration was 100 and 1000 μM, TIMP-1 and TIMP-2 mRNA expression levels in HNPCECs significantly decreased compared to the control levels.

We performed gelatin zymography to measure the enzymatic activity of MMP-2 and MMP-9 in HNPCECs treated with 10, 100, or 1000 μM bimatoprost, latanoprost, or tafluprost (Fig. 2). MMP-2 and MMP-9 controls were used to identify the location of each band (Fig. 2, arrowheads). We detected active MMP-2 forms, but not pro-MMP-9 or pro-MMP-2 forms. We performed a quantitative analysis of the band densities to evaluate active MMP-2 activity in HNPCECs treated with 10, 100, or 1000 μM of bimatoprost, latanoprost, or tafluprost. When the band density of active MMP-2 in HNPCECs treated with 1000 μM bimatoprost was defined as 100, the relative band densities of active MMP-2 in HNPCECs treated with 100 and 1000 μM latanoprost and tafluprost were calculated as 18 and 63 and 31 and 47, respectively. No band was detected in HNPCECs

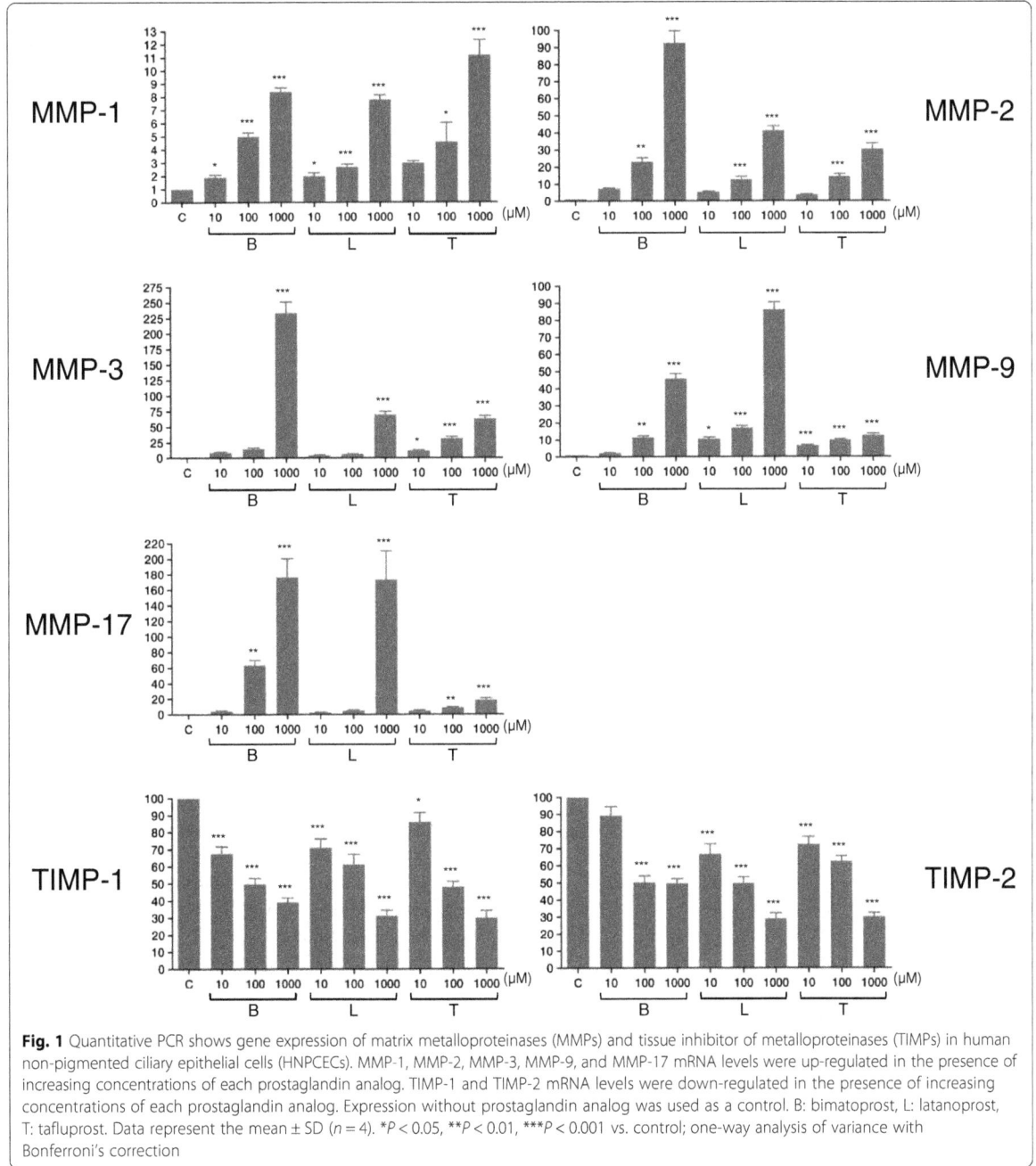

Fig. 1 Quantitative PCR shows gene expression of matrix metalloproteinases (MMPs) and tissue inhibitor of metalloproteinases (TIMPs) in human non-pigmented ciliary epithelial cells (HNPCECs). MMP-1, MMP-2, MMP-3, MMP-9, and MMP-17 mRNA levels were up-regulated in the presence of increasing concentrations of each prostaglandin analog. TIMP-1 and TIMP-2 mRNA levels were down-regulated in the presence of increasing concentrations of each prostaglandin analog. Expression without prostaglandin analog was used as a control. B: bimatoprost, L: latanoprost, T: tafluprost. Data represent the mean ± SD ($n = 4$). *$P < 0.05$, **$P < 0.01$, ***$P < 0.001$ vs. control; one-way analysis of variance with Bonferroni's correction

treated with 10 and 100 μM bimatoprost or 10 μM latanoprost and tafluprost. The relative mRNA expression levels of MMP-2 in HNPCECs treated with 1000 μM bimatoprost and with 100 or 1000 μM latanoprost or tafluprost were calculated as 100:14:45:16:33, respectively (Fig. 1), and this relationship appeared similar to the relative band densities of activeMMP-2 in HNPCECs analyzed by gelatin zymography.

Discussion

Previous studies showed that PGAs induce expression of MMP-1, −2, −3, −9, and −17 and TIMP-1 and −2 in the human ciliary body [7, 10–15]. Here, we investigated the expression levels of MMPs and TIMPs in HNPCECs cultured with various concentrations of bimatoprost, latanoprost, or tafluprost, demonstrating different profiles with respect to increases

Table 1 Comparison with control group

Response	Drug	Dose	Mean	SD	P
MMP-1	B	10	1.9	0.4	0.044
	B	100	5.0	0.6	<0.001
	B	1000	8.4	0.6	<0.001
	L	10	2.0	0.5	0.018
	L	100	2.7	0.4	<0.001
	L	1000	7.8	0.7	<0.001
	T	10	3.0	0.3	0.273
	T	100	4.6	2.9	0.023
	T	1000	11.2	2.3	<0.001
MMP-2	B	10	7.5	0.6	0.501
	B	100	23.1	4.5	0.002
	B	1000	92.5	14.2	<0.001
	L	10	5.5	0.6	0.100
	L	100	12.7	3.4	<0.001
	L	1000	41.2	5.2	<0.001
	T	10	3.6	0.6	0.706
	T	100	14.4	3.0	<0.001
	T	1000	30.5	6.4	<0.001
MMP-3	B	10	8.9	0.9	1.000
	B	100	14.9	3.8	0.604
	B	1000	234.0	34.7	<0.001
	L	10	4.2	0.8	1.000
	L	100	6.1	0.7	0.432
	L	1000	69.8	10.9	<0.001
	T	10	11.4	2.2	0.030
	T	100	31.6	5.8	<0.001
	T	1000	63.3	9.2	<0.001
MMP-9	B	10	2.3	0.3	1.000
	B	100	11.5	1.6	0.001
	B	1000	45.8	5.7	<0.001
	L	10	10.6	1.9	0.019
	L	100	17.0	2.5	<0.001
	L	1000	86.2	8.9	<0.001
	T	10	6.5	0.6	<0.001
	T	100	9.8	0.9	<0.001
	T	1000	12.6	2.1	<0.001
MMP-17	B	10	3.9	2.2	1.000
	B	100	63.2	13.4	0.006
	B	1000	176.5	47.9	<0.001
	L	10	2.3	1.1	1.000
	L	100	4.9	1.7	1.000
	L	1000	173.1	74.7	<0.001
	T	10	4.8	1.7	0.105
	T	100	8.8	1.7	0.002
	T	1000	18.5	4.8	<0.001
TIMP-1	B	10	67.6	8.3	<0.001
	B	100	49.8	6.7	<0.001
	B	1000	39.2	5.2	<0.001
	L	10	71.0	10.2	<0.001
	L	100	61.3	11.9	<0.001
	L	1000	31.3	6.5	<0.001
	T	10	85.9	11.5	0.038
	T	100	48.1	6.3	<0.001
	T	1000	30.0	8.7	<0.001
TIMP-2	B	10	89.2	10.8	0.082
	B	100	50.2	7.5	<0.001
	B	1000	49.6	5.3	<0.001
	L	10	66.7	11.6	<0.001
	L	100	49.7	7.1	<0.001
	L	1000	29.0	6.6	<0.001
	T	10	72.2	9.1	<0.001
	T	100	62.4	6.2	<0.001
	T	1000	30.1	4.6	<0.001

P one-way ANOVA with Bonferroni's post hoc test for multiple comparisons
B bimatoprost, *L* latanoprost, *T* tafluprost
Dose: µM

in MMP and decrease in TIMP expression by each PGA.

Each PGA elicited a unique MMP and TIMP expression profile in HNPCECs. At a concentration of 1000 µM, bimatoprost induced greater expression of MMP-2 and MMP-3 than latanoprost and tafluprost. Bimatoprost has a greater effect on lowering IOP than latanoprost [16, 17]. The ability of PGAs to lower IOP may involve MMP-2 and -3. At a concentration of 1000 µM, tafluprost and latanoprost increased the expression MMP-1 and MMP-9, respectively, more than bimatoprost. Some reports showed no significant difference between bimatoprost and latanoprost [18, 19]. Furthermore, Alm showed no clinically significant difference in efficacy between latanoprost and tafluprost [18]. The MMP and TIMP expression profiles of each PGA may be different in individual patients. Thus, the decrease IOP by PGAs may be determined by several diverse factors.

The ratio of infiltration of each PGA from the ophthalmic solution into the aqueous humor and the concentration of each PGA may be essential for the efficacy of each agent. We investigated PGAs at 10, 100, and 1000 µM, concentrations intentionally ranged within those of commercial ophthalmic solutions. In clinical use, 0.03 % bimatoprost, 0.005 % latanoprost, and 0.0015 % tafluprost ophthalmic solutions are available, corresponding to 720 µM, 110 µM, and 33 µM,

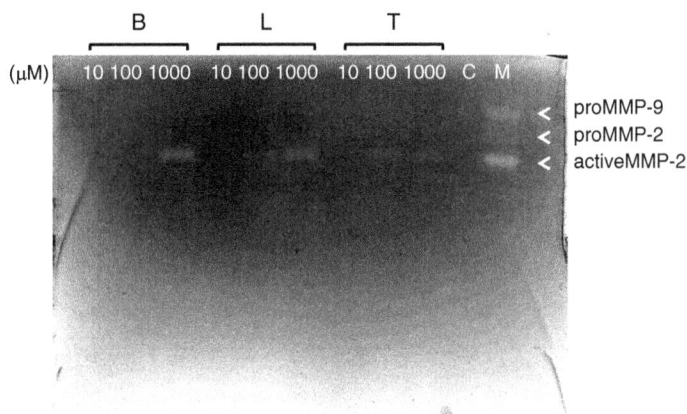

Fig. 2 Gelatin zymogram showing the band densities of MMP-2 and MMP-9. Only bands of activeMMP-2 were detected after treatment with the prostaglandin analogs. No bands were detected without treatment (control lane). Samples containing 20 μg of protein were analyzed. B: bimatoprost, L: latanoprost, T: tafluprost. C: control, M: molecular weight marker. Molecular weights of proMMP-9, proMMP-2, and activeMMP-2 are 92 kDa, 72 kDa, and 62 kDa, respectively

respectively. The concentration of each PGA in the aqueous humor is lower than that in the ophthalmic solution. In an in vitro study, peak aqueous concentrations after topical administration were 0.009 μg/ml, 0.028 μg/ml, and 0.00875 μg/ml, respectively [20–22], with each concentration corresponding to 22 nM, 65 nM, and 19 nM for bimatoprost, latanoprost, and tafluprost, respectively. The relative infiltration ratios of bimatoprost, latanoprost, and tafluprost from ophthalmic solutions into the aqueous humor are calculated as 1.00:19.3:18:8, respectively. This suggests a more favorable infiltration ratio of the ester prodrugs latanoprost and tafluprost than the free acid form of bimatoprost.

To measure the MMP and TIMP expression levels in HNPCECs in the present study, we did not use the ester prodrugs of latanoprost and tafluprost, but rather used the free acid forms to avoid differences in efficacy owing to hydrolysis by esterases. We obtained scattered MMP and TIMP expression levels when the ester forms of latanoprost and tafluprost were used in the experiments. The varying efficacy of PGAs due to hydrolysis by esterases in the cornea, depending on levels expressed in each patient, may consequently determine the effectiveness of latanoprost and tafluprost.

Our results showed a consistency in the expression levels of MMP-2 mRNA and MMP-2 enzyme activity as measured by qPCR and gelatin zymography, respectively. On the other hand, we did not detect other MMP bands by gelatin zymography, possibly because the levels were beyond the sensitivity of the assay. As a consequence, we estimated the enzymatic level of the other MMPs by the mRNA levels of each MMP.

Claudin-1 and occludin in HNPCECs and nonpigmented ciliary epithelial cells, which comprise the BAB in the uvea, are candidate substrates of MMPs. We previously showed that MMP-1, MMP-3, and MMP-9 degraded claudin-1 and occludin in HNPCECs and in non-pigmented ciliary epithelial cells of a swine ciliary body and showed increased expression of MMP-1, MMP-3, and MMP-9 in the presence of TNF-α in HNPCECs [9]. Interestingly MMP-17 can activate TNF-α [23]. These data suggest that inflammation in the ciliary body, like in iridocyclitis, may be involved in the reduction of IOP.

Fibrillin-1, versican, and hyaluronan (FiVerHy) in the ciliary nonpigmented epithelium are other candidate substrates of MMPs expressed in HNPCECs [24]. Versican was digested by MMP-3 [25], and fibrillin-1 was digested by MMP-2 and MMP-9 [26]. The increased expression levels of MMP-2, MMP-3, and MMP-9 in HNPCECs induced by PGAs may lead the degradation of the physiological complex of FiVerHy in the ciliary nonpigmented epithelium. The precise function of FiVerHy is still unknown, but the dense localization of hyaluronan in this high molecular complex on the surface of the ciliary nonpigmented epithelium may exhibit a protective effect of the ciliary nonpigmented epithelium from the MMPs in the vitreous humor [27–30], and the destruction of FiVerHy by MMPs may induce mild iridocyclitis.

Conclusion

In conclusion, unique expression profiles of MMPs and TIMPs induced by bimatoprost, latanoprost, and tafluprost, as shown in HNPCECs, may contribute to clinically different effects on intraocular pressure decreases in patients with glaucoma or ocular hypertension. This information may be important in the selection of the best PGA for individual patients.

Abbreviations
BAB: blood-aqueous barrier; DMSO: dimethyl sulfoxide; FBS: fetal bovine serum; FiVerHy: fibrillin-1, versican, and hyaluronan; HNPCEC: human non-pigmented ciliary epithelial cell; IOP: intraocular pressure; MMP: matrix metalloproteinase; PGA: prostaglandin analog; TIMP: tissue inhibitor of metalloproteinase; TNF: tumor necrosis factor.

Competing interests
The authors declare that they have no competing interest.

Authors' contributions
HY was responsible for, collection of data, analysis and interpretation of results and wrote the first draft of the manuscript. MY participated in its design and supervised the experiments. MG performed the statistical analysis. TK was involved in data collection. MZ conceived the study. All authors reviewed and approved the final manuscript.

Acknowledgement
This study was supported by Strategic Research Foundation Grant-Aided Project for Private Universities from the Ministry of Education, Culture, Sports, Science, and Technology, Japan (MEXT), 2011–2015 (S1101027).

Author details
[1]Department of Opthalmology, Aichi Medical University, Nagakute, Aichi 480-1195, Japan. [2]Department of Biochemistry and Molecular Biology, School of Nursing and Health, Aichi Prefectural University, Nagakute, Aichi 463-8502, Japan. [3]Department of Clinical Trial and Clinical Epidemiology, Faculty of Medicine, University of Tsukuba, Tsukuba, Ibaraki 305-8575, Japan.

References
1. Winkler NS, Fautsch MP. Effects of prostaglandin analogues on aqueous humor outflow pathways. J Ocul Pharmacol Ther. 2014;30:102–9.
2. Toris CB, Gabelt BT, Kaufman PL. Update on the mechanism of action of topical prostaglandins for intraocular pressure reduction. Surv Ophthalmol. 2008;53:S107–20.
3. Ooi YH, Oh DJ, Rhee DJ. Effect of bimatoprost, latanoprost, and unoprostone on matrix metalloproteinases and their inhibitors in human ciliary body smooth muscle cells. Invest Ophthalmol Vis Sci. 2009;50:5259–65.
4. Woodward DF, Wang JW, Poloso NJ. Recent progress in prostaglandin F2α ethanolamide (prostamide F2α) research and therapeutics. Pharmacol Rev. 2013;65:1135–47.
5. Woodward DF, Regan JW, Lake S, Ocklind A. The molecular biology and ocular distribution of prostanoid receptors. Surv Ophthalmol. 1997;41:S15–21.
6. Ishida N, Odani-Kawabata N, Shimazaki A, Hara H. Prostanoids in the therapy of glaucoma. Cardiovasc Drug Rev. 2006;24:1–10.
7. Oh DJ, Martin JL, Williams AJ, Peck RE, Pokorny C, Russell P, Birk DE, Rhee DJ. Analysis of expression of matrix metalloproteinases and tissue inhibitors of metalloproteinases in human ciliary body after latanoprost. Invest Ophthalmol Vis Sci. 2006;47:953–63.
8. Gablet B, Kiland JA, Tian B, Kaufman PL, Aqueous humor: Secretion and dynamics, Kiel JW. Physiology of the eye and visual system. In: Tasman W, Jaeger EA, editors. Duane's ophthalmology on CD-ROM. 2006th ed. Philadelphia: Lippincott Williams & Wilkins; 2006. http://www.eyecalcs.com/DWAN/index.html.
9. Yamada H, Yoneda M, Inaguma S, Watanabe D, Banno S, Yoshikawa K, Mizutani K, Iwaki M, Zako M. Infliximab counteracts tumor necrosis factor-α-enhanced induction of matrix metalloproteinases that degrade claudin and occludin in non-pigmented ciliary epithelium. Biochem Pharmacol. 2013;85:1770–82.
10. Oh DJ, Martin JL, Williams AJ, Russell P, Birk DE, Rhee DJ. Effect of latanoprost on the expression of matrix metalloproteinases and their tissue inhibitors in human trabecular meshwork cells. Invest Ophthalmol Vis Sci. 2006;47:3887–95.
11. Weinreb RN, Kashiwagi K, Kashiwagi F, Tsukahara S, Lindsey JD. Prostaglandins increase matrix metalloproteinase release from human ciliary smooth muscle cells. Invest Ophthalmol Vis Sci. 1997;38:2772–80.
12. Ocklind A. Effect of latanoprost on the extracellular matrix of the ciliary muscle. A study on cultured cells and tissue sections. Exp Eye Res. 1998;67:179–91.
13. el-Shabrawi Y, Eckhardt M, Berghold A, Faulborn J, Auboeck L, Mangge H, Ardjomand N. Synthesis pattern of matrix metalloproteinases (MMPs) and inhibitors (TIMPs) in human explant organ cultures after treatment with latanoprost and dexamethasone. Eye (Lond). 2000;14:375–83.
14. Lindsey JD, Kashiwagi K, Boyle D, Kashiwagi F, Firestein GS, Weinreb RN. Prostaglandins increase proMMP-1 and proMMP-3 secretion by human ciliary smooth muscle cells. Curr Eye Res. 1996;15:869–75.
15. Anthony TL, Lindsey JD, Weinreb RN. Latanoprost's effects on TIMP-1 and TIMP-2 expression in human ciliary muscle cells. Invest Ophthalmol Vis Sci. 2002;43:3705–11.
16. Simmons ST, Dirks MS, Noecker RJ. Bimatoprost versus latanoprost in lowering intraocular pressure in glaucoma and ocular hypertension: results from parallel-group comparison trials. Adv Ther. 2004;21:247–62.
17. Noecker RS, Dirks MS, Choplin NT, Bernstein P, Batoosingh AL, Whitcup SM, Bimatoprost/Latanoprost Study Group. A six-month randomized clinical trial comparing the intraocular pressure-lowering efficacy of bimatoprost and latanoprost in patients with ocular hypertension or glaucoma. Am J Ophthalmol. 2003;135:55–63.
18. Alm A. Latanoprost in the treatment of glaucoma. Clin Ophthalmol. 2014;8:1967–85.
19. Parrish RK, Palmberg P, Sheu WP, XLT Study Group. A comparison of latanoprost, bimatoprost, and travoprost in patients with elevated intraocular pressure: a 12-week, randomized, masked-evaluator multicenter study. Am J Ophthalmol. 2003;135:688–703.
20. Fukano Y, Odani-Kawabata N, Nakamura M, Kawazu K. Intraocular penetration and intraocular pressure-lowering effect of new formulation 0.0015 % tafluprost ophthalmic solution with reduced benzalkonium chloride. Atarashii Ganka. 2010;27:691–4.
21. Camras CB, Toris CB, Sjoquist B, Milleson M, Thorngren JO, Hejkal TW, Patel N, Barnett EM, Smolyak R, Hasan SF, Hellman C, Meza JL, Wax MB, Stjernschantz J. Detection of the free acid of bimatoprost in aqueous humor samples from human eyes treated with bimatoprost before cataract surgery. Ophthalmology. 2004;111:2193–8.
22. Sjöquist B, Stjernschantz J. Ocular and systemic pharmacokinetics of latanoprost in humans. Surv Ophthalmol. 2002;47:S6–12.
23. English WR, Puente XS, Freije JM, Knauper V, Amour A, Merryweather A, Lopez-Otin C, Murphy G. Membrane type 4 matrix metalloproteinase (MMP17) has tumor necrosis factor-alpha convertase activity but does not activate pro-MMP2. J Biol Chem. 2000;275:14046–55.
24. Ohno-Jinno A, Isogai Z, Yoneda M, Kasai K, Miyaishi O, Inoue Y, Kataoka T, Zhao JS, Li H, Takeyama M, Keene DR, Sakai LY, Kimata K, Iwaki M, Zako M. Versican and fibrillin-1 form a major hyaluronan-binding complex in the ciliary body. Invest Ophthalmol Vis Sci. 2008;49:2870–7.
25. Muir EM, Adcock KH, Morgenstern DA, Clayton R, von Stillfried N, Rhodes K, Ellis C, Fawcett JW, Rogers JH. Matrix metalloproteases and their inhibitors are produced by overlapping populations of activated astrocytes. Brain Res Mol Brain Res. 2002;100:103–17.
26. Ashworth JL, Murphy G, Rock MJ, Sherratt MJ, Shapiro SD, Shuttleworth CA, Kielty CM. Fibrillin degradation by matrix metalloproteinases: implications for connective tissue remodelling. Biochem J. 1999;340:171–81.
27. Takeyama M, Yoneda M, Takeuchi M, Isogai Z, Ohno-Jinno A, Kataoka T, Li H, Sugita I, Iwaki M, Zako M. Increase in matrix metalloproteinase-2 level in the chicken retina after laser photocoagulation. Lasers Surg Med. 2010;42:433–41.
28. Vaughan-Thomas A, Gilbert SJ, Duance VC. Elevated levels of proteolytic enzymes in the aging human vitreous. Invest Ophthalmol Vis Sci. 2000;41:3299–304.
29. De La Paz MA, Itoh Y, Toth CA, Nagase H. Matrix metalloproteinases and their inhibitors in human vitreous. Invest Ophthalmol Vis Sci. 1998;39:1256–60.
30. Plantner JJ, Smine A, Quinn TA. Matrix metalloproteinases and metalloproteinase inhibitors in human interphotoreceptor matrix and vitreous. Curr Eye Res. 1998;17:132–40.

Permissions

All chapters in this book were first published in Ophthalmology, by BioMed Central; hereby published with permission under the Creative Commons Attribution License or equivalent. Every chapter published in this book has been scrutinized by our experts. Their significance has been extensively debated. The topics covered herein carry significant findings which will fuel the growth of the discipline. They may even be implemented as practical applications or may be referred to as a beginning point for another development.

The contributors of this book come from diverse backgrounds, making this book a truly international effort. This book will bring forth new frontiers with its revolutionizing research information and detailed analysis of the nascent developments around the world.

We would like to thank all the contributing authors for lending their expertise to make the book truly unique. They have played a crucial role in the development of this book. Without their invaluable contributions this book wouldn't have been possible. They have made vital efforts to compile up to date information on the varied aspects of this subject to make this book a valuable addition to the collection of many professionals and students.

This book was conceptualized with the vision of imparting up-to-date information and advanced data in this field. To ensure the same, a matchless editorial board was set up. Every individual on the board went through rigorous rounds of assessment to prove their worth. After which they invested a large part of their time researching and compiling the most relevant data for our readers.

The editorial board has been involved in producing this book since its inception. They have spent rigorous hours researching and exploring the diverse topics which have resulted in the successful publishing of this book. They have passed on their knowledge of decades through this book. To expedite this challenging task, the publisher supported the team at every step. A small team of assistant editors was also appointed to further simplify the editing procedure and attain best results for the readers.

Apart from the editorial board, the designing team has also invested a significant amount of their time in understanding the subject and creating the most relevant covers. They scrutinized every image to scout for the most suitable representation of the subject and create an appropriate cover for the book.

The publishing team has been an ardent support to the editorial, designing and production team. Their endless efforts to recruit the best for this project, has resulted in the accomplishment of this book. They are a veteran in the field of academics and their pool of knowledge is as vast as their experience in printing. Their expertise and guidance has proved useful at every step. Their uncompromising quality standards have made this book an exceptional effort. Their encouragement from time to time has been an inspiration for everyone.

The publisher and the editorial board hope that this book will prove to be a valuable piece of knowledge for researchers, students, practitioners and scholars across the globe.

List of Contributors

Nevin Hande Dikel and Kemal Ornek
Department of Ophthalmology, Kırıkkale University School of Medicine, Kırıkkale, Turkey

Erhan Yumusak
Department of Ophthalmology, Kırıkkale University School of Medicine, Kırıkkale, Turkey
Kirikkale University Medical Faculty Hospital District Tahsin Duru Akdeniz Caddesi No: 14, Yahsihan/Kırıkkale 71450, Turkey

Aydin Ciftci
Department of Internal Medicine, Kırıkkale University School of Medicine, Kırıkkale, Turkey

Selim Yalcin
Department of Medical Oncology, Kırıkkale University School of Medicine, Kırıkkale, Turkey

Cemile Dayangan Sayan
Department of Obstetrics and Gynecology, Kırıkkale University School of Medicine, Kırıkkale, Turkey

Xiaowen Zhao, Yao Wang, Suxia Li and Peng Chen
State Key Laboratory Cultivation Base, Shandong Provincial Key Laboratory of Ophthalmology, Shandong Eye Institute, Shandong Academy of medical Sciences, No. 5 Yanerdao Rd, Qingdao 266071, China

Ye Wang
State Key Laboratory Cultivation Base, Shandong Provincial Key Laboratory of Ophthalmology, Shandong Eye Institute, Shandong Academy of medical Sciences, No. 5 Yanerdao Rd, Qingdao 266071, China
Current affiliation: Central Laboratory of the Second Affiliated Hospital, Medical College of Qingdao University, Qingdao 266042, China

Min Tang, Yang Fu and Xun Xu
Department of Ophthalmology, Shanghai General Hospital of Nanjing Medical University, No.100 Haining Road, Hongkou District, Shanghai 200080, China

Ying Wang, Zhi Zheng, Ying Fan and Xiaodong Sun
Department of Ophthalmology, Shanghai General Hospital, Shanghai Jiao Tong University, School of Medicine, Shanghai 200080, China

Francesco Sofi
Department of Experimental and Clinical Medicine, University of Florence, Florence, Italy
Agency of Nutrition, University Hospital of Careggi, Florence, Italy
Don Carlo Gnocchi Foundation Italy, Onlus IRCCS, Florence, Italy

Andrea Sodi, Fabrizio Franco, Vittoria Murro, Alba Miele, Ugo Menchini, Stanislao Rizzo and Giacomo Abbruzzese
Department of Surgery and Translational Medicine, Eye Clinic, University of Florence, Florence, Italy

Dania Biagini
Agency of Nutrition, University Hospital of Careggi, Florence, Italy

Dario Pasquale Mucciolo
Department of Experimental and Clinical Medicine, University of Florence, Florence, Italy

Gianni Virgili
Department of Experimental and Clinical Medicine, University of Florence, Florence, Italy
Don Carlo Gnocchi Foundation Italy, Onlus IRCCS, Florence, Italy

Alessandro Casini
Department of Experimental and Clinical Medicine, University of Florence, Florence, Italy
Agency of Nutrition, University Hospital of Careggi, Florence, Italy

Na Liao, Chaohong Li, Huilv Jiang, Aiwu Fang, Shengjie Zhou and Qinmei Wang
School of Optometry and Ophthalmology and Eye Hospital, Wenzhou Medical University, Wenzhou, Zhejiang, China

Zhaotian Zhang, Shaochong Zhang, Xintong Jiang, Suo Qiu and Yantao Wei
State Key Laboratory of Ophthalmology, Zhongshan Ophthalmic Center, Sun Yat-sen University, No.54, South Xianlie Road, Guangzhou 510060, China

Ozlem Sahin
Department of Ophthalmology/Uveitis, Dunya Goz Hospital Ltd., Ankara, Turkey

Alireza Ziaei
Department of Ophthalmology, Boston University School of Medicine, Boston, MA, USA

Eda Karaismailoğlu
Department of Biostatistics, Hacettepe University Medical Faculty, Ankara, Turkey

Nusret Taheri
Department of Biochemistry, Middle East Technical University, Health Sciences, Ankara, Turkey

Nan Jiang, Guiqiu Zhao, Shanshan Yang, Jing Lin, Liting Hu, Chengye Che, Qian Wang and Qiang Xu
Department of Ophthalmology, the Affiliated Hospital of Qingdao University, Qingdao, Shandong Province, China

Tso-Ting Lai and Tzyy-Chang Ho
Department of Ophthalmology, National Taiwan University Hospital, No. 7, Chun-Shan S. Rd., Taipei City 100, Taiwan

Chung-May Yang
Department of Ophthalmology, National Taiwan University Hospital, No. 7, Chun-Shan S. Rd., Taipei City 100, Taiwan
College of Medicine, National Taiwan University, No.1 Jen-Ai Rd. Sec. 1, Taipei City 100, Taiwan

Hui Song, Xiaoyong Yuan and Xin Tang
Tianjin Eye Hospital, Tianjin Key Laboratory of Ophthalmology and Vision Science, Clinical College of Ophthalmology, Tianjin Medical University, No. 4 Gansu Rd, Heping District, Tianjin 300020, China

Ibrahim Elaraoud, Walter Andreatta and Ajay Bhatnagar
Wolverhampton Eye Infirmary, New Cross Hospital, Wednesfield Road, Wolverhampton WV10 0QP, UK

Andrej Kidess and Marie Tsaloumas
Queen Elizabeth University Hospital Birmingham, Birmingham B15 2TH, UK

Fahad Quhill
Royal Hallamshire Hospital, Glossop Road, Sheffield S10 2JF, UK

Yit Yang
Wolverhampton Eye Infirmary, New Cross Hospital, Wednesfield Road, Wolverhampton WV10 0QP, UK
School of Life and Health Sciences, Aston University, Birmingham B4 7ET, UK

Oriel Spierer, Yitzhak Golan, Hadas Newman and Rony Rachmiel
Department of Ophthalmology, Tel Aviv Sourasky Medical Center, Sackler Faculty of Medicine, Tel Aviv University, 6 Weizmann Street, Tel Aviv 64239, Israel

Michael Waisbourd
Wills Eye Hospital, Philadelphia, PA, USA

Yanwei Chen, Jianfang Li, Yan Yan and Xi Shen
The Department of Ophthalmology, RuiJin Hospital Affiliated Shanghai Jiao Tong University School of Medicine, Shanghai, China

Semra Acer, Ebru Nevin Çetin , Gökhan Pekel, Alper Kaşıkçı and Ramazan Yağcı
Department of Ophthalmology, Kinikli Kampusu, Pamukkale University, Denizli, TR 20100, Turkey

Attila Oğuzhanoğlu and Nedim Ongun
Department of Neurology, Kinikli Kampusu, Pamukkale University, Denizli, Turkey

Leonardo Colombo, Paolo Fogagnolo, Giovanni Montesano, Stefano De Cillà, Nicola Orzalesi and Luca Rossetti
Eye Clinic, San Paolo Hospital, University of Milan, Via A. Di Rudinì 8, 20142 Milan, Italy

Shaolin Du
Zhongshan Ophthalmic Center, State Key Laboratory of Ophthalmology, Sun Yat-Sen University, Guangzhou, China
Tungwah Hospital of Sun Yat-Sen University, Dongguan, China

Wenbin Huang, Xiulan Zhang, Jiawei Wang, Wei Wang and Dennis S. C. Lam
Zhongshan Ophthalmic Center, State Key Laboratory of Ophthalmology, Sun Yat-Sen University, Guangzhou, China

Salvatore Cillino, Francesco Di Pace, Lucia Lee Ferraro and Giovanni Cillino
Department of Experimental Biomedicine and Clinical Neuroscience,Ophthalmology Section, University of Palermo (Italy), via Liborio Giuffrè, 13, 90127 Palermo, Italy

Alessandra Casuccio
Department of Sciences for Health Promotion and Mother-Child Care "G. D'Alessandro", University of Palermo, Via del Vespro 127, I, 90127 Palermo, Italy

Carlo Cagini
Department of Surgical and Biomedical Sciences, Section of Ophthalmology, University of Perugia, Piazza Menghini 1. S. Andrea delle Fratte, 06156 Perugia, Italy

Bruno Simonazzi and Yan Guex-Crosier
Jules-Gonin Eye Hospital, University of Lausanne, FAA, Av. de France 15, CH-1004 Lausanne, Switzerland

Konstantinos Balaskas
Jules-Gonin Eye Hospital, University of Lausanne, FAA, Av. de France 15, CH-1004 Lausanne, Switzerland
Manchester Royal Eye Hospital, Manchester, UK

Ferial M. Al-Zeraid
Department of Optometry & Vision Sciences, College of Applied Medical Sciences, King Saud University, Riyadh, P.O Box 10219, Riyadh 11433, Saudi Arabia

Uchechukwu L. Osuagwu
Department of Optometry & Vision Sciences, Faculty of Health, Ophthalmic and Visual Optics Laboratory Group (Chronic Disease & Ageing), Institute of Health and Biomedical Innovation, Q Block, Room 5WS36 60 Musk Avenue Kelvin Grove, Brisbane, QLD 4059, Australia

Yao Chen and Xiaobo Xia
Department of Ophthalmology, Xiangya Hospital, Central South University, Changsha, Hunan, China

Daisuke Nagasato and Toshihiko Nagasawa
Department of Ophthalmology, Saneikai Tsukazaki Hospital, Himeji, Japan
Department of Ophthalmology and Visual Sciences, Graduate School of Biomedical Sciences, Hiroshima University, Hiroshima, Japan

Yoshinori Mitamura, Kentaro Semba and Kei Akaiwa
Department of Ophthalmology, Institute of Biomedical Sciences, Tokushima University Graduate School, 3-18-15 Kuramoto, Tokushima 770-8503, Japan

Yuki Yoshizumi and Hitoshi Tabuchi
Department of Ophthalmology, Saneikai Tsukazaki Hospital, Himeji, Japan

Yoshiaki Kiuchi
Department of Ophthalmology and Visual Sciences, Graduate School of Biomedical Sciences, Hiroshima University, Hiroshima, Japan

Cheolmin Yun, Jaeryung Oh, Kwang-Eon Choi, Seong-Woo Kim and Kuhl Huh
Department of Ophthalmology, Korea University College of Medicine, 126-1 Anam-dong 5-ga, Sungbuk gu, Seoul 136-705, South Korea

Soon-Young Hwang
Department of Biostatistics, Korea University College of Medicine, Seoul, South Korea

Kenji Fujitani, Neha Gadaria, Kyu-In Lee, Brendan Barry and Penny Asbell
Department of Ophthalmology, Icahn School of Medicine at Mount Sinai, New York, NY 10029, USA

Hyo Seok Lee, Sang Woo Park and Hwan Heo
Department of Ophthalmology, Chonnam National University Medical School and Hospital, 42 Jebong-ro, Dong-Gu, Gwang-Ju 61469, South Korea

Maria Teresa Zocher, Nicole Oertel, Jens Dawczynski, Peter Wiedemann and Franziska G. Rauscher
Department of Ophthalmology, Leipzig University Hospital, Liebigstrasse 10-14, 04103 Leipzig, Germany

Jos J. Rozema
Department of Ophthalmology, Antwerp University Hospital, Wilrijkstraat 10, 2650 Edegem, Belgium
Department of Medicine and Health Science, University of Antwerp, Universiteitsplein 1, 2610 Wilrijk, Belgium

Selam Yekta Sendul, Burcu Dirim, Mehmet Demir, Zeynep Acar, Atilla Gokce Demir, Ali Olgun, Semra Tiryaki and Dilek Guven
Department of Ophthalmology, Sisli Hamidiye Etfal Training and Research Hospital, Etfal Street 34280, Sisli, Istanbul, Turkey

Cemile Ucgul
Department of Ophthalmology, Ulucanlar Eye Training and Research Hospital, Ulucanlar street, 06030, Altındag, Ankara, Turkey

Hiroshi Yamada, Tomohiro Kato and Masahiro Zako
Department of Opthalmology, Aichi Medical University, Nagakute, Aichi 480-1195, Japan

Masahiko Yoneda
Department of Biochemistry and Molecular Biology, School of Nursing and Health, Aichi Prefectural University, Nagakute, Aichi 463-8502, Japan

Masahiko Gosho
Department of Clinical Trial and Clinical Epidemiology, Faculty of Medicine, University of Tsukuba, Tsukuba, Ibaraki 305-8575, Japan

Index

www.ingramcontent.com/pod-product-compliance
Lightning Source LLC
Chambersburg PA
CBHW061948190326
41458CB00009B/2816